I.V. Therapy

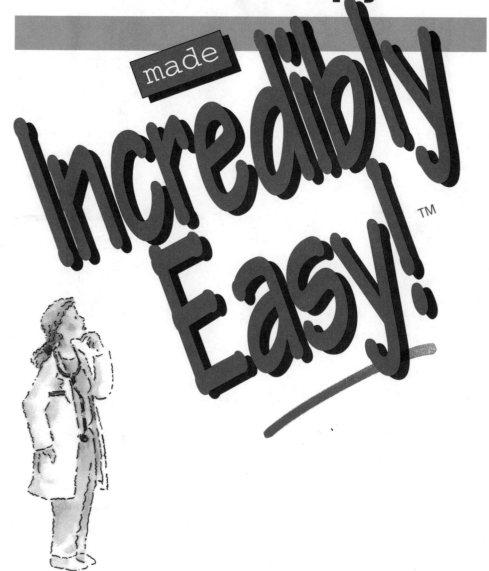

made Incredibly Easy!™

Springhouse Corporation
Springhouse, Pennsylvania

Staff

Executive Director
Matthew Cahill

Clinical Director
Judith A. Schilling McCann, RN, MSN

Art Director
John Hubbard

Managing Editor
Michael Shaw

Clinical Editors
Carla M. Roy, RN, BSN, CCRN (project manager); Joanne M. Bartelmo, RN, MSN, CCRN; Beverly Tscheschlog, RN; Tracy L. Yeomans, RN, BSN, BA, CCRN;

Editors
Kevin Howarth, Anthony Prete, Patricia Wittig

Copy Editors
Cynthia C. Breuninger (manager), Mary T. Durkin, Brenna H. Mayer, Pamela Wingrod

Designers
Arlene Putterman (associate art director), Mary Ludwicki (book designer), Joseph Clark

Illustrators
Bot Roda, Jackie Facciolo, Betty Winnberg, Jean Gardener, Bob Jackson, Judy Newhouse

Typography
Diane Paluba (manager), Joyce Rossi Biletz, Valerie Molettiere

Manufacturing
Deborah Meiris (director), Pat Dorshaw (manager), Otto Mezei

Editorial Assistant
Beverly Lane

Indexer
Barbara Hodgson

Printed in the United States of America.

IEP-010898

R A member of the Reed Elsevier plc group

Library of Congress Cataloging-in Publication Data

I.V. Therapy made incredibly easy.
   p. cm.
   Includes index.
   1. Intravenous therapy. 2. Nursing. I. Springhouse Corporation.
   [DNLM: 1. Infusions, Intravenous nurses' instruction. 2. Drug therapy nurses' instruction
   WB 354193 1998]
RM170.I25 1998
615'.6—dc21
DNLM/DLC
ISBN 0-87434-958-3 (alk. paper)   98-21797
                         CIP

Contents

Contributors and consultants

Deborah B. Benvenuto, RN, CRNI
Nurse Educator, Intravenous Therapy
Intravenous Nurses Society
Cambridge, Mass.

Peggi Guenter, RN, PhD, CNSN
Clinical Director, Nutrition Support Services
Allegheny University Hospitals, Graduate Department of Surgery
Philadelphia

Ann Helm, RN, BSN, MS, JD
Nurse-Attorney
Clinical Associate Professor
School of Medicine
Oregon Health Sciences University
Portland

Susan K. Markel-Poole, RN, BSN, MS, CRNI, CNSN
Senior Director, Professional Services
Option Care, Inc.
Chicago

Robert Rauch
Medical Economics Manager
Amgen, Inc.
Maple Glen, Pa.

Foreword

Hey, I'm a multidimensional guy.

Ah, the pleasures of being a nurse. There's nothing so satisfying as cannulating a vein on the first attempt. Between you and me, I feel a deep — if unspoken — pride each time I achieve successful venous access. So, when the clinical experts at Springhouse asked me to write the foreword for a revolutionary new book on I.V. therapy, I couldn't refuse.

Of course, there's a lot more to I.V. therapy than performing venipuncture. Administering I.V. therapy is a multidimensional nursing skill. Consider the following:

• I.V. lines are used for a multitude of purposes, including administering solutions and medications, transfusing blood, and providing parenteral nutrition.

• I.V. therapy is practiced in all patient care settings, including hospitals, long-term care facilities, and at home.

• I.V. administration requires a variety of skills — for example, starting infusions, assessing patients during therapy, knowing the advantages and disadvantages of different delivery methods, and much more.

Indeed, contemporary nursing practice and patient care couldn't exist without I.V. therapy. A book devoted to a topic so vital to nursing must be approached with enthusiasm, developed with special care and, allow me to say it, treated with love. That's why the clinical experts at Springhouse created *I.V. Therapy Made Incredibly Easy.* It's utterly different from the run-of-the-mill nursing books that currently populate bookstores and libraries. It's lively, fun to read, and filled with surprises. You'll love reading it and, in the process, find everything you need to practice I.V. therapy with skill and confidence.

The first chapter of *I.V. Therapy Made Incredibly Easy* discusses the basics, introducing such topics as purpose, delivery methods, I.V. flow rates, legal issues, professional standards, documentation, and more.

Chapter 2 is devoted to peripheral I.V. therapy and chapter 3 discusses central venous therapy. In each chapter, you'll learn about appropriate venous access sites, selecting equipment, preparing for therapy, maintaining and ending the infusion, and potential complications.

Chapter 4 covers I.V. medications, including the advantages and disadvantages of I.V. drug delivery, administration rates, preparing medications, equipment selection, complications, special considerations for pediatric, elderly, and home care patients, and much more.

Chapter 5 is devoted to transfusion therapy. It covers such topics as blood composition and physiology; administration of whole blood, blood components, plasma, and plasma fractions; and potential complications.

Chapter 6 covers chemotherapy infusions, including the types of chemotherapeutic drugs, administration guidelines, adverse effects of chemotherapy, and how to avoid dangerous drug exposure.

The last chapter, chapter 7, discusses parenteral nutrition. It features information on basic nutritional needs, performing a nutritional assessment, administering parenteral nutrition, and potential complications.

Within each chapter, you'll find many special features to enhance your understanding and make learning enjoyable. Each chapter begins with an at-a-glance summary of key topics. *Memory joggers* provide novel ways to remember the most important points, and cartoon characters help turn learning about I.V. therapy into a joy. A *Quick quiz* at the end of each chapter helps you assess what you've learned.

Special logos throughout each chapter alert you to essential information:

The *Running smoothly* logo alerts you to equipment malfunctions in I.V. therapy and what to do about them.

Advice from the experts provides tips, pointers, and guidelines galore that will make I.V. therapy easier than ever.

My favorite feature is the full-color illustrations on pages 27 to 30 explaining the different types of I.V. solutions. Take a look and you'll see that *I.V. Therapy Made Incredibly Easy* is unique.

Please take the time to explore this clinically useful and refreshingly original book. I am confident that *I.V. Therapy Made Incredibly Easy* will strengthen your clinical skills and keep you smiling. Enjoy learning.

Susan K. Markel-Poole, RN, BSN, MS, CRNI, CNSN
Senior Director of Professional Services
Option Care, Inc.
Chicago
Editorial Board Member
Journal of Intravenous Nurses

Introduction to I.V. therapy

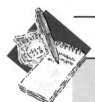

Just the facts

In this chapter you'll learn:

♦ the purposes of I.V. therapy

♦ delivery methods

♦ I.V. flow rates

♦ legal and professional standards

♦ patient teaching

♦ documentation.

Purposes of I.V. therapy

One of your most important nursing responsibilities is to administer fluids, medications, and blood products to patients. In I.V. therapy, liquid solutions are introduced directly into the bloodstream.

The main objectives of I.V. therapy are to:
• restore and maintain fluid and electrolyte balance
• provide medications and chemotherapeutic agents
• transfuse blood and blood products
• deliver parenteral nutrients and nutritional supplements.

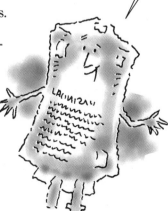

That's me, fast and accurate.

Benefits of I.V. therapy

I.V. therapy has great benefits. For example, it can be used to administer fluids, drugs, nutrients, and other solutions when a patient is unable to take oral substances.

On target and fast

I.V. drug delivery also allows more accurate dosing. Because the entire amount of a drug given I.V. reaches the bloodstream immediately, the drug begins to act almost instantaneously.

Risks of I.V. therapy

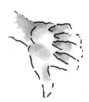

Like other invasive procedures, I.V. therapy has its downside. Risks include bleeding, infiltration (infusion of the I.V. solution into surrounding tissues rather than the blood vessel), infection, overdose (because response to I.V. drugs is more rapid), incompatibility between drugs or I.V. solutions when mixed together, and the potential for an adverse or allergic response to an infused substance.

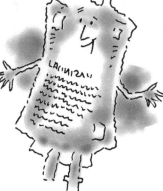

Well, nobody's perfect.

Sit still, please

Patient activity can be problematic. Simple tasks, such as transferring to a chair, ambulating, and washing oneself, can become complicated when the patient must cope with I.V. poles, I.V. lines, and dressings.

Everything costs

Finally, I.V. therapy is more costly than oral, subcutaneous, or intramuscular methods of delivering medications.

Fluids, electrolytes, and I.V. therapy

One of the primary objectives of I.V. therapy is to restore and maintain fluid and electrolyte balance. To understand how I.V. therapy works to restore fluid and electrolyte balance, let's first review some basics of fluids and electrolytes.

Two-thirds of the total

The human body is composed largely of liquid. These fluids account for about two-thirds of total body weight in an adult who weighs 155 lb (70 kg) and about three-fourths of total body weight in an infant.

Water plus

Body fluids are composed of water (a solvent) and dissolved substances (solutes). The solutes in body fluids include electrolytes, such as sodium, and nonelectrolytes, such as proteins.

Fluid functions

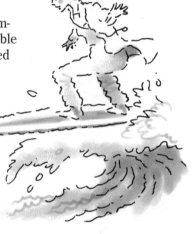

When fluid levels are optimal, you can just ride the wave.

What functions do body fluids provide? They:
- help regulate body temperature
- transport nutrients and gases throughout the body
- carry wastes to excretion sites
- maintain cell shape.

Optimal levels are where it's at

When fluid levels are optimal, the body performs swimmingly, but when fluid levels deviate from the acceptable range, organs and systems can quickly become bogged down.

Inside and outside

Body fluids exist in two major compartments: inside the cells and outside the cells. The fluid inside the cells—about 55% of the total body fluid—is called intracellular fluid (ICF). The rest is called extracellular fluid (ECF). Normally, the distribution of fluids between the two compartments is constant. (See *Understanding body fluid distribution,* page 4.)

Extra! Extra!

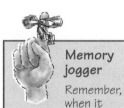

Memory jogger

Remember, when it comes to body fluids, two i's make an e. The two i's (*intravascular* and *interstitial* fluid) are part of the e (*extracellular* fluid), not the i (*intracellular* fluid).

Here's some extra information about ECF, which occurs in two forms:
- interstitial fluid (ISF)
- intravascular fluid.

Interstitial fluid surrounds each cell of the body; even bone cells are bathed in it. Intravascular fluid is blood plasma, the liquid component of blood. It surrounds red blood cells and accounts for most of the blood volume.

In an adult, about 5% of the body fluid is intravascular ECF; about 15% is interstitial ECF. Part of that interstitial ECF is transcellular fluid, which includes cerebrospinal fluid, lymph, and fluid in such spaces as the pleural and abdominal cavities.

Now I get it!

Understanding body fluid distribution

Body fluid is distributed between two main compartments — extracellular and intracellular. Extracellular fluid has two components — interstitial fluid and intravascular fluid (plasma). This illustration shows body fluid distribution for a 155-lb (70-kg) adult.

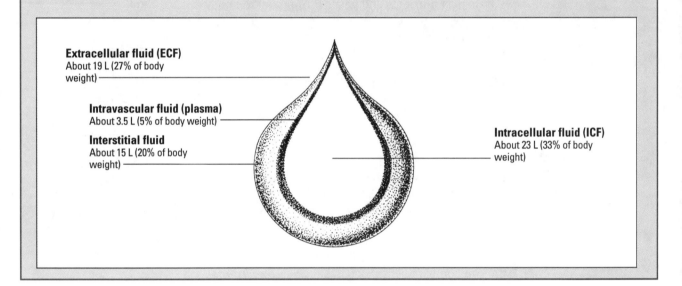

Extracellular fluid (ECF)
About 19 L (27% of body weight)

Intravascular fluid (plasma)
About 3.5 L (5% of body weight)

Interstitial fluid
About 15 L (20% of body weight)

Intracellular fluid (ICF)
About 23 L (33% of body weight)

Balancing act

Maintaining fluid balance in the body involves the kidneys, heart, liver, adrenal and pituitary glands, and nervous system. This balancing act is affected by:
- fluid volume
- distribution of fluids in the body
- concentration of solutes in the fluid.

You win some and you lose some

Every day, the body gains and loses fluid. To maintain fluid balance, the gains must equal the losses. (See *Daily fluid gains and losses.*)

Hormones at work

Fluid volume and concentration are regulated by the interaction of two hormones:
- antidiuretic hormone (ADH)
- aldosterone.

ADH affects fluid volume and concentration by regulating water retention. It's secreted when plasma osmolarity increases or circulating blood volume decreases and blood pressure drops. Aldosterone acts to retain sodium and water. It's secreted when the serum sodium is low, potassium is high, or the circulating volume of fluid decreases.

The thirst mechanism also regulates water volume and participates with hormones in maintaining fluid balance. Thirst is experienced whenever water loss equals 2% of body weight, or when osmolarity (solute concentration) increases. Drinking water restores plasma volume and dilutes ECF osmolarity.

> Water level is down — down 2% of body weight to be precise. Time for a drink.

Daily fluid gains and losses

Each day the body gains and loses fluid through several different processes. The illustration below shows the main sites involved. The amounts shown apply to adults; infants exchange a greater amount of fluid than adults.

Note: Gastric, intestinal, pancreatic, and biliary secretions total about 8,200 ml, but they are almost completely reabsorbed, so they're not usually counted in daily fluid gains and losses.

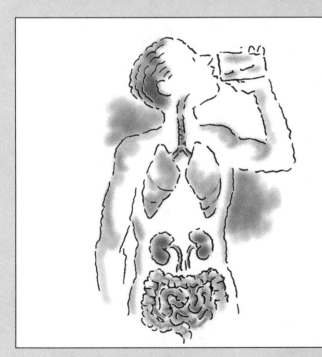

Daily total intake — 2,400 to 3,200 ml
Liquids — 1,400 to 1,800 ml
Water in foods (solid) — 700 to 1,000 ml
Water of oxidation (combined water and oxygen in the respiratory system) — 300 to 400 ml

Daily total output — 2,400 to 3,200 ml
Lungs (respiration) — 600 to 800 ml
Skin (perspiration) — 300 to 500 ml
Kidneys (urine) — 1,400 to 1,800 ml
Intestines (feces) — 100 ml

There's gonna be some changes

Nurses need to anticipate changes in fluid balance that may take place during I.V. therapy. Therefore, it's important to establish the patient's baseline fluid status before starting any fluid replacement therapy. During I.V. therapy, changes in fluid status alert the nurse to impending fluid imbalances. (See *Identifying fluid imbalances.*)

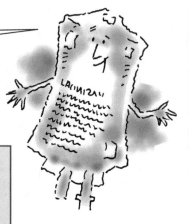

Don't start with me until you've established the patient's baseline fluid status.

Identifying fluid imbalances

By carefully assessing a patient before and during I.V. therapy, you can identify fluid imbalances early — before serious complications develop. The following assessment findings and test results indicate fluid deficit or excess.

Fluid deficit	Fluid excess
• Weight loss	• Weight gain
• Increased, thready pulse rate	• Elevated blood pressure
• Diminished blood pressure, often with postural hypotension	• Bounding pulse that's not easily obliterated
• Decreased central venous pressure	• Jugular vein distention
• Sunken eyes, dry conjunctivae, decreased tearing	• Increased respiratory rate
• Poor skin turgor (not a reliable sign in elderly patients)	• Dyspnea
• Lack of moisture in groin and axillae	• Moist crackles or rhonchi on auscultation
• Thirst	• Edema of dependent body parts; sacral edema in patients on bed rest
• Decreased salivation	• Generalized edema
• Dry, cracked lips	• Puffy eyelids
• Furrows in tongue	• Fuller-than-normal cheeks
• Difficulty forming words (patient needs to moisten mouth first)	• Periorbital edema
• Mental status changes	• Slow emptying of hand veins when arm is raised
• Weakness	• Decreased hematocrit
• Diminished urine output	• Decreased serum electrolyte levels
• Increased hematocrit	• Decreased BUN levels
• Increased serum electrolyte levels	• Reduced serum osmolarity
• Increased blood urea nitrogen (BUN) levels	
• Increased serum osmolarity	

Electrolytes

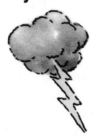

Electrolytes are another major component of body fluids. There are six major electrolytes:
- sodium
- potassium
- calcium
- chloride
- phosphate
- magnesium.

You'll get a charge outta this

As the name implies, electrolytes are associated with electricity. These vital substances are chemical compounds that dissociate in solution into electrically charged particles called ions. Like wiring for the body, the electrical charges of ions conduct current that is necessary for normal cell function. (See *Understanding electrolytes,* pages 8 and 9.)

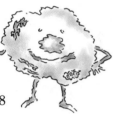

Without electrolytes, I'd be unplugged. I just wouldn't be able to function.

Fluid and electrolyte balance

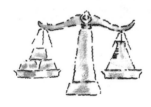

Fluids and electrolytes are usually discussed in tandem, especially where I.V. therapy is concerned, because fluid balance and electrolyte balance are interdependent. Any change in one alters the other and any solution given I.V. can affect a patient's fluid and electrolyte balance.

Electrolyte balance

All electrolytes aren't distributed evenly. The major intracellular electrolytes are:
- potassium
- phosphorus.

The major extracellular electrolytes are:
- sodium
- chloride.

The ICF and ECF contain different electrolytes because the cell membranes separating the two compartments have selective permeability. That is, only certain ions can cross those membranes. Although the ICF and ECF contain different solutes, the concentration levels of the two fluids are about equal when balance is maintained.

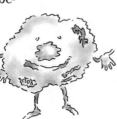

I practice selective permeability. Some electrolytes get through my membranes, some don't.

Now I get it!

Understanding electrolytes

Six major electrolytes play important roles in maintaining chemical balance: sodium, potassium, calcium, chloride, phosphorus, and magnesium. Electrolyte concentrations are expressed in milliequivalents per liter (mEq/L) and milligrams per deciliter (mg/dl).

Electrolyte	Principal functions	Signs and symptoms of imbalance
Sodium (Na⁺) • Major cation in extracellular fluid (ECF) • Normal serum level: 135 to 145 mEq/L	• Maintains appropriate ECF osmolarity • Influences water distribution (with chloride) • Affects concentration, excretion, and absorption of potassium and chloride • Helps regulate acid-base balance • Aids nerve- and muscle-fiber impulse transmission	*Hyponatremia:* muscle weakness, decreased skin turgor, headache, tremor, seizures *Hypernatremia:* thirst, fever, flushed skin, oliguria, and dry, sticky membranes
Potassium (K⁺) • Major cation in intracellular fluid (ICF) • Normal serum level: 3.5 to 5.0 mEq/L	• Maintains cell electroneutrality • Maintains cell osmolarity • Assists in conduction of nerve impulses • Directly affects cardiac muscle contraction • Plays major role in acid-base balance	*Hypokalemia:* decreased GI, skeletal muscle, and cardiac muscle function; decreased reflexes; rapid, weak, irregular pulse; muscle weakness or irritability; decreased blood pressure; nausea and vomiting; paralytic ileus *Hyperkalemia:* muscle weakness, nausea, diarrhea, oliguria
Calcium (Ca⁺⁺) • Major cation in teeth and bones • Normal serum level: 8.9 to 10.1 mg/dl	• Enhances bone strength and durability (along with phosphorus) • Helps maintain cell-membrane structure, function, and permeability • Affects activation, excitation, and contraction of cardiac and skeletal muscles • Participates in neurotransmitter release at synapses • Helps activate specific steps in blood coagulation • Activates serum complement in immune system function	*Hypocalcemia:* muscle tremor, muscle cramps, tetany, tonic-clonic seizures, paresthesia, bleeding, arrhythmias, hypotension *Hypercalcemia:* lethargy, headache, muscle flaccidity, nausea, vomiting, anorexia, constipation, polydipsia, hypertension, polyuria
Chloride (Cl⁻) • Major anion in ECF • Normal serum level: 96 to 106 mEq/L	• Maintains serum osmolarity (along with Na⁺) • Combines with major cations to create important compounds, such as sodium chloride (NaCl), hydrogen chloride (HCl), potassium chloride (KCl), and calcium chloride (CaCl$_2$)	*Hypochloremia:* increased muscle excitability, tetany, decreased respirations *Hyperchloremia:* stupor, rapid deep breathing, muscle weakness

Understanding electrolytes *(continued)*

Electrolyte	Principal functions	Signs and symptoms of imbalance
Phosphorus (P) • Major anion in ICF • Normal serum level (phosphate level): 2.5 to 4.5 mg/dl	• Helps maintain bones and teeth • Helps maintain cell integrity • Plays major role in acid-base balance (as a urinary buffer) • Promotes energy transfer to cells • Plays essential role in muscle, red blood cell, and neurologic functions	*Hypophosphatemia:* paresthesia (circumoral and peripheral), lethargy, speech defects (such as stuttering or stammering) *Hyperphosphatemia:* renal failure, vague neuroexcitability to tetany and seizures, arrhythmias and muscle twitching with sudden rise in phosphate level
Magnesium (Mg++) • Major cation in ICF (closely related to Ca++ and P) • Normal serum level 1.5 to 2.5 with 33% bound protein and remainder as free cations	• Activates intracellular enzymes; active in carbohydrate and protein metabolism • Acts on myoneural vasodilation • Facilitates Na+ and K− movement across all membranes • Influences Ca++ levels	*Hypomagnesemia:* dizziness, confusion, seizures, tremor, leg and foot cramps, hyperirritability, arrhythmias, vasomotor changes, anorexia, nausea *Hypermagnesemia:* drowsiness, lethargy, coma, arrhythmias, hypotension, vague neuromuscular changes (such as tremor), vague GI symptoms (such as nausea), and slow, weak pulse

Extra extracellular info

The two ECF components — ISF and intravascular fluid (plasma) — have identical electrolyte compositions. Because of pores in the capillary walls, electrolytes can move freely between the ISF and plasma, allowing for equal distribution of electrolytes in both substances.

The protein contents of ISF and plasma differ, however. ISF doesn't contain proteins because protein molecules are too large to pass through capillary walls. Plasma has a high concentration of proteins.

Body fluids are in constant motion.

Fluid movement

Fluid movement is another mechanism that regulates fluid and electrolyte balance.

Ebb and flow

Body fluids are in constant motion; although separated by membranes, they continually move between the major fluid compartments. Besides regulating fluid and electrolyte balance, this is how nutrients, waste products, and other substances get into and out of cells, organs, and systems.

Fluid movement is influenced by membrane permeability and by colloid osmotic and hydrostatic pressure. Balance is maintained when solutes and fluids are distributed evenly on each side of the membrane. When this scale is tipped, solutes and fluids are able to restore balance by crossing membranes as needed.

Solutes and fluids have several modes for moving through membranes. Solutes move between compartments mainly by:
- diffusion (passive transport)
- active transport.

Fluids move between compartments by:
- osmosis
- capillary filtration and reabsorption.

Passive but effective

Most solutes move by diffusion; that is, they move from areas of higher concentration to areas of lower concentration. This change is referred to as moving down the concentration gradient. The result is an equal distribution of solutes. Because diffusion doesn't require energy, it's considered a form of passive transport.

Against the gradient

By contrast, in active transport, solutes move from areas of lower concentration to areas of higher concentration. This change, referred to as moving against the concentration gradient, requires energy in the form of adenosine triphosphate.

In active transport, solutes are moved by physiologic pumps. You're probably familiar with one active transport pump — the sodium-potassium pump. It moves sodium ions out of cells to the ECF and potassium ions into cells from the ECF. This balances sodium and potassium concentrations.

Oh, osmosis

Fluids move by osmosis. Movement of water is caused by the existence of a concentration gradient. Water flows passively across the membrane, from an area of higher water concentration to an area of lower water concentration.

Memory jogger

Remember, diffusion is a descender; active transport is an ascender:

Diffusion descends (high to low)

In Diffusion, solutes **descend** the concentration gradient. Movement is from an area of **higher** concentration to one of **lower** concentration.

Active transport ascends (low to high)

In Active transport, solutes **ascend** against the gradient. Movement is from an area of **lower** concentration to an area of **higher** concentration, as if Ascending.

This dilution process stops when the solute concentrations on both sides of the membrane are equal.

Osmosis between the ECF and the ICF depends on the osmolarity (concentration) of the compartments. Normally, the osmotic (pulling) pressures of ECF and ICF are equal.

Equal but unbalanced

Osmosis can create a fluid imbalance between the ECF and ICF compartments despite equal concentrations of solute if the concentrations aren't optimal. This can cause complications such as tissue edema.

Up against the capillary wall

Of all the vessels in the vascular system, only capillaries have walls thin enough to let solutes pass. Water and solutes move across capillary walls by two opposing processes:

 capillary filtration

capillary reabsorption.

Filtration is the movement of substances from an area of high hydrostatic pressure to an area of lower hydrostatic pressure (hydrostatic pressure is the pressure at any level on water at rest due to weight of water above it). Capillary filtration forces fluid and solutes through capillary wall pores and into the ISF.

Left unchecked, capillary filtration would cause plasma to move in only one direction — out of the capillaries. This movement would cause severe hypovolemia and shock.

Fortunately, capillary reabsorption keeps capillary filtration in check. During filtration, albumin, a protein that can't pass through capillary walls, remains behind in the diminishing volume of water. As the albumin concentration inside the capillaries increases, the albumin begins to draw water back in by osmosis. Water is thus reabsorbed by capillaries.

COP story

The osmotic, or pulling, force of albumin in capillary reabsorption is called colloid osmotic pressure (COP), or oncotic pressure. As long as capillary blood pressure exceeds COP, water and diffusible solutes can leave the cap-

Memory jogger

Think *O* is for osmosis: *O*smosis is *O*ngoing when *O*smolarity is *O*ff balance.

Capillary filtration is a pushy process . . .

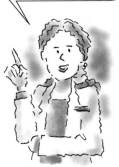

. . . and capillary reabsorption has a lot of pull.

illaries and circulate into the ISF. When capillary blood pressure falls below COP, water and diffusible solutes return to the capillaries.

Up to the midpoint

In any capillary, blood pressure normally exceeds COP up to the vessel's midpoint, then falls below COP along the rest of the vessel. That's why capillary filtration takes place along the first half of a capillary, and reabsorption occurs along the second half. As long as capillary blood pressure and plasma albumin levels remain normal, no net movement of water occurs.

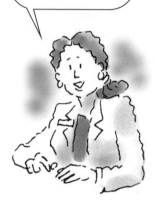

Tiny but tireless, capillaries expel and reabsorb fluids concurrently.

Correcting imbalances

The effect an I.V. solution has on fluid compartments depends on how the solution's osmolarity compares with the patient's serum osmolarity.

Serum osmolarity normally at parity

Osmolarity is the concentration of a solution. It's expressed in milliosmols of solute per liter of solution (mOsm/L). Normally, serum has the same osmolarity as other body fluids, about 300 mOsm/L. A lower serum osmolarity suggests fluid overload; a higher osmolarity suggests hemoconcentration and dehydration.

Restoring the balance

When serum osmolarity increases or decreases, the doctor may order I.V. solutions to maintain or restore fluid balance. There are three basic types of I.V. solutions:

 isotonic

 hypotonic

 hypertonic.

(See *Understanding I.V. solutions*.)

Isotonic solutions

An isotonic I.V. solution has the same osmolarity (or tonicity) as serum and other body fluids. Because the solution doesn't alter serum osmolarity, it stays where it's infused, inside the blood vessel (the intravascular compartment).

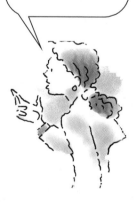

An isotonic solution stays where it's infused, inside the blood vessel.

Now I get it!

Understanding I.V. solutions

Solutions used for I.V. therapy may be isotonic, hypotonic, or hypertonic. The type you give a patient depends on whether you want to change or maintain his body fluid status.

Isotonic solution

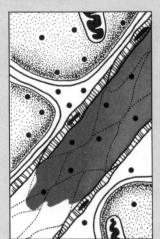

Hypotonic solution

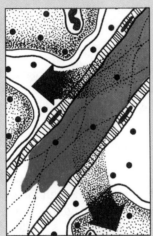

Hypertonic solution

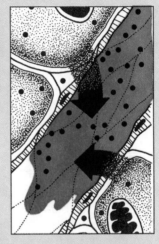

An isotonic solution has an osmolarity about equal to that of serum. Because it stays in the intravascular space, it expands the intravascular compartment and is an excellent choice for hydration.

A hypotonic solution has an osmolarity lower than that of serum. It shifts fluid out of the intravascular compartment, hydrating the cells and the interstitial compartments.

A hypertonic solution has an osmolarity higher than that of serum. It draws fluid into the intravascular compartment from the cells and the interstitial compartments.

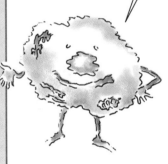

For more information on I.V. solutions, see pages 27 to 29.

The solution expands this compartment without pulling fluid from other compartments.

One indication for an isotonic solution is hypotension due to hypovolemia. Common isotonic solutions include lactated Ringer's and normal saline.

Hypertonic solutions

A hypertonic I.V. solution has an osmolarity higher than serum osmolarity. When a patient receives a hypertonic I.V. solution, serum osmolarity initially increases, causing fluid to be pulled from the interstitial and intracellular compartments into the blood vessels.

Don't get hyper about it

Hypertonic solutions may be ordered for patients postoperatively. That's because the shift of fluid into the blood vessels caused by a hypertonic solution has several beneficial effects for these patients. For example, it:
- reduces the risk of edema
- stabilizes blood pressure
- regulates urine output.

Examples

Some examples of hypertonic solutions are dextrose 5% in half-normal saline (405 mOsm/L), dextrose 5% in normal saline (560 mOsm/L), and dextrose 5% in lactated Ringer's solution (527 mOsm/L).

Hypotonic solutions

A hypotonic I.V. solution has an osmolarity lower than serum osmolarity. When a patient receives a hypotonic solution, fluid shifts out of the blood vessels and into the cells and interstitial spaces, where osmolarity is higher. A hypotonic solution hydrates cells while reducing fluid in the circulatory system.

Hypotonic solutions may be ordered when diuretic therapy dehydrates cells. Other indications include hyperglycemic conditions, such as diabetic ketoacidosis and hyperosmolar hyperglycemic nonketotic syndrome. In these conditions, high serum glucose levels draw fluid out of cells. Examples of hypotonic solutions include: half-normal saline, 0.33% sodium chloride, dextrose 5% in water, and dextrose 2.5%.

Not for everyone

Because hypotonic solutions flood cells, certain patients shouldn't receive them. For example, patients with cerebral edema or increased intracranial pressure shouldn't receive hypotonic solutions because the increased extracellular fluid can cause further tissue damage and edema.

A few common solutions can be used to illustrate the role of I.V. therapy in restoring and maintaining fluid and electrolyte balance. (See *Quick guide to I.V. solutions.*)

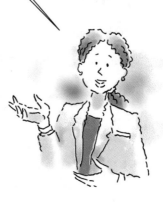

A hypertonic solution causes fluid to be pulled from the interstitial and intracellular compartments into the blood vessels.

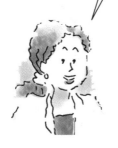

Note that the osmolarity of all these hypertonic solutions is greater than the osmolarity of body fluids, which is about 300 mOsm/L.

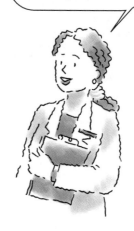

A hypotonic solution causes fluid to shift out of the blood vessels and into the cells and interstitial spaces.

Quick guide to I.V. solutions

A solution is isotonic if its osmolarity falls within (or near) the normal range for serum (275 to 295 mOsm/L). A hypotonic solution has a lower osmolarity; a hypertonic solution, a higher osmolarity.

   This chart lists common examples of the three types of I.V. solutions and provides key considerations for administering them.

Solution	Examples	Nursing considerations
Isotonic	• Lactated Ringer's (275 mOsm/L) • Ringer's (275 mOsm/L) • Normal saline (308 mOsm/L) • Dextrose 5% in water (D_5W) (260 mOsm/L) • 5% albumin (308 mOsm/L) • Hetastarch (310 mOsm/L) • Normosol (295 mOsm/L)	• Because these solutions expand the intravascular compartment, closely monitor your patient for signs of fluid overload, especially if he has hypertension or heart failure. • Because the liver converts lactate to bicarbonate, don't give lactated Ringer's solution if the patient's blood pH exceeds 7.5. • Don't give lactated Ringer's solution if the patient has liver disease because he won't be able to metabolize lactate. • Avoid giving D_5W to a patient at risk for increased intracranial pressure (ICP), because it acts like a hypotonic solution. (Although usually considered isotonic, D_5W is actually isotonic only in the container. After administration, dextrose is quickly metabolized, leaving only water — a hypotonic fluid.)
Hypotonic	• Half-normal saline (154 mOsm/L) • 0.33% sodium chloride (103 mOsm/L) • Dextrose 2.5% in water (126 mOsm/L)	• Administer cautiously. These solutions will cause a fluid shift from blood vessels into cells. This could cause cardiovascular collapse from intravascular fluid depletion and increased ICP from fluid shift into brain cells. • Don't give hypotonic solutions to patients at risk for increased ICP from cerebrovascular accident, head trauma, or neurosurgery. • Don't give hypotonic solutions to patients at risk for third-space fluid shifts (abnormal fluid shifts into the interstitial compartment or a body cavity) — for example, patients suffering from burns, trauma, or low serum protein levels from malnutrition or liver disease.
Hypertonic	• Dextrose 5% in half-normal saline (406 mOsm/L) • Dextrose 5% in normal saline (560 mOsm/L) • Dextrose 5% in lactated Ringer's (575 mOsm/L) • 3% sodium chloride (1,025 mOsm/L) • 25% albumin (1,500 mOsm/L) • 7.5% sodium chloride (2,400 mOsm/L)	• Because these solutions greatly expand the intravascular compartment, closely monitor your patient for circulatory overload. • Hypertonic solutions pull fluid from the intracellular compartment, so don't give them to a patient with a condition that causes cellular dehydration — for example, diabetic ketoacidosis. • Don't give hypertonic solutions to a patient with impaired heart or kidney function — his system can't handle the extra fluid.

Additional uses of I.V. therapy

Besides restoring and maintaining fluid and electrolyte balance, I.V. therapy is used to administer drugs, transfuse blood and blood products, and deliver parenteral nutrition.

Drug administration

The I.V. route provides a rapid, effective way of administering medications. Commonly infused drugs include antibiotics, thrombolytics, histamine-receptor antagonists, and antineoplastic, cardiovascular, and anticonvulsant drugs.

Drugs may be delivered long-term by continuous infusion, over a short period, or directly as a single dose.

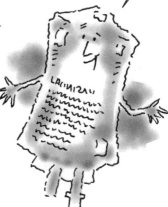

Leave it to me to deliver drugs rapidly and effectively.

Blood administration

Your nursing responsibilities also may include giving blood and blood components and monitoring patients receiving transfusion therapy. Blood products can be given through a peripheral or central I.V. line. Various blood products are given to:
• restore and maintain adequate blood volume
• prevent cardiogenic shock
• increase the blood's oxygen-carrying capacity
• maintain hemostasis.

Parts of the whole

Whole blood is composed of cellular elements and plasma. Cellular elements include:
• erythrocytes, or red blood cells (RBCs)
• leukocytes, or white blood cells (WBCs)
• thrombocytes, or platelets.
Each of these elements is packaged separately for transfusion. Plasma may be delivered intact or separated into several components that may be given to correct various deficiencies. Whole blood transfusions are unnecessary unless the patient has lost massive quantities of blood in a short period.

Parenteral nutrition

Parenteral nutrition provides essential nutrients to the blood, organs, and cells by the I.V. route. It's not the same as a seven-course meal in a fine restaurant, but I.V. nutrients can contain the essence of a balanced diet.

You wouldn't call it gourmet cooking but...

The ingredients in solutions developed for total parenteral nutrition (TPN) provide all of a patient's energy and nutrient requirements:
- proteins
- carbohydrates
- fats
- electrolytes
- vitamins
- trace elements
- water.

A patient can receive TPN indefinitely.

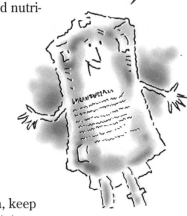

Would you like to hear today's specials?

Tracking changes

When your patient is receiving parenteral nutrition, keep close track of changes in his fluid and electrolyte status and glucose levels. You'll also need to assess your patient's response to the nutrient solution to detect early signs of complications, such as alterations in the pancreatic enzymes (lipase, amylase trypsin, and chymotrypsin) or in the albumin.

A limited menu

Peripheral parenteral nutrition (PPN) is delivered by peripheral veins. PPN is used in limited nutritional therapy. The solution contains fewer nonprotein calories and lower amino acid concentrations than TPN solutions. It may also include lipid emulsions. A patient can receive PPN for approximately 3 weeks. It can be used to support the nutritional status of a patient who doesn't require total nutritional support.

I.V. delivery

Depending in part on how concentrated an I.V. solution is, it may be delivered by one of two routes:

 through a peripheral vein

 through a central vein.

Usually, a low-concentration solution is infused through a peripheral vein in the arm or hand; a more concentrated solution may be given through a central vein. (See *Veins used in I.V. therapy.*)

Delivery methods

There are three basic methods for delivering I.V. therapy:

 continuous infusion

 intermittent infusion

 direct injection.

Prolonged, short-term, or single dose

Continuous I.V. therapy allows you to give a carefully regulated amount of fluid over a prolonged period. In intermittent I.V. therapy, a solution (often a medication) is given for shorter periods at set intervals. Direct injection (sometimes called I.V. push) is used to deliver a single dose (bolus) of a drug or other substance.

Choosing a method

The choice of I.V. delivery method depends not only on the purpose and duration of therapy, but also on the patient's condition, age, and health history.

At times, a patient may receive I.V. therapy by more than one delivery method. Also, variations of each delivery method may be used. Some therapies also require extra equipment. For example, in some long-term chemotherapy, an implanted central venous access device is needed. (See *Comparing I.V. delivery methods,* pages 20 to 22.)

Which I.V. delivery method? That depends on the purpose and duration of therapy and the patient's condition, age, and health history.

Continuous infusion

A continuous I.V. infusion helps maintain a constant therapeutic drug level. It's also used to provide I.V. fluid therapy or parenteral nutrition.

Veins used in I.V. therapy

This illustration shows the veins commonly used for peripheral I.V. and central venous therapy.

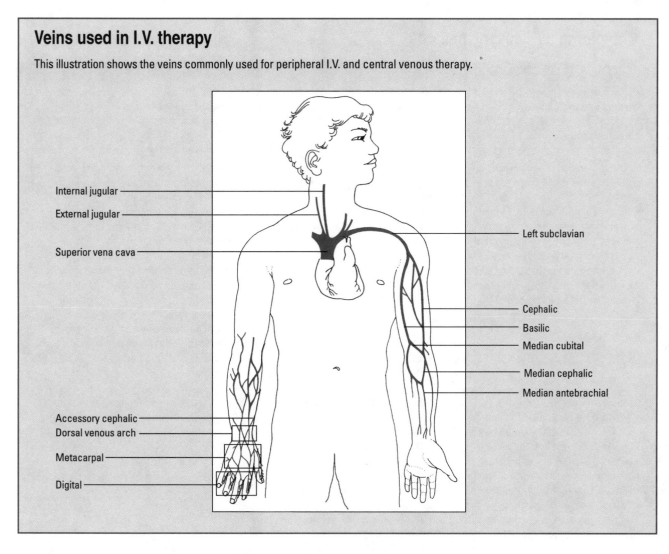

- Internal jugular
- External jugular
- Superior vena cava
- Left subclavian
- Cephalic
- Basilic
- Median cubital
- Median cephalic
- Median antebrachial
- Accessory cephalic
- Dorsal venous arch
- Metacarpal
- Digital

Upside

Continuous I.V. infusion has its advantages. For example, less time is spent mixing solutions and hanging containers than with the intermittent method. You'll also handle less tubing and access the patient's I.V. device less often, decreasing the risk of infection.

Downside

Continuous administration has some disadvantages, too. For example, the patient may become annoyed if the

(Text continues on page 22.)

Comparing I.V. delivery methods

This chart gives you the indications, advantages, and disadvantages of methods commonly used to administer I.V. medications.

Method and indications	Advantages	Disadvantages
Direct injection		
Into a vein, which doesn't involve any infusion line and is often referred to as I.V. push • When a nonirritating drug with low risk of immediate adverse reaction is required for a patient with no other I.V. needs (for example, outpatients requiring I.V. contrast injections for radiologic examinations or cancer patients receiving chemotherapeutic agents)	• Eliminates risk of complications from implanted (indwelling) venipuncture device. • Eliminates inconvenience of indwelling venipuncture device.	• Can only be given by doctor or specially certified nurse. • Requires venipuncture, which can cause patient anxiety. • Requires two syringes — one to administer medication and one to flush vein after administration. • Risks infiltration (puncture of the vein, allowing the solution to enter the surrounding tissue) from steel needle. • It isn't possible to dilute drug or interrupt delivery when irritation occurs. • Risks clotting with administration of drug over a long period and with a small volume.
Through existing infusion line • When drug required is incompatible with I.V. solution and must be given as bolus injection for therapeutic effect • When patient requires immediate high blood levels of a medication (for example, regular insulin, dextrose 50%, atropine, and antihistamines) • In emergencies, when drug must be given quickly for immediate effect	• Doesn't require time or authorization to perform venipuncture because vein is already accessed. • Doesn't require needle puncture, which can cause patient anxiety. • Allows use of I.V. solution to test patency of venipuncture device before drug administration. • Allows continued venous access in case of adverse reactions. • Reduces risk of infiltration with irritating drugs because most continuous infusions are started with an over-the-needle catheter.	• Carries same inconveniences and complication risks associated with an indwelling venipuncture device.

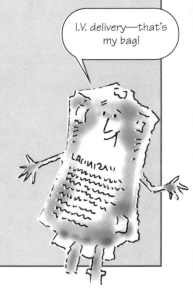

I.V. delivery—that's my bag!

Comparing I.V. delivery methods *(continued)*

Method and indications	Advantages	Disadvantages
Intermittent infusion		
Piggyback method, which requires plugging a second administration set into a primary line • Often used with drugs given over short periods at varying intervals (for example, antibiotics and gastric secretion inhibitors)	• Avoids multiple needle injections required for I.M. injections. • Permits repeated administration of drugs through single I.V. site. • Provides high drug blood levels for short periods without causing drug toxicity.	• May cause periods when drug level becomes too low to be clinically effective (for example, when peak and trough times aren't considered in the medication order).
Heparin (or saline) lock, which allows for maintaining venous access • When patient requires constant venous access but not continuous infusion	• Provides venous access for patients with fluid restrictions. • Allows better patient mobility between doses. • Preserves veins by reducing venipuncture. • Lowers cost.	• Requires close monitoring during administration so device can be flushed on completion. • Can't use heparin flush if patient has heparin sensitivity; sterile saline flush most commonly used in adults with peripheral I.V. access devices.
Volume-control set, which has a medication chamber that allows it to deliver small doses over an extended period • When patient requires low volume of fluid	• Requires only one large-volume container; prevents fluid overload from runaway infusion. • Chamber is reusable.	• Costs for equipment may be high. • Risk of contamination is high. • If set doesn't contain membrane to block air passage when empty, must close flow clamp when set empties.
Continuous infusion		
Through primary line, which provides direct access to the vein • When continuous serum levels are needed and there's little chance infusion will be stopped abruptly	• Maintains steady serum levels. • Less risk of rapid shock and vein irritation from large volume of fluid diluting drug.	• Increases risk of incompatibility with drugs administered by piggyback infusion. • Patient is connected to I.V. system, restricting mobility. • Increases risk of undetected infiltration because slow infusion makes it difficult to see swelling in area of infiltration.

(continued)

Comparing I.V. delivery methods (continued)

Method and indications	Advantages	Disadvantages
Continuous infusion (continued)		
Through secondary line, which is piggybacked onto a primary line • When patient requires continuous infusion of two or more compatible admixtures administered at different rates • When there is moderate to high chance of abruptly stopping one admixture without infusing the drug remaining in the I.V. tubing	• Permits primary infusion and each secondary infusion to be given at different rates. • Permits primary line to be shut off and kept standing by to maintain venous access in case secondary line must be abruptly stopped.	• Increases risk of incompatibility with piggyback infusion. • Patient is connected to I.V. system, restricting mobility. • Increases risk of undetected infiltration because slow infusion makes it difficult to see swelling in area of infiltration. • Eliminates use of drugs with immediate incompatibility. • Increases risk of phlebitis or vein irritation from increased number of drugs. • Uses multiple I.V. systems (for example, primary lines with secondary lines attached), which can create physical barriers to patient care and limit patient mobility, especially those with electronic pumps or controllers.

equipment hinders mobility and interferes with other activities of daily living. Also, the drip rate must be carefully monitored to ensure that the I.V. fluid and medication don't infuse too rapidly or too slowly.

Intermittent infusion

The most common and flexible method of administering I.V. medications is by intermittent infusion.

On again, off again

In intermittent I.V. infusion, drugs are administered over a specified period at varying intervals, thereby maintaining therapeutic blood levels. A small volume (1 to 250 ml) may be delivered over several minutes or a few hours, depending on the infusion prescription. You can deliver an intermittent infusion through a primary line (the most common method) or a secondary line. The secondary line is usually piggybacked into the primary line by way of a Y-

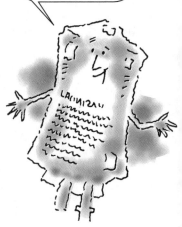

I can be flexible. Use intermittent infusion to administer drugs over short periods at varying intervals.

site (a Y-shaped section of tubing with a self-sealing rubber diaphragm).

Direct injection

You might say that I.V. therapy by direct injection gets right to the point. You can access a vein directly for a single dose of a prescribed drug or other substance, removing the needle when the bolus is completed. You may also give a bolus injection through an intermittent infusion device (called a heparin or saline lock) that is already in place.

Administration sets

You need to choose the correct administration set for your patient's infusion. Your choice depends on the type of infusion to be provided, the infusion container, and whether you're using a volume-control device.

Vented and unvented

I.V. administration sets come in two forms: vented and unvented. The vented set is for containers that have no venting system (I.V. plastic bags and some bottles). The unvented are for those bottles that have their own venting system.

Various other features

I.V. administration sets come with various other features as well, including ports for infusing secondary medications and filters for blocking microbes, irritants, or large particles. The tubing also varies. Some types are designed to enhance the proper functioning of devices that help regulate the flow rate. Other tubing is used specifically for continuous or intermittent infusion, for infusing parenteral nutrition and blood, or for monitoring blood pressure.

I.V. flow rates

A key aspect of administering I.V. therapy is maintaining accurate flow rates for the I.V. solutions. If an infusion runs too fast or too slow, your patient may suffer complications, such as phlebitis, infiltration, circulatory overload (possibly leading to heart failure and pulmonary edema), and adverse drug reactions.

Volume-control devices and the correct I.V. tubing help prevent such complications. You can help too by being familiar with all of the information in doctors' orders and being able to recognize orders for I.V. therapy that are incomplete or written incorrectly. (See *Reading an I.V. order.*)

Calculating flow rates

There are two basic types of flow rates available with I.V. administration sets:

 macrodrip

 microdrip.

Each set delivers a specific number of drops per milliliter (gtt/ml). Macrodrip delivers 10, 15, or 20 gtt/ml; microdrip delivers 60 gtt/ml. Regardless of the type of set you use, the formula for calculating flow rates is the same. (See *Calculating flow rates.*)

Regulating flow rates

When a patient's condition requires you to maintain precise I.V. flow rates, use an infusion control device, such as:
• clamps
• volumetric controllers
• nonvolumetric controllers (rely on gravity)
• volumetric pumps
• rate minders.

ml/hour or gtt/minute?

When you regulate I.V. flow rate with a clamp or a nonvolumetric controller, the rate is usually measured in

Reading an I.V. order

Orders for I.V. therapy may be standardized for different illnesses and therapies (such as burn treatment) or individualized for a particular patient. Some hospital policies dictate an automatic stop order for I.V. fluids. For example, I.V. orders are good for 24 hours from the time they're written, unless otherwise specified.

It's complete
A complete order for I.V. therapy should specify the following:
• type and amount of solution
• any additives and their concentrations (such as 10 mEq potassium chloride in 500 ml dextrose 5% in water)
• rate and volume of infusion
• duration of infusion.

It's not complete
If you find that an order isn't complete or you think an I.V. order is inappropriate because of the patient's condition, consult the doctor.

drops per minute (gtt/minute). If you use a volumetric
controller or pump, the flow rate is measured in milliliters
per hour (ml/hour).

Advice from the experts

Calculating flow rates

When calculating the flow rate (drops per minute) of I.V. solutions, remember that the number of drops required to deliver 1 ml varies with the type of administration set used and its manufacturer.
• Administration sets are of two types — macrodrip (the standard type) and microdrip. Macrodrip delivers 10 to 20 gtt/ml; microdrip usually delivers about 60 gtt/ml (see illustrations).
• Manufacturers calibrate their devices differently, so be sure to look for the "drip factor" — expressed in drops per milliliter, or gtt/ml — in the packaging that accompanies the device you're using. (This packaging also has crucial information about such things as special infusions and blood transfusions.)
   Once you know your device's drip factor, use the following formula to calculate specific flow rates:

$$\frac{\text{volume of infusion (in milliliters)}}{\text{time of infusion (in minutes)}} \times \text{drip factor (in drops per milliliter)} = \text{flow rate (in drops per minute)}$$

After you calculate the flow rate for the I.V. set you're using, remove your watch or position your wrist so you can look at your watch and the drops at the same time. Next, adjust the clamp to achieve the ordered flow rate and count the drops for 1 full minute. Readjust the clamp, as necessary, and count the drops for another minute. Keep adjusting the clamp and counting the drops until you have the correct rate.

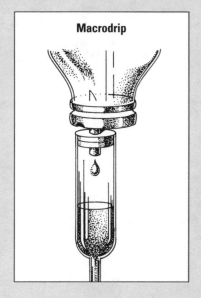

Macrodrip

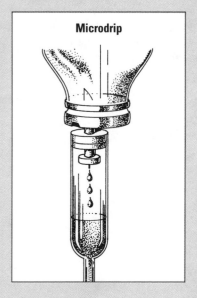

Microdrip

I.V. clamps

You can regulate the I.V. flow rate with two types of clamps:

 screw clamp

 roller clamp.

The screw clamp offers greater accuracy but the roller clamp, used for standard fluid therapy, is faster and easier to manipulate. A third type, the slide clamp, can stop or start the flow but can't regulate the rate. (See *Using I.V. clamps.*)

Controllers and pumps

New controllers and pumps are being developed all the time; be sure to attend instruction sessions to learn how to use them. On your unit, keep a file of instruction manuals (provided by the manufacturers) for each piece of equipment used.

(Text continues on page 31.)

Running smoothly

Using I.V. clamps

You may use a roller or a screw clamp to regulate the flow of an I.V. solution. With these clamps, a wheel or screw increases or decreases the flow through the I.V. line. The slide clamp moves horizontally to open and close the I.V. line. It can stop and start the flow but doesn't allow fine adjustments to regulate the flow. The illustrations below show each type of clamp, with arrows to indicate the direction you turn or push to open the clamp.

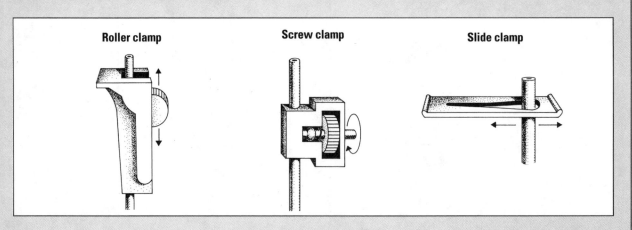

Roller clamp **Screw clamp** **Slide clamp**

Incredibly Easy miniguide: Isotonic solutions

How isotonic solutions affect cells

An isotonic solution has the same solute concentration (or osmolarity) as serum and other body fluids. Infusing the solution doesn't alter the concentration of serum; therefore, osmosis doesn't occur. (For osmosis to occur, there must be a difference in solute concentration between serum and the interstitial fluid.)

The isotonic solution stays where it's infused, inside the blood vessel, and doesn't affect the size of cells.

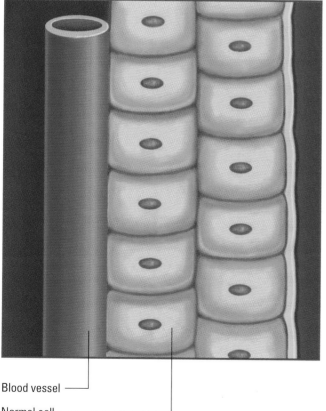

Blood vessel

Normal cell

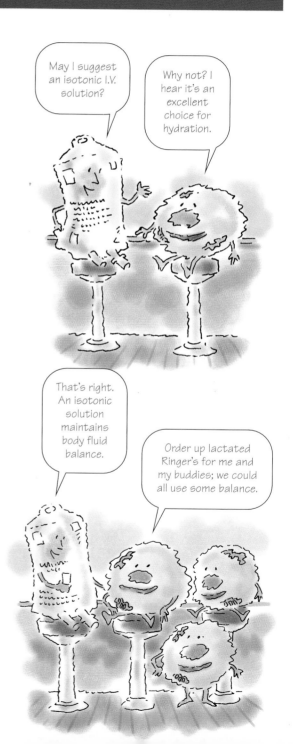

Incredibly Easy miniguide: Hypertonic solutions

How hypertonic solutions affect cells

A hypertonic I.V. solution has a solute concentration higher than the solute concentration of serum. Infusing a hypertonic solution increases the solute concentration of serum. Because the solute concentration of serum is now different from the interstitial fluid, osmosis occurs. Fluid is pulled from the cells and the interstitial compartment into the blood vessels.

Many patients receive hypertonic fluids postoperatively. The shift of fluid into the blood vessels reduces the risk of edema, stabilizes blood pressure, and regulates urine output.

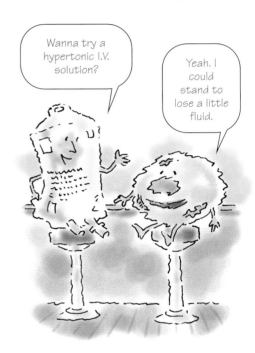

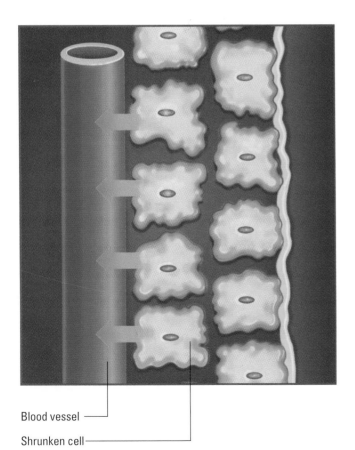

Blood vessel

Shrunken cell

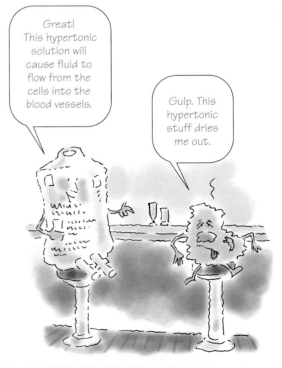

Incredibly Easy miniguide: Hypotonic solutions

How hypotonic solutions affect cells

A hypotonic I.V. solution is the opposite of a hypertonic solution. It has a lower solute concentration than serum. Infusion of a hypotonic solution causes the solute concentration of serum to decrease. Because the solute concentration of serum is now different from the interstitial fluid, osmosis occurs.

This time, the fluid shift is in the opposite direction than that of a hypertonic fluid. Fluid shifts out of the blood vessels and into the cells and interstitial spaces, where the solute concentration is higher.

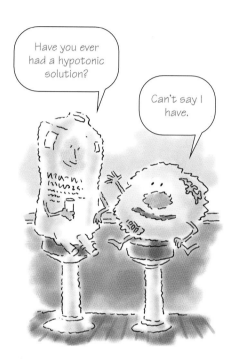

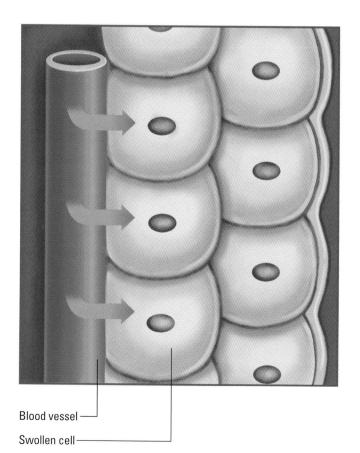

Blood vessel —
Swollen cell —

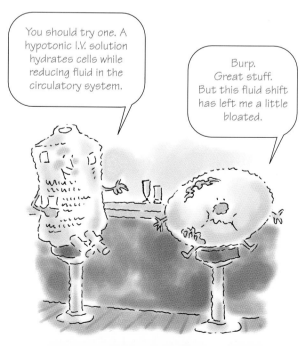

Incredibly Easy miniguide: Common catheter insertion sites

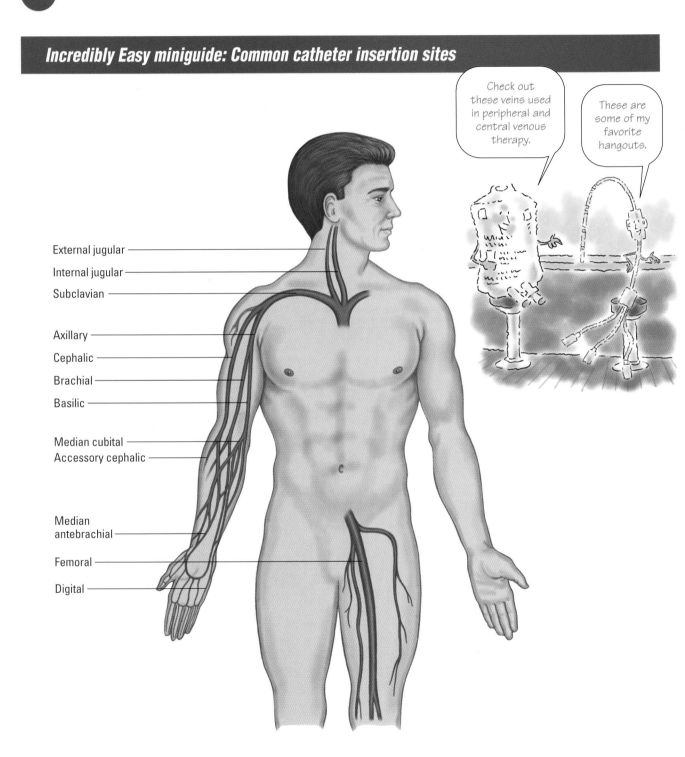

Rate minder

Another type of flow control device is the rate minder, which resembles a roller clamp. This device is added to the I.V. tubing. By setting the rate minder to the desired flow rate, you adjust the clamp to deliver that rate. Be sure you label the infusion bag with the rate in milliliters per hour.

Limitations

Rate minders have some limitations. The flow rate may vary by as much as 5%, so the infusion must be checked frequently to prevent a too-rapid infusion or nonflow situations. The other drawback is that the rate minders don't usually deliver infusions at rates lower than 5 to 10 ml/hour. For this reason, they're used mainly in adult patients and only with noncritical infusions.

Factors that affect flow rate

When you're using a clamp for flow regulation, you must monitor the flow rate closely and adjust as needed. Factors such as vein spasm, vein pressure changes, patient movement, manipulations of the clamp, and bent or kinked tubing can cause the rate to vary markedly. For easy monitoring, use a time tape, which marks the prescribed solution level at hourly intervals. (See *Using a time tape*.)

Other factors that affect I.V. flow rate include the type of I.V. fluid and its viscosity, the height of the infusion container, the type of administration set, and the size and position of the venous access device.

Checking flow rates

Flow rates can be fickle; they need to be checked and adjusted regularly. The frequency at which I.V. flow rates are checked depends on the patient's condition and age and the I.V. solution or medication being administered.

I'll be back soon!

Many nurses check the I.V. flow rate every time they're in a patient's room and after each position change. The flow rate should be assessed more frequently for some patients, such as:

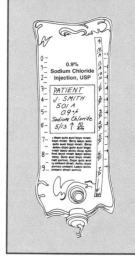

- critically ill patients
- patients with conditions that might by exacerbated by fluid overload
- pediatric patients
- elderly patients
- patients receiving a drug that can cause tissue damage if infiltration occurs.

Back on schedule

If the infusion rate slows significantly, you can usually get it back on schedule by adjusting the rate slightly. Don't make a major adjustment, though. If the rate must be increased by more than 30%, check with the doctor.

You should also time an infusion control device or rate minder for 1 to 2 hours per shift. (These devices have an error rate ranging from 2% to 10%.) Before using any infusion control device, become thoroughly familiar with its features. Attend instruction sessions and perform return demonstrations until you learn the system.

Memory jogger

To remind yourself of the need to check and adjust flow rates, remember the following tongue twister:

Fight fickle flow with frequent follow-up.

Professional and legal standards

Administering drugs and solutions to patients is one of the most legally significant tasks nurses perform. Unfortunately, the number of lawsuits directed against nurses who are involved in I.V. therapy is increasing. For example, a 1995 Missouri study reported a high incidence of errors involving I.V. solution administration, with the wrong solution used or administered by an incorrect route. Many lawsuits centered on errors in infusion pump use.

Lawsuits may also result from administration of the wrong medication dosage, inappropriate placement of an I.V. line, and failure to monitor for adverse reactions, infiltration, dislodgment of I.V. equipment, or other mishaps.

Court cases

The following are examples of lawsuits involving I.V. therapy.

Versed verdict

In a 1990 Los Angeles case, a nurse administered Versed (midazolam) through a port in an I.V. line to an infant,

The court determines liability based on the standards of care required of nurses when administering I.V. medications.

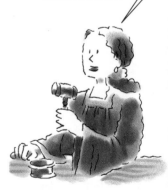

leading to the infant's death. This nurse had never administered I.V. Versed to an infant or child before. A hospital protocol prohibited the use of Versed on the pediatric floor. The manufacturer recommended a dosage of 0.1 mg/kg, and the infant weighed 9 kg. The hospital record indicated 5 mg had been administered. A settlement awarded the plaintiff $225,000.

Still accountable

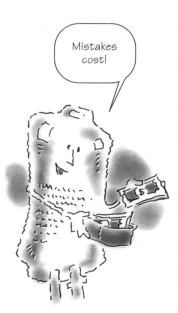

Mistakes cost!

In a 1993 Los Angeles case, continuous infusion of 145 mg of morphine over 18 hours led to a patient's death. The doctor failed to limit the amount to be infused. Nevertheless, the charge nurse and staff nurse were held accountable for failing to recognize a "gross overdose." The patient's widow and children were awarded over $2 million for lost wages and general damages.

Syringe confusion

In a 1992 Illinois case, a nurse administered the wrong dose of Xylocaine (lidocaine). The order was for 100 mg; the nurse injected 2 g. The packaging caused confusion: the Xylocaine was provided in a 2-g syringe for mixing into an I.V. solution and in a 100-mg syringe for direct injection. The nurse accidentally used the 2-g syringe. However, information about previous overdose incidents from the FDA and medical literature had been available to the hospital.

Clamp error

In a 1992 Ohio case, a nurse failed to clamp a pump regulating the flow of antibiotic through a central line to a child. This resulted in delivery of nearly seven times the prescribed dosage of gentamicin, causing the child to become totally deaf.

Infiltration injury

In Pennsylvania, an emergency department nurse misplaced an I.V. line, which infiltrated into the patient's hand, resulting in reflex sympathetic dystrophy. The patient couldn't return to work and won a $702,000 award.

Striking a nerve

Several recent lawsuits have involved allegations that a nurse struck a patient's radial nerve during insertion of an I.V. line. Such injuries can cause compartment syndrome and may require emergency fasciotomy, skin grafts, and other surgery. Uncorrected compartment syndrome can progress to gangrene and amputation of fingers. One New York case involving finger amputation resulted in a $40 million jury verdict, later reduced to $5 million.

Listen up

When monitoring an I.V. line, listening to the patient is as important as monitoring the site, pump, and tubing. In the Tampa, Florida, case of *Frank v. Hillsborough County Hospital*, a patient's frequent complaints of pain were ignored. The patient suffered permanent nerve damage and, in 1997, obtained an award of almost $60,000.

Know your responsibility

As a nurse, you have a legal and ethical responsibility to your patients. The good news is that if you honor these duties and meet the appropriate standards of care, you will be able to hold your own in court.

By becoming aware of professional standards and laws related to administering I.V. therapy, you can both provide the best care for your patients and protect yourself legally. Professional and legal standards are defined by state nurse practice acts, federal regulations, and institutional policies.

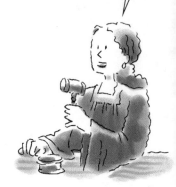

When monitoring an I.V. line, listening to the patient is as important as monitoring the site, pump, and tubing.

State nurse practice acts

Each state has a nurse practice act that broadly defines the legal scope of nursing practice. Your state's nurse practice act is the most important law affecting your nursing practice.

Within the limits

Every nurse is expected to care for patients within defined limits. If a nurse gives care beyond those limits, she becomes vulnerable to charges of violating her state nurse practice act. For a copy of your state nurse practice act, contact your state nurse's association or your state board of nursing.

Many state nurse practice acts don't specifically address scope of practice issues with regard to I.V. therapy for RNs. However, many state nurse practice acts do address whether LPNs or LVNs can administer I.V. therapy.

This is important for LPNs and LVNs, and for RNs who are supervising or training LPNs or LVNs.

Federal regulations

The federal government issues regulations and establishes policies related to administration of I.V. therapy. For example, the federal government mandates adherence to standards of I.V. therapy practice for health care facilities to be eligible to receive reimbursement under Medicare, Medicaid, and other programs.

75 million served

Medicare and Medicaid, the two major federal health care programs, serve about 75 million Americans. They are run by the Health Care Financing Administration (HCFA), which is part of the Department of Health and Human Services. HCFA formulates national Medicare policy, including policies related to I.V. therapy, but contracts with private insurance companies to oversee claims and make payment for services and supplies provided under Medicare. These agencies, in turn, enforce HCFA policy by accepting or denying claims for reimbursement. When reviewing claims, agencies may evaluate practices and quality of care — an important factor underlying the emphasis on proper documentation in health care.

Medicaid, which serves certain low income people, is a state-federal partnership administered by a state agency. There are broad federal requirements for Medicaid, but states have a wide degree of flexibility to design their own programs.

One patient, many regulators

To be eligible for reimbursement, health care agencies must comply with the standards of a complex network of regulators. Consider, for example, a patient receiving I.V. medications at home with a reusable pump. This patient is primarily covered by Medicare with secondary Medicaid coverage. A variety of carriers, fiscal intermediaries, and agencies share responsibility for reimbursement and regulatory oversight of the patient's care:
• An insurance carrier contracts with Medicare to cover services such as refilling the pump.

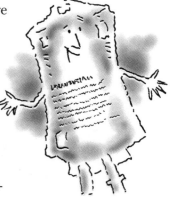

Big Brother is watching me!

• A separate insurance carrier (a durable medical equipment carrier designated by HCFA) covers administered drugs, the pump itself, and pump supplies.

• Another insurance carrier (called a fiscal intermediary) contracts with Medicare to cover preliminary in-hospital training of the patient in I.V. therapy techniques.

• A Medicaid agency also covers a portion of the patient's care.

Nursing documentation must be complete enough to meet the requirements of all these different agencies. The underlying (though unstated) philosophy of these agencies is that "if it's not documented, it's not done." The regulatory network is becoming more complicated as many Medicare and Medicaid patients are being covered by managed care organizations that have their own rules and procedures.

Institutional policy

Every health care facility has I.V. therapy policies for nurses. Such policies are required to obtain accreditation from the Joint Commission on Accreditation of Healthcare Organizations and other accrediting bodies. These policies can't go beyond what a state's nurse practice act permits but they more specifically define your duties and responsibilities.

Awareness of institutional policy is particularly important in rapidly developing areas of practice, such as home care, where the intensity of service and patient needs is increasing dramatically. For example, home health nurses need to be acutely aware of patient and family education policies because I.V. lines are being used in the home 24 hours a day without the presence of full-time nursing staff.

INS (not the Immigration and Naturalization Service)

The Intravenous Nurses Society (INS) has developed a set of standards, the *Revised Intravenous Nursing Standards of Practice*, that are used by many committees when developing institutional policy. According to the INS, the goals of these standards are to "protect and preserve the patient's right to safe, quality care and protect the nurse who administers infusion therapy." These standards address all aspects of I.V. nursing. For more information, contact the INS at (617) 441-3008.

Documentation

You need to document I.V. therapy for several reasons. Proper documentation provides:
• an accurate description of care that can serve as legal protection such as evidence that a prescribed treatment was administered
• a mechanism for recording and retrieving information
• a record for health care insurers of equipment and supplies used.

Forms, forms, forms

I.V. therapy may be documented on progress notes, a special I.V. therapy sheet or flow sheet, a nursing care plan on the patient's chart, or an intake and output sheet.

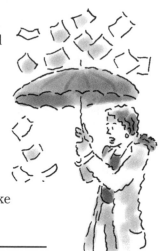

Documenting initiation of I.V. therapy

When documenting the insertion of a venipuncture device or the beginning of therapy, specify the following:
• size and type of device
• name of the person who inserted the device
• date and time
• I.V. site
• type of solution
• any additives
• flow rate
• use of any electronic infusion device
• complications, patient response, and nursing interventions
• patient teaching and evidence of patient understanding (for example, ability to explain instructions or perform a return demonstration).

Labeling dressings and equipment

In addition to documentation in the patient's chart, you need to label the dressing on the insertion site. Whenever you change the dressing, label the new one. (See *How to label a dressing,* page 38.)

You should also label the I.V. fluid container and place a time tape on it. With a child, you may need to label the volume-control set as well. In labeling the container and the set, follow your facility's policy and procedures. (See *How to label an I.V. bag.*)

Documenting I.V. therapy maintenance

When documenting I.V. therapy maintenance, specify the following:
- condition of the site
- site care provided
- dressing changes
- site changes
- tubing and solution changes
- your teaching and evidence of patient's understanding.

Sequential system

One way to document I.V. solutions throughout therapy is to number each container sequentially. For example, if a patient is to receive normal saline at 125 ml/hour (3,000 ml per day) on day 1, number the 1,000-ml containers as 1, 2, 3. If another 3,000 ml is ordered on day 2, number those containers as 4, 5, 6. This system may reduce administration errors. Also, check your facility's policy and procedures; some facilities require beginning the count again if the type of fluid changes, while others keep the count sequential regardless of the type of fluid.

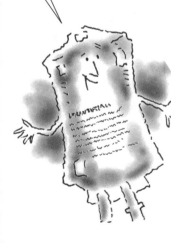

Count me in! Sequential numbering may help to reduce administration errors.

Flow sheets

Flow sheets highlight specific patient information according to preestablished parameters of nursing care. They have spaces for recording dates, times, and specific interventions. When you use an I.V. flow sheet, record the following:
- date
- flow rate
- use of an electronic flow device
- type of solution
- sequential solution container
- date and time of dressing and tubing changes.

Intake and output sheets

When you're documenting I.V. therapy on an intake and output sheet, follow these guidelines:

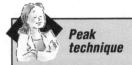

Peak technique

How to label a dressing

To label a new dressing over an I.V. site, include:
- the date of insertion
- the type of venipuncture device
- the date and time of the dressing change
- your initials.

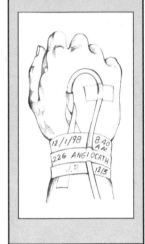

• If the patient is a child, note fluid levels on the I.V. containers hourly. If the patient is an adult, note these levels at least twice per shift.

• With children and critical care patients, record intake of all I.V. infusions, including fluids, medications, flush solutions, blood and blood products, and other infusates, every 1 to 2 hours.

• Document the total amount of each infusate and totals of all infusions at least every shift, so you can monitor fluid balance.

• Note output hourly or less often (but at least each shift), depending on the patient's condition. Output includes urine, stool, vomitus, and gastric drainage. For an acutely ill or unstable patient, you may need to assess urine output every 15 minutes.

• Read fluid levels from the infusate containers or electronic volume-control device to estimate the amounts infused and the amounts remaining to be infused.

Documenting discontinuation of I.V. therapy

All things come to an end, and when that time comes in I.V. therapy, make sure you have a record of it. When you document the discontinuation of I.V. therapy, be sure to specify the following:

• time and date

• reason for discontinuing therapy

• assessment of venipuncture site before and after venous access device is removed

• patient reactions and complications, and nursing interventions

• integrity of the venous access device on removal

• follow-up actions (for example, applying a bandage to the site or restarting the I.V. infusion in another limb).

Patient teaching

Although you may be accustomed to I.V. therapy, many patients aren't. Your patient may be apprehensive about the procedure and concerned that his condition has worsened. A child may be even more afraid. He may imagine he's about to be poisoned or that the needle will never be removed.

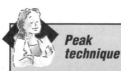

Peak technique

How to label an I.V. bag

To properly label an I.V. solution container, include the following (in addition to the time tape):

• patient's name, identification number, and room number

• date and time the container was hung

• any additives and their amounts

• the rate at which the solution is to run

• sequential container number

• expiration date and time of infusion

• your name.

When you place the label on the bag, be sure not to cover the name of the I.V. solution.

Teaching the patient and, when appropriate, members of his family will help him relax and take the mystery out of I.V. therapy.

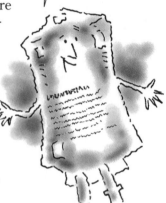

Good teaching will help me appear less mysterious.

Based on past experience

Begin by assessing your patient's previous infusion experience, his expectations, and his knowledge of venipuncture and I.V. therapy. Then base your teaching on this assessment:

• Describe the procedure. Tell the patient that *I.V.* means inside the vein and that a plastic catheter or needle will be placed in his vein.

• Explain that fluids containing certain nutrients or medications will flow from a bag or bottle through a length of tubing, then through the catheter or needle into his vein.

• Tell the patient how long the catheter or needle may stay in place, and explain that his doctor will decide how much and what type of fluid and medication he needs.

The whole story

Give the patient as much information as possible. Consider providing pamphlets, sample catheters and I.V. equipment, slides, videotapes, and other appropriate information. Make sure you tell the whole story:

• Tell the patient that although he may feel transient pain as the needle goes in, the discomfort will stop once the catheter or needle is in place.

• Explain why I.V. therapy is needed and how the patient can help by holding still when the needle is inserted and not withdrawing if there's pain.

• Explain that the I.V. fluids may feel cold at first, but the sensation should last only a few minutes.

• Instruct the patient to report any discomfort after therapy begins.

• Explain any activity restrictions such as those regarding bathing and ambulating.

Easing anxiety

Give the patient time to express his concerns and fears, and take the time to provide reassurance. Also, encourage the patient to use stress-reduction techniques such as deep, slow breathing. Allow the patient and his family to participate in his care as much as possible.

But did they get it?

Make sure you evaluate how well your patient and members of the patient's family understand your instruction. Evaluate their understanding while you're teaching and when you're done. You can do this by asking frequent questions and having them explain or demonstrate what you've taught.

Don't forget the paperwork

Document all your teaching in the patient's records. Note what you taught and how well the patient understood it.

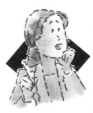

Quick quiz

1. Purposes of I.V. therapy include all of the following except:
   A. to provide enteral nutrition.
   B. to maintain fluid and electrolyte balance.
   C. to administer medications.

Answer: A. I.V. therapy is used to maintain fluid and electrolyte balance, provide parenteral nutrition, and administer medications. Enteral nutrition provides nutrients through the GI tract.

2. A solution that raises serum osmolarity and pulls fluid and electrolytes from the intracellular and the interstitial compartments into the intravascular compartment is:
   A. isotonic.
   B. hypertonic.
   C. hypotonic.

Answer: B. Hypertonic solutions draw fluids into the intravascular compartment due to the higher osmolarity of the solution.

3. All of the following affect I.V. flow rates except:
   A. osmolarity of the fluid.
   B. container height.
   C. gauge of the venipuncture device.

Answer: A. Osmolarity refers to the concentration of a solution, expressed in milliosmols of solute per liter of solution. Osmolarity doesn't affect the I.V. flow rate. Other factors that do affect the flow rate include viscosity of the solution and size of the venous access device.

4. Intravascular infections can be prevented by all of the following precautions except:
   A. taping the venipuncture device securely to prevent motion.
   B. changing insertion sites according to institutional policy.
   C. applying the tourniquet 6" to 8" (15 to 20 cm) above the insertion site.

Answer: C. Placement of the tourniquet has no effect on preventing infection.

5. When capillary blood pressure exceeds colloid osmotic pressure (COP):
   A. water and diffusible solutes leave the capillaries and circulate into the ISF.
   B. water and diffusible solutes return to the capillaries.
   C. there is no change.

Answer: A. When capillary blood pressure exceeds COP, water and diffusible solutes leave the capillaries and circulate into the ISF. When capillary blood pressure falls below COP, water and diffusible solutes return to the capillaries.

Scoring

☆☆☆ If you answered all five questions correctly, congratulations. Clearly, reading this chapter has infused you with a great deal of knowledge.

☆☆ If you answered three or four questions correctly, good job. Whether hypertonic, hypotonic, or isotonic, you have most of the solutions.

☆ If you answered fewer than two questions correctly, don't fret. Put this book under your pillow at night and see if you can absorb the material by osmosis.

Peripheral I.V. therapy

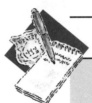

Just the facts

In this chapter you'll learn:

♦ how to prepare for a peripheral I.V. venipuncture

♦ how to perform a peripheral I.V. venipuncture

♦ how to maintain peripheral infusions

♦ how to recognize and respond to signs of complications of peripheral I.V. therapy

♦ how to discontinue a peripheral infusion.

Understanding peripheral I.V. therapy

Few nursing responsibilities require more time, knowledge, and skill than administering peripheral I.V. therapy. At the bedside, you need to assemble the equipment, prepare the patient, insert the venous access device, regulate the I.V. flow rate, and monitor the patient for possible adverse effects. You also have behind-the-scenes responsibilities, such as checking the doctor's orders, ordering or preparing supplies and equipment, labeling solutions and tubing, and documenting your nursing interventions.

Practice, practice, practice

Perhaps the most challenging aspect of peripheral I.V. therapy is performing the venipuncture itself. You need good hands and a sharp eye, plus lots of practice. Even so, it's worth the effort, especially in terms of positive outcome and patient satisfaction. As you gain experience, you'll learn to perform even difficult venipunctures confidently and successfully.

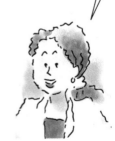

Peripheral I.V. therapy requires time, knowledge, and skill — at the bedside and behind the scenes.

Basics of peripheral I.V. therapy

Peripheral I.V. therapy is ordered whenever venous access is needed — for example, when a patient requires surgery, transfusion therapy, or emergency care. You may also use peripheral I.V. therapy to maintain hydration, restore fluid and electrolyte balance, provide fluids for resuscitation, or administer I.V. drugs, blood and blood components, and nutrients for metabolic support.

Benefits

Peripheral I.V. therapy offers easy access to veins and rapid administration of solutions, blood, and drugs. It allows continuous administration of drugs to produce rapid systemic changes. It's also easy to monitor.

Risks

Peripheral I.V. therapy is an invasive vascular procedure that carries such associated risks as bleeding, infiltration, and infection. Rapid infusion of some drugs can produce hearing loss, bone marrow depression, kidney or heart damage, and other irreversible adverse effects. Finally, peripheral I.V. therapy can't be used indefinitely and costs more than oral, subcutaneous, or I.M. drug therapy.

> Face it. Any invasive procedure carries certain risks.

Mainstay of modern medicine

Despite its risks, peripheral I.V. therapy remains a mainstay of modern medicine and a crucial contribution that nurses make to their patients' well-being. The key is to do it well, and that starts with preparation.

Preparing for venipuncture and infusion

Before performing a venipuncture, talk with the patient, select and prepare the proper equipment, and choose the best access site and venipuncture device.

Preparing the patient

Before approaching the patient, check his medical record for allergies and his disease history for diagnosis and care plan. Review the doctor's orders, noting pertinent laboratory studies that might affect the administration or outcome of the prescribed therapy.

Careful and confident = relaxed and cooperative

Many patients will be apprehensive. Among other things, this anxiety may cause vasoconstriction, making the venipuncture more difficult for you and more painful for the patient. Careful patient teaching and a confident, understanding attitude will help your patient relax and cooperate during the procedure. (See *Teaching your patient about I.V. therapy*, page 46.)

After completing your teaching, ensure your patient's privacy by asking visitors to leave and drawing the curtains around the bed if another patient is present. Have him put on a gown if he isn't already wearing one, and remove any jewelry from the arm where the I.V. will be inserted. As soon as he is ready, position him comfortably in the bed, preferably on his back. Make sure that the area is well lit and the bed is in a position that allows you to maneuver easily when inserting the device.

Selecting the equipment

Besides the venipuncture device, peripheral I.V. therapy requires a solution container, an administration set (usually with an in-line filtration system) and, if needed, an infusion pump or controller.

Solution containers

Some health care facilities always use glass I.V. solution containers, but many use plastic bags for routine administration of I.V. fluids. Glass must be used to deliver medications that are absorbed by plastic, such as nitroglycerin, and for albumin and immune globulin preparations.

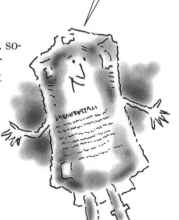

Plastic bags may be okay for routine administration of I.V. fluids.

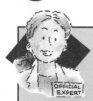

Advice from the experts

Teaching your patient about I.V. therapy

Many patients feel apprehensive about peripheral I.V. therapy. So before you begin therapy, teach your patient what to expect before, during, and after the procedure. Thorough patient teaching can reduce his anxiety, making therapy easier. Follow the guidelines below.

Describe the procedure

• Tell the patient that "intravenous" means inside the vein and that a plastic catheter or needle will be placed in his vein. Explain that fluids containing certain nutrients or medications will flow from an I.V. bag or bottle through a length of tubing, then through the plastic catheter or needle into his vein.

• Tell the patient approximately how long the catheter or needle will stay in place. Explain that the doctor will decide how much and what type of fluid he needs.

• Mention that he may feel some pain during insertion but that the discomfort will stop once the catheter or needle is in place.

• Tell him that the I.V. fluid may feel cold at first but this should last only a few minutes.

Do's and Don'ts

• Tell the patient to report any discomfort after the catheter or needle has been inserted and the fluid has begun to flow.

• Explain any restrictions, as ordered. If appropriate, tell the patient he can walk while receiving I.V. therapy. Depending on the insertion site and the device, he may also be able to shower or take a tub bath during therapy.

• Teach the patient how to assist in the care of the I.V. system. Tell him not to pull at the insertion site or tubing and not to remove the container from the I.V. pole. Also, tell him not to kink the tubing or lie on it. Explain that he should call a nurse if the flow rate suddenly slows down or speeds up.

Just about finished

• Explain that removing a peripheral I.V. line is a simple procedure. Tell the patient that pressure will be applied to the site until the bleeding stops. Reassure him that once the device is out and the bleeding stops, he'll be able to use his arm normally.

Plastic or glass

Because they're available in soft, flexible bags or semi-rigid rectangular containers, plastic solution containers allow easy storage, transportation, and disposal. Unlike glass bottles, they collapse as fluid flows out and don't require air venting, thus reducing the risk of air embolism or airborne contamination.

By contrast, glass containers don't collapse as fluid flows out and require vented tubing. A vented I.V. administration set has an extra filtered port near the spike that allows air to enter and displace fluid. This helps the solution flow correctly.

Administration sets

The three major types of I.V. administration set are basic, add-a-line, and volume-control. (See *Comparing I.V. administration sets*.) All three have drip chambers that may be vented or nonvented (glass containers require venting, plastic ones don't) and two drip systems: macrodrip and microdrip.

Comparing I.V. administration sets

I.V. administration sets come in three major types: basic, add-a-line, and volume-control. The basic set is used to administer most I.V. solutions. An add-a-line set delivers an intermittent secondary infusion through one or more additional Y-sites, or Y-ports. A volume-control set delivers small, precise amounts of solution. All three types come with vented or nonvented drip chambers.

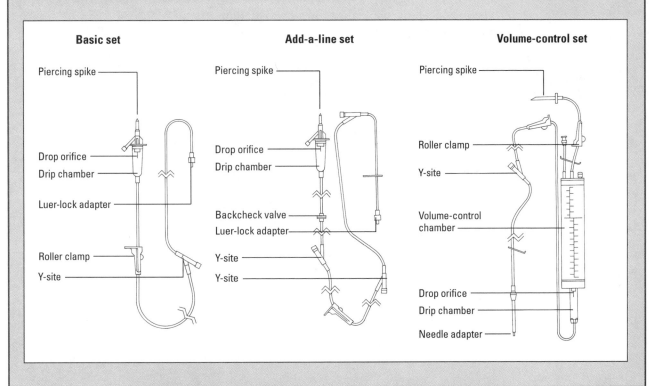

Basic set

Piercing spike
Drop orifice
Drip chamber
Luer-lock adapter
Roller clamp
Y-site

Add-a-line set

Piercing spike
Drop orifice
Drip chamber
Backcheck valve
Luer-lock adapter
Y-site
Y-site

Volume-control set

Piercing spike
Roller clamp
Y-site
Volume-control chamber
Drop orifice
Drip chamber
Needle adapter

Comparing drips

A macrodrip system delivers a solution in large quantities at rapid rates. A microdrip system delivers a smaller amount of solution with each drop and is used for pediatric patients and for adults who need small or closely regulated amounts of I.V. solution.

A macrodrip system delivers a solution in large quantities at rapid rates.

A microdrip system delivers a smaller amount of solution with each drop.

Sizing up the situation

Selecting the correct set requires knowing the type of solution container and comparing the set's flow rate with the nature of the I.V. solution — the more viscous the solution, the larger the drops and, thus, the fewer drops per milliliter. Also, make sure the intended solution can be infused using a filtration system; otherwise, you'll need an infusion set without the filtration component. Depending on the type of therapy ordered, you may need to supplement the administration set with such equipment as a flow regulator, a T-connector, an I.V. loop, and extension tubing. (See *Supplemental I.V. equipment*, pages 50 and 51.)

Back to basics

Basic I.V. administration sets range from 70″ to 110″ (178 to 279 cm) long. They're used to deliver any I.V. solution or to infuse solutions through an intermittent infusion device. The Y-site provides a secondary injection port for separate or simultaneous infusion of two compatible solutions. A macrodrip set generally delivers 10, 15, or 20 gtt/ml. A microdrip set always delivers 60 gtt/ml.

Solutions — primary and secondary

Add-a-line sets can deliver intermittent secondary infusions through one or more additional Y-sites. A backcheck valve prevents backflow of the secondary solution into the primary solution. After the secondary solution has been infused, the set automatically resumes infusing the primary one.

Down to the milliliter

Volume-control sets — used primarily for pediatric patients — deliver small, precise amounts of fluids and medications from a volume-control chamber that is calibrated in milliliters. This chamber is placed at the top of the I.V. tubing, just above the drip chamber. Also called burette sets, Buretrols, or Metrisets, volume-control sets are available with or without an in-line filter. They may be attached directly to the venipuncture device or connected to the Y-site of a primary I.V. administration set. Macrodrip and microdrip systems are available.

> Volume-control sets deliver small, precise amounts of fluids and medications.

In-line filters

In-line filters are located in a segment of the I.V. tubing through which the fluid passes. In-line filters remove pathogens and particles, thus reducing the risk of infection and phlebitis. Filters also help prevent air from entering the patient's vein by venting it through the filter housing.

Filters range in size from 0.22 micron (the most common) to 170 microns. Some are built into the line; others need to be added. The Intravenous Nurses Society (INS) recommends routine use of a 0.22-micron, in-line, air-eliminating bacterial retention filter.

> I don't like pathogens and particles. That's why I hooked up with an in-line filter.

Cracking under pressure

Most facilities have guidelines for using in-line filters; they usually include the following:

• If you're using a filter with an infusion pump, make sure it can withstand the pump's infusion pressure. Some filters are made for use only with gravity flow and may crack if the pressure exceeds a certain level.

• Carefully prime the in-line filter to eliminate all the air from it, following the manufacturer's directions.

• Be sure to change the filter according to the manufacturer's recommendation. This helps prevent bacteria from accumulating and releasing endotoxins and pyrogens small enough to pass through the filter into the bloodstream.

Supplemental I.V. equipment

When administering I.V. therapy, you may use certain additional pieces of equipment — including extension tubing, T-connectors, I.V. loops, and flow regulators. Examples of these devices are illustrated below. Before attaching this equipment to the venipuncture device, you must purge the add-on tubing of air.

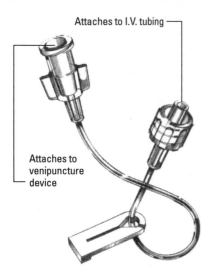

Attaches to I.V. tubing

Attaches to venipuncture device

Extension tubing
Extending 6″ to 12″ (15 to 30 cm), this small-bore tubing can be attached to any I.V. tubing. Unlike large-bore tubing, it allows a smaller loop tubing to adjoin the venipuncture device. It also allows I.V. tubing to be changed away from the insertion site, thereby reducing the risk of contamination.

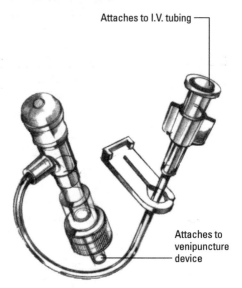

Attaches to I.V. tubing

Attaches to venipuncture device

T-connector
Useful for simultaneous administration of fluids and drugs, this small-bore extension tubing is 3″ to 6″ (7.5 to 15 cm) long and has an injection site near its luer-lock adapter. Attach the luer end to the venipuncture device and the opposite end to the I.V. tubing. Then another I.V. needle can be inserted into the latex injection cap. The added injection site can also serve as an intermittent infusion device — for example, a heparin lock — while the primary I.V. solution infuses. This device frequently eliminates the need for inserting a second venipuncture device.

Is there a filter in your future?

When can you can expect to use an in-line filter? Usually in the following situations:
- when treating an immunosuppressed patient
- when administering total parenteral nutrition
- when using additives composed of many separate parti-

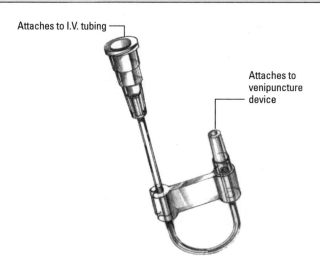

Attaches to I.V. tubing

Attaches to venipuncture device

I.V. loop
Shaped like a small horseshoe and made of small-bore tubing, an I.V. loop connector fits between the venipuncture device and the I.V. tubing. It enables the tubing to be changed away from the device and facilitates stabilization of the device.

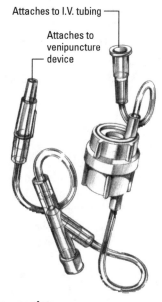

Attaches to I.V. tubing

Attaches to venipuncture device

Flow regulator
By delivering a specific number of milliliters per hour, flow regulators help ensure accurate delivery of I.V. fluids, although they're not as accurate as infusion pumps or controllers.

cles (such as antibiotics that require reconstitution) or when administering several additives
• when the risk of phlebitis is high.

Don't expect to use a 0.22-micron filter if you're administering blood or its components or lipid emulsions; the larger particles in these could clog the filter. The same is true of low-dose (less than 5 µg/ml), low-volume medications because the filter membrane may absorb them.

Preparing the equipment

After you've selected and gathered the infusion equipment, you need to prepare it for use. This involves inspecting the I.V. container and solution, preparing the solution, attaching and priming the administration set, and setting up the controller or infusion pump.

Inspecting the container and solution

Check that the container size and the type of I.V. solution are correct. Note the expiration date; discard an outdated solution.

When in doubt, throw it out

Make sure that the solution container is intact. Examine a glass container for cracks or chips and a plastic container for tears or leaks. (Plastic bags often come with an outer wrapper, which you must remove before inspecting the container.) Discard a damaged container, even if the solution appears clear. If the solution isn't clear, discard the container and notify the pharmacy or dispensing department. Solutions may vary in color, but they should never appear cloudy, turbid, or separated.

Preparing the solution

Make sure the container is labeled with the following information: your name; the patient's name, identification number, and room number; the date and time the container was hung; any additives; and the container number. For pediatric patients, you may label the volume-control set instead of the container. Once the container is labeled, use sterile technique to remove the cap or the pull tab. Be careful not to contaminate the port.

Attaching the administration set

Make sure the administration set is correct for the patient and the type of I.V. container and solution you're using. Also make sure the set has no cracks, holes, or missing clamps. If the solution container is glass, check whether it's vented or nonvented. This will determine how you prepare it to attach to the administration set. Plastic containers are prepared differently.

Nonvented bottle

When attaching a nonvented bottle to an administration set, take the following steps:

Remove the metal cap and inner disk, if necessary.

Place the bottle on a stable surface and wipe the rubber stopper with an alcohol swab.

Close the flow clamp on the administration set.

Remove the protective cap from the spike.

Push the spike through the center of the rubber stopper. Avoid twisting or angling the spike to prevent pieces of the stopper from breaking off and falling into the solution. If the vacuum is intact you should hear a "swoosh" sound, indicating that the solution hasn't been contaminated. (You may not hear this sound if a medication has been added to the bottle.)

Invert the bottle. If the vacuum isn't intact, discard the bottle. If it is intact, hang the bottle on the I.V. pole, about 36″ (91 cm) above the venipuncture site.

Listen for that swoosh. It lets you know the infusate hasn't been contaminated.

Vented bottle

When attaching a vented bottle to an administration set, take the following steps:

Remove the metal cap and latex diaphragm to release the vacuum. If the vacuum isn't intact, discard the bottle (unless a medication has been added).

Place the bottle on a stable surface and wipe the rubber stopper with an alcohol swab.

Close the flow clamp on the administration set.

Remove the protective cap from the spike.

Push the spike through the insertion port, which is located next to the air vent.

Hang the bottle on the I.V. pole about 36″ above the venipuncture site.

Plastic bag

When attaching a plastic bag to an administration set, take the following steps:

Place the bag on a flat, stable surface or hang it on an I.V. pole.

Remove the protective cap or tear the tab from the tubing insertion port.

Slide the flow clamp up close to the drip chamber and close the clamp.

Remove the protective cap from the spike.

Holding the port carefully and firmly with one hand, quickly insert the spike with your other hand.

Hang the bag about 36″ above the venipuncture site.

Priming the administration set

Before you prime any administration set, label it with the date and time you opened it. Make sure you've also labeled the container. When priming a set with an electronic infusion device, the procedure is similar to priming other infusion sets. (See *Electronic infusion devices.*)

Priming a basic set

When priming a basic set, take the following steps:

Close the roller clamp.

Squeeze the drip chamber until it's half full.

Aim the distal end of the tubing at a receptacle.

Open the roller clamp and allow the solution to flow through the tubing to remove air. (Most distal tube coverings allow the solution to flow without having to remove the protective end.)

Close the clamp after the solution has run through

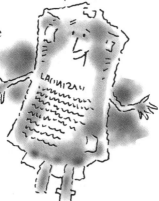

That's where I like to hang. About 36″ above the venipuncture site.

the line and all the air has been purged from the system.

Priming an add-a-line set

Follow the same steps you'd use to prime a basic set, along with these additional steps:

☝ As the solution flows through the tubing, tap the backcheck valve to release trapped air bubbles.

✌ Straighten the tubing and continue purging air in the usual manner.

Priming a volume-control set

To prime a volume-control set, take the following steps:

☝ Attach the set to the solution container and close the lower clamp on the I.V. tubing.

✌ Open the clamp between the solution container and the fluid chamber, and allow about 50 ml of the solution to flow into the chamber.

🤟 Close the upper clamp.

🖖 Open the lower clamp and allow the solution in the chamber to flow through the remainder of the tubing. Make sure that some fluid remains in the chamber so that air won't fill the tubing below it.

🖐 Close the lower clamp.

🖐 ✌ Fill the chamber with the desired amount of solution.

A few facts about filters

If you're using a filter on any of these sets and it's not an integral part of the infusion path, attach it to the primed distal end of the I.V. tubing and follow the manufacturer's instructions for filling and priming it. Most filters are positioned with the distal end of the tubing facing upward so the solution will wet the filter membrane completely and the line will be purged of all air bubbles.

Additional steps

For more information on setting up peripheral I.V. equipment, see *Setting up and monitoring an infusion pump, page 57.* You'll also need to change the tubing according

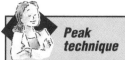

Peak technique

Electronic infusion devices

Electronic infusion devices help regulate the rate and volume of infusions. This improves the safety and accuracy of drug and fluid administration. Examples of electronic infusion devices are pumps and controllers.

Priming the set

Follow the steps below to prime an infusion set with an electronic infusion device:

1. Fill the drip chamber to the halfway mark.
2. Slowly open the roller clamp.
3. As gravity assists the flow, invert the distal end of the tubing to expel air and fill the chambered sections of the tubing with infusate. The chambered sections fit into the pump of the electronic infusion device; they must be filled exactly so they won't activate the air-in-line alarm during use.
4. Re-invert the tubing, continuing to purge the air along the fluid path.

to the manufacturer's instructions and your facility's policy, once the equipment is up and running.

Selecting the insertion site

Here are general suggestions for selecting the vein:
• Keep in mind that the most prominent veins aren't necessarily the best veins — they're frequently sclerotic from previous use.
• Never select a vein in an edematous or impaired arm.
• Never select a vein in the arm closest to an area that is surgically compromised — for example, veins compromised by a mastectomy or placement of dialysis access.
• Never select a vein in the affected arm of a patient following a cerebrovascular accident (CVA).
• Select a vein in the nondominant arm or hand.
• For subsequent venipunctures, select sites above the previously used or injured vein.
• Make sure you rotate access sites.

Commonly used veins

The veins commonly used for placement of venipuncture devices include the metacarpal, cephalic, and basilic veins, along with the branches or accessory branches that merge with them. (See *Comparing peripheral venipuncture sites,* pages 58 and 59.)

Superficial advice: Try the hand and forearm

Generally, the superficial veins in the dorsum of the hand and forearm offer the most choices. The dorsum of the hand is well supplied with small, superficial veins that can be dilated easily and usually accommodate either a needle or a catheter. The dorsum of the forearm has long, straight veins with fairly large diameters, making them convenient sites for introducing the large-bore needles and long I.V. catheters used in prolonged I.V. therapy.

Alternatives: Upper arms, legs, feet, and more

Veins of the hand and forearm are suitable for most drugs and solutions. For irritating drugs and solutions with a high osmolarity, the cephalic and basilic veins in the upper arm are more suitable. When leg or foot veins must be used, the saphenous vein of the inner aspect of the ankle and the veins of the dorsal foot network are best — but

Memory jogger

In selecting the best site for a venipuncture, keep in mind *VIP*:

V   vein

I   infusion

P   patient.

For the vein, consider its location, condition, and physical path along the extremity.

For the infusion, consider its purpose and duration.

For the patient, consider his degree of cooperation and compliance, along with his preference.

Peak technique

Setting up and monitoring an infusion pump

Infusion pumps help maintain a steady flow of liquid at a set rate over a specified period of time. After gathering your equipment, follow these step-by-step directions to smoothly set up an infusion pump for peripheral I.V. therapy.

Attach the controller to the I.V. pole. Insert the administration spike into the I.V. container.

Fill the drip chamber completely to prevent air bubbles from entering the tubing. To avoid fluid overload, clamp the tubing whenever the pump door is open.

Follow the manufacturer's instructions for priming the tubing and for placing the I.V. tubing.

Be sure to flush all air out of the tubing before connecting it to the patient; this lowers the risk of air embolism.

Place the infusion pump on the same side of the bed as the I.V. setup and the intended venipuncture site.

Set the appropriate controls to the desired infusion rate or volume.

Check the patency of the I.V. device, watch for infiltration, and monitor the accuracy of the infusion rate.

Be sure to explain the alarm system to the patient, so he isn't frightened when a change in the infusion rate triggers the alarm.

Be prepared to disengage the device if infiltration occurs, otherwise the pump will continue to infuse medication in the infiltrated area.

Frequently check the infusion pump to make sure it's working properly — specifically, note the flow rate. Monitor the patient for signs of infiltration and other complications, such as infection and air embolism.

only as an absolute last resort. Venous access in the lower extremities can cause thrombophlebitis. In infants under age 6 months, scalp veins are frequently used.

The lowdown on the upper arm

An upper arm vein may seem like an excellent site for a venous access device — it's comfortable for the patient and reasonably safe from accidental dislodging. Even so, it has a serious drawback. When an upper arm vein has an I.V. device in place, this compromises the use of sites dorsal to the upper arm. Moreover, upper arm veins can be difficult to locate in obese patients and in those with shorter arms such as pediatric patients.

You aren't an artery, are you?

Before choosing a vein as an I.V. site, make sure it's actually a vein — not an artery. (See *Reviewing anatomy of the skin and veins*, page 60.) Arteries are located deep in soft

Comparing peripheral venipuncture sites

Venipuncture sites located in the hand, forearm, foot, and leg offer various advantages and disadvantages. The following chart includes some of the major benefits and drawbacks of several common venipuncture sites.

Site	Advantages	Disadvantages
Digital veins Run along lateral and dorsal portions of fingers	• May be used for short-term therapy • May be used when other means aren't available	• Splinting fingers with a tongue blade required, which decreases ability to use hand • Uncomfortable for patient • Significant risk of infiltration • Not used if veins in dorsum of hand already used
Metacarpal veins On dorsum of hand; formed by union of digital veins between knuckles	• Easily accessible • Lies flat on back of hand; more difficult to dislodge • In adult or large child, bones of hand act as splint	• Wrist movement decreased unless short catheter is used • Painful insertion likely because of large number of nerve endings in hands • Phlebitis likely at site
Accessory cephalic vein Runs along radial bone as a continuation of metacarpal veins of thumb	• Large vein excellent for venipuncture • Readily accepts large-gauge needles • Doesn't impair mobility • Doesn't require an arm board in an older child or adult	• Some difficulty positioning catheter flush with skin • Discomfort during movement due to device located at bend of wrist
Cephalic vein Runs along radial side of forearm and upper arm	• Large vein excellent for venipuncture • Readily accepts large-gauge needles • Doesn't impair mobility	• Decreased joint movement due to proximity of device to elbow • Tendency of vein to roll during insertion
Median antebrachial vein Arises from palm and runs along ulnar side of forearm	• Holds winged needles well • A last resort when no other means are available	• Painful insertion or infiltration damage possible due to large number of nerve endings in area • High risk of infiltration in this area
Basilic vein Runs along ulnar side of forearm and upper arm	• Takes large-gauge needle easily • Straight, strong vein suitable for large-gauge venipuncture devices	• Uncomfortable position for patient during insertion • Painful insertion due to penetration of dermal layer of skin where nerve endings are located • Tendency of vein to roll during insertion

Comparing peripheral venipuncture sites (continued)

Site	Advantages	Disadvantages
Antecubital veins Located in antecubital fossa (median cephalic, on radial side; median basilic, on ulnar side; median cubital, which rises in front of elbow joint)	• Large vein; facilitates drawing blood • Often visible or palpable in children when other veins won't dilate • May be used in an emergency or as a last resort	• Difficult to splint elbow area with arm board • Veins may be small and scarred if blood has been drawn frequently from this site
Dorsal venous network Located on dorsal portion of foot	• Suitable for infants and toddlers	• Difficult to see or find vein if edema is present • Difficult to walk with device in place • Increased risk of deep vein thrombosis

tissue and muscles; veins are superficial. Arteries contain bright red blood that flows away from the heart; veins contain dark red blood that flows toward the heart. A single artery supplies a large area; many veins supply and remove blood from the same area. If you puncture an artery (which is difficult to do because of the arteries' depth), the blood pulsates from the site; if you puncture a vein, the blood flows slowly.

Avoid valves

All major veins have valves, but they're usually apparent only in long, straight arm veins or in large, well-developed veins that have good tone. If possible, don't let the tip of the venipuncture device terminate near a valve; such placement might affect the flow rate.

Selection guidelines

When selecting an I.V. site, choose distal veins first, unless the solution is very irritating (for example, 40 mEq or more of potassium chloride). Generally, your best choice is a peripheral vein that is full and pliable and appears long enough to accommodate the length of the intended catheter. It should be large enough to allow blood flow around the catheter; this will minimize venous lumen irritation. If the patient has an area that is bruised, tender, or phlebitic, choose a vein proximal to it. Avoid flexion areas.

Reviewing anatomy of the skin and veins

Understanding the anatomy of the skin and veins can help you locate appropriate venipuncture sites and perform venipunctures with minimal patient discomfort.

Layers of the skin

Epidermis

• Top layer that forms a protective covering for the dermis
• Varied thickness in different parts of the body — usually thickest on palms of hands and soles of feet, thinnest on inner surface of limbs
• Varied thickness depending on age; possibly thin in elderly people

Dermis

• Highly sensitive and vascular because it contains many capillaries
• Location of thousands of nerves, which react to temperature, touch, pressure, and pain
• Varied number of nerve fibers throughout the body; some I.V. sites more painful than others (For example, the inner aspect of the wrist is more painful than the dorsum of the hand or the forearm.)

Subcutaneous tissue

• Located below the two layers of skin
• Site of superficial veins
• Varied thickness that loosely covers muscles and tendons
• Potential site of cellulitis if strict aseptic technique not observed during venipuncture and care of I.V. site

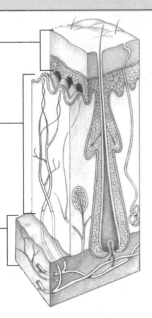

Layers of the veins

Tunica intima (inner layer)

• Inner elastic endothelial lining made up of layers of smooth, flat cells, which allow blood cells and platelets to flow smoothly through the blood vessels. (Unnecessary movement of the venipuncture device may scratch or roughen this inner surface, causing thrombus formation.)
• Valves in this layer located in the semilunar folds of the endothelium (Valves prevent backflow and ensure the flow of blood toward the heart.)

Tunica media (middle layer)

• Muscular and elastic tissue
• Location of vasoconstrictor and vasodilator nerve fibers that stimulate the veins to contract and relax (These fibers are responsible for venous spasm that can occur as the result of anxiety or infusion of I.V. fluids that are too cold.)

Tunica externa (outer layer)

• Connective tissue that surrounds and supports the vessel and holds it together

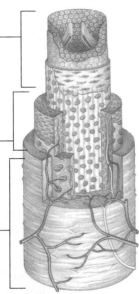

Veins to avoid

Some veins are best to avoid. These include:
• veins in the legs. (Circulation may be easily compromised.)
• veins in the inner wrist and arm. (They're small and uncomfortable for the patient.)
• veins in the affected arm of a mastectomy patient
• veins in an arm with an arteriovenous shunt or fistula or in an arm being treated for thrombosis or cellulitis.

How long?

The size and health (tone) of the vein help determine how long the venipuncture device can remain in place before irritation develops. However, the key to determining how long the venous access device will remain functional is the effect of the fluid or drug on the vein. Drugs and solutions with high osmolarity and high or low pH will cause vein irritation sooner. Concentrated solutions of drugs and rapid infusion rates can also affect how long the I.V. site remains symptom-free.

Selecting the venipuncture device

Basically, you should select the device with the shortest length and the smallest diameter that allows for proper administration of the therapy. Other considerations include:
• length of time the device will stay in place
• type of therapy
• type of procedure or surgery to be performed
• patient's age and activity level
• type of solution used (blood, for instance, will require a larger-gauge device)
• available veins.

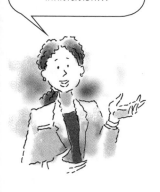

Plastic catheters allow more patient movement and activity and are less prone to infiltration...

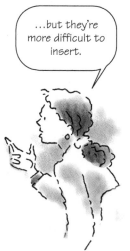

...but they're more difficult to insert.

Venipuncture devices

The three available devices are over-the-needle plastic catheter sets, through-the-needle plastic catheter sets, and winged steel needle infusion sets. (See *Comparing basic venipuncture devices,* page 62.) As a rule, plastic catheters allow more patient movement and activity and are less prone to infiltration than steel needles. However, they're more difficult to insert.

Comparing basic venipuncture devices

Use the chart below to compare three major types of venipuncture devices.

Over-the-needle catheter
Purpose
• Long-term therapy for the active or agitated patient
Advantages
• Inadvertent puncture of vein less likely than with a winged steel needle set
• More comfortable for the patient
• Radiopaque thread for easy location
• Syringe attached to some units that permits easy check of blood return and prevents air from entering the vessel on insertion
• Activity-restricting device, such as arm board, rarely required
Disadvantages
• Difficult to insert
• Extra care required to ensure that needle and catheter are inserted into vein

Through-the-needle catheter
Purpose
• Long-term therapy for the active or agitated patient
Advantages
• Infiltration less likely than with a winged steel needle set
• More comfortable for the patient
• Available in many lengths
• Radiopaque thread (in most) for easy location
• Activity-restricting device, such as arm board, rarely required
Disadvantages
• Leaking at site, especially in elderly patient, because needle produces skin puncture that is larger than catheter
• Severed catheter possible if needle guard not used

Winged steel needle set
Purpose
• Short-term therapy for any cooperative adult patient
• Therapy of any duration for an infant or child or for an elderly patient with fragile or sclerotic veins
Advantages
• Easiest intravascular device to insert because needle is thin-walled and extremely sharp
• Ideal for I.V. push drugs
• Available with catheter that can be left in place like over-the-needle catheter
Disadvantage
• Infiltration easily caused if rigid needle winged infusion device is used

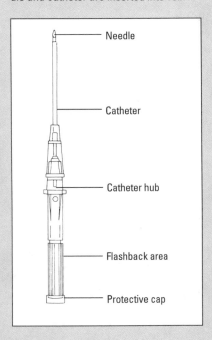

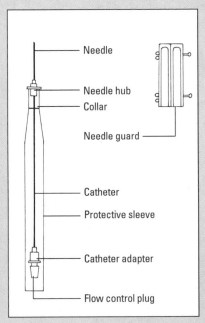

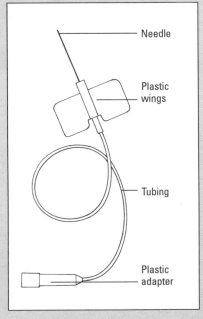

Over the needle

Over-the-needle catheters are the most commonly used device for peripheral I.V. therapy. They consist of a plastic outer tube and an inner needle that extends just beyond the catheter. They're available in lengths of 1″ and 1¼″, with gauges ranging from 14 to 26. (See *Guide to needle and catheter gauges*, page 64.) Longer-length models, used mainly in the operating room, are for insertion into a deep vein.

The needle is removed after insertion, leaving the catheter in place. Typically, you should change over-the-needle catheters every 2 to 3 days, depending on the facility's policy and procedures. But it may stay in place longer if a patient has poor venous access and the device isn't causing any problems. Be sure to have a doctor's order for such a deviation from standard practice, and document it thoroughly.

Through the needle

Through-the-needle catheters are generally used for placement in long veins, such as the antecubital or upper arm veins, or when venous access is poor and the device must stay in place for up to 4 weeks. They're usually 6″ to 10″ long and 18G to 24G. One type combines an 8″ to 12″ (20.3- to 30.5-cm) catheter with a 1½″ introducer needle, which must be guarded by an enclosed shield after insertion.

Despite their length and use, through-the-needle catheters are still considered peripheral devices. Maintain and monitor them as you would a shorter catheter. They should be inserted only by trained personnel.

Give it wings

Winged infusion sets come in two basic types — an over-the-needle catheter and a steel needle. Both have flexible wings you can grasp when inserting the device. Once the device is in place, the wings lie flat and can be taped to the surrounding skin.

Winged over-the-needle catheters have short, small-bore tubing between the catheter and the hub. The catheter stays in place after the needle is removed. This type of catheter is available in a ¾″ (2-cm)

Guide to needle and catheter gauges

How do you know which gauge needle and catheter to use for your patient? The answer depends on your patient's age and condition, and on the type of infusion he's receiving. The following chart lists the uses and nursing considerations for the various gauges.

Gauge	Uses	Nursing considerations
16	• Adolescents and adults • Major surgery • Trauma • Whenever large amounts of fluids must be infused	• Painful insertion • Requires large vein
18	• Older children, adolescents, and adults • Administration of blood and blood components and other viscous infusions	• Painful insertion • Requires large vein
20	• Children, adolescents, and adults • Suitable for most I.V. infusions, blood, blood components, and other viscous infusions	• Commonly used
22	• Infants, toddlers, children, adolescents, and adults (especially elderly) • Suitable for most I.V. infusions	• Easier to insert into small, thin, fragile veins • Slower flow rates must be maintained • Difficult to insert into tough skin
24, 26	• Neonates, infants, toddlers, school-age children, adolescents, and adults (especially elderly) • Suitable for most infusions, but flow rates are slower • Painful insertion • Requires large vein	• For extremely small veins — for example, small veins of fingers or veins of inner arms in elderly patients • Possible difficulty inserting into tough skin

length for wider gauges and is especially useful for hard veins.

Commonly called butterfly needles, winged steel needle catheters have no hub and lie flat on the skin, which makes taping easy. These devices range in size from 19G

Venipuncture variations

Here are some common variations on venipuncture devices.

Winged infusion sets with catheter

Winged infusion sets sometimes have an over-the-needle catheter plus short, small-bore tubing between the catheter and the hub. These catheters are available in a ¾" (2-cm) length for smaller gauges and a 1" (2.5-cm) length for larger ones. They're especially useful for hand veins or areas that require angled insertions.

The Intima

The Intima is a winged infusion set that has a Y-shaped design with a latex cap and is available in 16G to 24G. Because it has two ports, this set can be used for intermittent infusion while a continuous I.V. solution is infusing, or for simultaneous infusion of two compatible solutions. Recent design changes have reduced the amount of latex in the Y-site, a consideration for individuals with latex allergies.

Dual-lumen catheter

For simultaneous infusion of two *incompatible* solutions, you might use the dual-lumen catheter. This set consists of side-by-side catheters that come together at a single tip. It's also useful for infusing multiple prescriptions over a short period of time and for drawing blood. Recommended only for arm veins, the dual-lumen catheter requires greater insertion skills than other venipuncture devices.

to 27G and are about ¾" long. Originally designed for pediatric and geriatric use, the winged steel needle should be used when a patient is in stable condition, has adequate veins, and requires I.V. fluids or medications for just a short time. They're also ideal for single I.V. push injections. For a description of this and other variations on I.V. devices, see *Venipuncture variations.*

Intermittent improvisation

Any venous access device that includes a catheter can be made into an intermittent infusion device by placing an access cap over the catheter's adapter end. These caps are commonly called "locks" because a saline or heparin solution is flushed into them to keep the device patent. Typically, the cap is a luer-locking attachment or add-on. Intermittent venous access devices should be flushed with saline solution or heparin before and after each use, at least once per day, or according to the facility's policy and procedures.

Any venous access device that includes a catheter can be made into an intermittent infusion device.

Just place an access cap over the catheter's adapter end.

Performing venipuncture

To perform a venipuncture, you need to dilate the vein, prepare the access site, and insert the device. After the infusion starts, you can complete the I.V. placement by securing the device with tape or a transparent semipermeable dressing.

Dilating the vein

To dilate or distend a vein effectively, you need to use a tourniquet, which traps blood in the veins by applying enough pressure to impede the venous flow. A properly distended vein should appear and feel round, firm, and fully filled with blood and should rebound when gently compressed. Because the amount of trapped blood depends on circulation, a patient who's hypotensive, very cold, or experiencing vasomotor changes (such as septic shock) may have inadequate filling of the peripheral blood vessels.

Pretourniquet prep

Before applying the tourniquet, place the patient's arm in a dependent position to increase capillary flow to the lower arm and hand. If his skin is cold, warm it by rubbing and stroking his arm or by covering the entire arm with warm moist towels for 5 to 10 minutes. As soon as you remove the warm towels, apply the tourniquet and continue to perform the insertion procedure.

Applying a tourniquet

The ideal tourniquet is one that can be secured easily, doesn't roll into a thin band, stays relatively flat, and releases easily. The most common type is a soft rubber band about 2″ (5 cm) wide. To tie it, follow the steps outlined in *Applying a tourniquet.* Other types use Velcro or a catch mechanism to anchor them.

Once you've applied the tourniquet about 6″ to 8″ (15 to 20 cm) above the intended site, have the patient open and close his fist tightly four to six times to distend the vein. If necessary, gently flick the skin over the vein with one or two short taps of your forefinger. This is less traumatic than slapping the skin, but it achieves the same re-

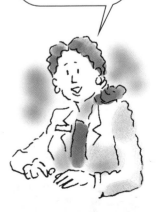

A properly distended vein should appear and feel round, firm, and full.

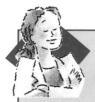

Peak technique

Applying a tourniquet

To safely apply a tourniquet, follow these steps:

1. Place the tourniquet under the patient's arm, about 6" (15 cm) above the venipuncture site. Position the arm on the middle of the tourniquet.

2. Bring the ends of the tourniquet together, placing one on top of the other.

3. Holding one end on top of the other, lift and stretch the tourniquet and tuck the top tail under the bottom tail. Don't allow the tourniquet to loosen.

4. Tie the tourniquet smoothly and snugly, being careful not to pinch the patient's skin or pull his arm hair.

No more than 2 minutes
Leave the tourniquet in place for no more than 2 minutes. If you can't find a suitable vein and prepare the venipuncture site in this amount of time, release the tourniquet for a few minutes. Then reapply it and continue the procedure. You may need to apply the tourniquet, find the vein, remove the tourniquet, prepare the site, and then reapply the tourniquet for the venipuncture.

As flat as possible
Keep the tourniquet as flat as possible. It should be snug but not uncomfortably tight. If it's too tight, it will impede arterial as well as venous blood flow. Check the patient's radial pulse. If you can't feel it, the tourniquet is too tight and must be loosened. Also loosen and reapply the tourniquet if the patient complains of severe tightness.

sult. If the vein still feels small and uniform, release the tourniquet, reapply it, and reassess the intended access site. If the vein still isn't well distended, remove the tourniquet; apply a warm, moist towel for 5 minutes; then reapply the tourniquet. This is especially helpful if the patient's skin feels cool.

Tourniquet technique

A tourniquet that is kept in place too long or is applied too tightly may cause increased bruising, especially in elderly patients whose veins are fragile. Release the tourniquet as soon as you've placed the venipuncture device in the vein. You'll know the device is in the vein when you see blood in the flashback chamber.

Infection control

Ideally, your facility's infection control guidelines will call for tourniquets to be discarded after use on one patient. When available, use latex-free tourniquets to reduce the chance of allergic reaction.

Preparing the access site

Before performing the venipuncture, you'll need to clean the site and stabilize the vein; you may also need to administer a local anesthetic.

Cleaning the venipuncture site

Wash your hands; then put on gloves. If necessary, clip the hair over the insertion site to make the veins and the site easier to see and reduce pain when the tape is removed. Avoid shaving the patient; irritation can occur with the use of povidone-iodine and alcohol.

Next, clean the skin with a thin coat of povidone-iodine solution. (If this solution is unavailable or the patient is allergic to iodine, use 70% alcohol. Other approved antimicrobial solutions include tincture of iodine 2% and 10% and chlorhexidine.) Using a swab stick or swab, start at the center of the insertion site and move outward with a circular motion. Be careful not to go over an area you've already cleaned. Allow the solution 30 to 60 seconds to dry thoroughly. (If you're using alcohol, do three successive scrubs, for at least 30 seconds each, or until the final applicator is virtually clean.)

Using a local anesthetic

Many doctors order a local anesthetic before venipuncture — though the practice isn't endorsed by the INS. If an anesthetic is ordered, first check with the patient and review his record for an allergy to lidocaine, iodine, or any other drugs. Then describe the procedure to him and explain that it will reduce the discomfort of the venipuncture.

Pressure, yes; pain, no

Now administer the local anesthetic, as ordered. You'll administer only a small amount, and the anesthetic will begin to work in 2 to 3 seconds. Lidocaine anesthetizes the site to pain but allows the patient to feel touch and pressure. (See *Administering a local anesthetic*.)

Transdermal analgesic cream may also be used before accessing a peripheral vein. Like injectable anesthetics, transdermal analgesic cream reduces pain, but the patient still feels pressure and touch. To be effective, a transdermal analgesic cream should be applied 60 minutes before insertion of the venous access device.

Stabilizing the vein

Stabilizing the vein helps ensure a successful venipuncture the first time and decreases the chances of bruising. If the tip of the venipuncture device repeatedly probes a moving vein wall, it can nick the vein and cause it to leak

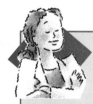

Peak technique

Administering a local anesthetic

A local anesthetic may be prescribed when starting peripheral I.V. therapy, although the Intravenous Nurses Society doesn't recommend the practice. If you'll be administering a local anesthetic, follow the steps below.

Using a U-100 insulin syringe with a 27G needle, draw up 0.1 ml of lidocaine 1% without epinephrine.

Clean the venipuncture site.

Insert the needle next to the vein, introducing about one-third of it into the skin at a 30-degree angle. The side approach carries less risk of accidental vein puncture (indicated by blood appearing in the syringe). If the vein is deep, however, inject the lidocaine over the top of it. To be sure you don't inject lidocaine into the vein — thus allowing it to circulate systemically — aspirate to check for a blood return. If this occurs, withdraw the needle and begin the procedure again.

Hold your thumb on the plunger of the syringe during insertion to avoid unnecessary movement once the needle is under the skin.

Without aspirating, quickly inject the lidocaine until a small wheal appears (as shown). You may not have to administer the entire amount in the syringe.

Quickly withdraw the syringe and massage the wheal with an alcohol swab. This will make the wheal disappear so the vein won't be hidden — although you'll see a small pinprick of blood. The skin numbness will last about 30 minutes.

Insert the venipuncture device into the vein.

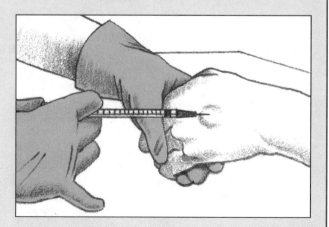

blood. When this happens, the vein can't be reused immediately and a new venipuncture site must be found. Thus, the patient will experience the discomfort of another needle puncture.

Stabilizing the vein helps ensure a successful venipuncture the first time...

...and also decreases the chances of bruising.

Hold still, vein

To stabilize the vein, stretch the skin and hold it taut, then lightly press it with your fingertips about 1½″ (3.8 cm) from the insertion site. (Never touch the prepared site or you'll recontaminate it.) The vein should feel round, firm, fully engorged, and resilient. Remove your fingertips. If the vein returns to its original position and appears larger than it did before you applied the tourniquet, it's adequately distended. (See *How to stabilize veins.*) To help prevent the vein from "rolling," apply adequate traction with your nondominant hand to hold the skin and vein in place. This is particularly helpful in elderly patients with loose skin and loosely anchored veins.

Insertion

Once you've prepared the venipuncture site, you're ready to insert the venipuncture device. The process involves three steps: positioning, inserting, and advancing. You might also need to add an intermittent infusion device, use deep veins rather than superficial, or collect a blood sample.

Positioning the venipuncture device

While still wearing gloves, use the appropriate method for the type of venipuncture device being used.

Over-the-needle catheter

Grasp the plastic hub with your dominant hand, remove the cover, and examine the device. If the edge isn't smooth, discard the device and obtain another. Insert the device, bevel up, through the skin and into the vein; then lower the hub portion until it's almost parallel to the skin. Advance the device to at least half its length, at which point you should see blood in the flashback

That's what I like: A round, firm, fully engorged, resilient vein.

Peak technique

How to stabilize veins

To help ensure successful venipuncture, you need to stabilize your patient's vein by stretching the skin and holding it taut. The stretching technique you'll use varies with the venipuncture site.

Vein	Stretching technique
Hand veins	Stretch the patient's hand and wrist downward, and hold the skin taut with your thumb.
Cephalic vein above wrist	Have the patient make a tight fist. Then stretch his fist laterally downward, and immobilize the skin with the thumb of your other hand.
Basilic vein at outer arm	Have the patient make a tight fist and flex his elbow. While standing behind the flexed arm, retract the skin away from the site, and anchor the vein with your thumb. As an alternative, rotate the patient's extended lower arm inward, and approach the vein from behind the arm. (This position may be difficult for the patient to maintain.)
Inner aspect of wrist	Extend the patient's open hand backward from the wrist. Anchor the vein with your thumb below the insertion site.
Inner arm	Extend the patient's closed fist backward from the wrist. Anchor the vein with your thumb above the wrist.
Antecubital fossa	Have the patient form a tight fist and extend his arm completely. Anchor the skin with your thumb, about 2″ to 3″ (5 to 7.5 cm) below the antecubital fossa.
Saphenous vein of ankle	Extend the patient's foot downward and inward. Anchor the vein with your thumb, about 2″ to 3″ below the ankle.
Dorsum of foot	Pull the patient's foot downward. Anchor the vein with your thumb, about 2″ to 3″ below the vein (usually near the toes).

chamber. If you're advancing the catheter before starting the infusion, leave the needle (stylette) in place. Advance the catheter to its hub; then withdraw the needle.

Through-the-needle catheter

Grasp the needle hub with one hand, and unsnap the needle cover with the other. Keeping the skin taut and anchored, position the device with the bevel up and the flashback chamber visible. Firmly hold this chamber, being careful not to touch the catheter.

Winged infusion set

Hold the edges of the wings between your thumb and forefinger, with the bevel facing upward. Then squeeze the wings together. Remove the protective cover from the needle, being careful not to contaminate the steel needle or over-the-needle catheter.

Inserting the venipuncture device

Tell the patient that you're about to insert the device. Ask him to remain still and to refrain from pulling away. Explain that the initial needle stick will hurt but will quickly subside. Then insert the device, using the direct or indirect approach. For the direct approach, place the bevel up and enter the skin directly over the vein at a 30- to 45-degree angle (deeper veins require a wider angle). For the indirect approach, enter the skin slightly adjacent to the vein; then direct the needle into the side of the vein wall. This approach reduces the risk of perforating the back vein wall. If the vein is bifurcated (looks like an inverted V), penetrate the skin about ½″ (1.25 cm) in front of the bifurcation; then proceed into the vein lumen.

Smooth and steady

When you insert the device, use a steady, smooth motion while keeping the skin taut. Usually, you'll know the device is in the vein because you'll meet resistance during insertion and see blood return in the flashback chamber. (You may not see a rapid blood return with a small vein.)

Pop precaution

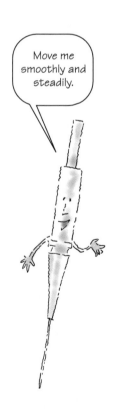

Move me smoothly and steadily.

Don't expect to always feel a "pop" or a sense of release when the device enters the vein. This usually occurs only when a larger-gauge venipuncture device (20G or more) enters a large, thick-walled vein or when the patient has good tissue tone.

As the device enters the vein

As soon as the device enters the vein, lower the distal portion of the adapter until it's almost parallel with the skin. This lifts the tip of the needle so it doesn't penetrate the opposite wall of the vein.

Advancing the venipuncture device

To advance the catheter before starting the infusion, first release the tourniquet. While stabilizing the vein with one hand, use the other to advance the catheter up to the hub. Next, remove the inner needle and, using aseptic technique, quickly attach the I.V. tubing. The advantage of this method is that it commonly results in less blood being spilled.

While infusing I.V. solution

To advance the catheter while infusing the I.V. solution, release the tourniquet and remove the inner needle (stylette). Using aseptic technique, attach the I.V. tubing and begin the infusion. While stabilizing the vein with one hand, use the other to advance the catheter into the vein. When the catheter is advanced, slow the I.V. flow rate. The advantage of using this method for advancing the catheter is that it reduces the risk of puncturing the vein wall because the catheter is advanced without the steel needle and the rapid flow dilates the vein.

Advancing the catheter while infusing I.V. fluids reduces the risk of puncturing the vein wall.

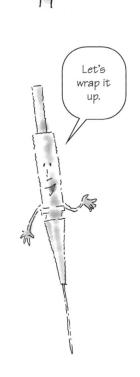

Winged infusion set

If you're using a steel needle winged infusion set, advance the needle fully, if possible, and hold it in place. Release the tourniquet, slightly open the administration set clamp, and check for free flow or infiltration. Next, tape the infusion set in place, using the wings as an anchor to prevent catheter movement, which could cause irritation and phlebitis. When using an over-the-needle winged infusion set, you can advance the catheter using the methods described above.

Finally...

After the venous access device has been successfully inserted and securely taped, clean the skin if necessary. Cover the access site with a transparent dressing or the dressing used by your facility. If your facility's policy and procedures require doing so, further stabilize the device. Dispose of the inner needle in a nonpermeable receptacle. Finally, regulate the flow rate; then remove your gloves and wash your hands.

Let's wrap it up.

Intermittent infusion device

Also called a heparin or saline lock, an intermittent infusion device may be used when venous access must be maintained for intermittent use and a continuous infusion isn't necessary. This device keeps the access device sterile and prevents blood and other fluids from leaking from an open end. Much like the administration set injection port, the intermittent injection cap is self-sealing after the needle or needleless injector is removed. The ends of these devices are universal in size and fit the female end of any catheter or tubing designed for infusion therapy. Most caps have a luer-lock design to prevent disconnections.

Continuous infusion not required

The intermittent infusion device can be filled with dilute heparin or saline solution to expel air from the equipment. This makes it possible to maintain venous access in patients who must receive I.V. medications regularly or intermittently but don't require continuous infusion.

Benefits

The intermittent infusion device has many benefits. It minimizes the risk of fluid overload and electrolyte imbalance that may be associated with a keep-vein-open infusion. By eliminating the continuous use of I.V. solution containers and administration sets, it reduces the risk of contamination and lowers costs. Finally, it allows for patient mobility, which helps reduce anxiety.

Risks

Occlusion is possible if the device is not flushed to ensure patency before and after medication is infused.

Two tips

Here are two tips related to intermittent infusion devices:

🖑 If the patient feels a burning sensation as you inject the heparin or saline solution, stop the injection and check the catheter placement. If it's in the vein, inject the solution at a slower rate to minimize irritation.

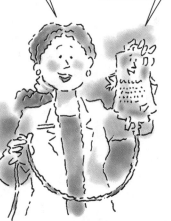

Don't use heparin if your patient has a clotting disorder or uncontrolled bleeding.

Use sterile normal saline solution instead.

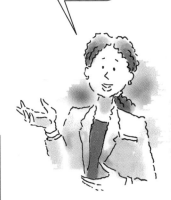

If the doctor orders discontinuation of an I.V. infusion, you can convert the existing line from a continuous to an intermittent venous access device. Just disconnect the I.V. tubing and insert an adapter plug into the device that's already in place. (See *From continuous to intermittent*.)

Insertion into deep veins

If a superficial vein isn't available, you may have to insert the venipuncture device into a deep vein that isn't visible. Here's how. First, put on gloves. Then, palpate the area with your fingertips until you feel the vein. Next, clean the skin over the vein with povidone-iodine solution or alcohol as you would for any other access procedure. Next, aim the device directly over the intended vein, stretch the skin

> If a superficial vein isn't available, you may have to insert the venipuncture device into a deep vein.

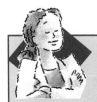

Peak technique

From continuous to intermittent

The two types of male adapter plugs shown below allow you to convert an existing I.V. line into an intermittent infusion device.

To make the conversion:
1. Prime the male adapter plug with dilute heparin or saline solution.
2. Clamp the I.V. tubing and remove the administration set from the catheter or needle hub.
3. Insert a short or long male adapter plug (see illustrations).
4. Flush the access with the remaining solution to prevent occlusion.

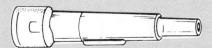

The long male adapter plug slides into place.

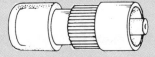

The short male luer-lock adapter plug twists into place.

with your gloved fingertips, and insert the venipuncture device about 1½″ (3.8 cm) distal to your fingertips.

Making sure

Expect to insert the device one-half to two-thirds its length; that way you'll be sure that both the needle and the catheter are in the vein lumen. When you see blood in the flashback chamber, remove the inner steel needle and advance the catheter with or without infusing fluid.

Collecting a blood sample

If a blood sample is ordered, you can collect it while performing the venipuncture. First, gather the necessary equipment: one or more evacuated tubes, a 19G needle, an appropriate-size syringe without a needle, and a protective pad. Then follow the steps outlined in *Collecting a blood sample*.

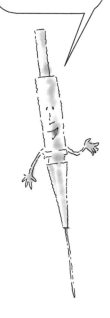

Insert the venous access device one-half to two-thirds its length.

Peak technique

Collecting a blood sample

To smoothly and safely collect a blood sample, follow these step-by-step techniques after assembling your equipment and making the venipuncture.

• Place a pad underneath the site to protect the bed linens.

• When the venipuncture device is correctly placed, remove the inner needle if you're using an over-the-needle device.

• Leave the tourniquet tied.

• Attach the syringe to the venipuncture device's hub, and withdraw the appropriate amount of blood.

• Release the tourniquet and disconnect the syringe.

• Quickly attach the saline or heparin lock or I.V. tubing, regulate the flow rate, and stabilize the device.

• Attach a 19G needle to the syringe, and insert the blood into the evacuated tubes. (Or, use equipment for drawing samples with evacuated devices.)

• Properly dispose of the needle and syringe; then complete I.V. line placement.

Needleless systems are available for collecting blood samples. Use them to reduce your risk of needle sticks.

Securing the venipuncture device

After the infusion begins, you need to secure the venipuncture device at the insertion site. You can do this with tape or a transparent semipermeable dressing.

Applying tape

If required by facility policy, apply a small amount of antiseptic ointment such as povidone-iodine to the insertion site. Then stabilize the device and keep the hub from moving by using a standard taping method, such as the chevron, U, or H method. (See *Taping techniques,* page 78.)

Taping technique

Use as little tape as possible, and don't let the tape ends meet. This reduces the risk of a tourniquet effect if infiltration occurs. Remove any hair from around the access area. Besides improving visibility and reducing pain when the tape is removed, this helps decrease colonization by bacteria present on the hair. Don't let the tape cover the patient's skin beyond the infusion device's entry site. This could obscure swelling and redness, signs of impending complications.

Nonallergenic but not paper

If the patient has had a previous sensitivity reaction to tape, use a nonallergenic tape, preferably one that is lightweight and easy to remove. Paper tape usually isn't satisfactory for I.V. sites because it shreds and is difficult to remove after prolonged contact with skin and body heat.

Applying a transparent dressing

To prevent infection, nurses in many health care facilities now cover the insertion site with a transparent, semipermeable dressing. This dressing allows air to pass through but is impervious to microorganisms. (For instructions, see *How to apply a transparent semipermeable dressing,* page 79.)

The benefits are transparent

If this dressing remains intact, daily changes aren't necessary. Other advantages include fewer skin reactions and a clearly visible insertion site (especially helpful in detecting

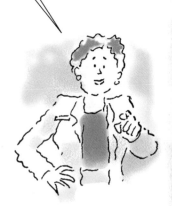

Don't let the tape cover the patient's skin beyond the infusion device's entry site.

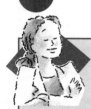

Peak technique

Taping techniques

If you use tape to secure the venipuncture device to the insertion site, use one of these methods.

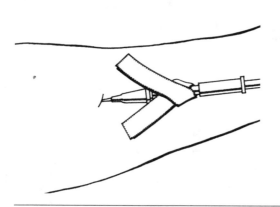

Chevron method

1. Cut a long strip of ½″ (1.25-cm) tape. Place it, sticky side up, under the hub.

2. Cross the ends of the tape over the hub, and secure the tape to the patient's skin on the opposite sides of the hub, as shown at left.

3. Apply a piece of 1″ (2.5-cm) tape across the two wings of the chevron. Loop the tubing and secure it with another piece of 1″ tape. Once a dressing is secured, apply a label. On the label, write the date and time of insertion, type and gauge of the needle, and your initials.

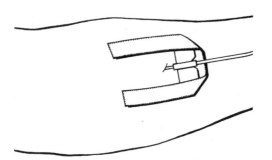

U method

1. Cut a strip of ½″ tape. With the sticky side up, place it under the hub of the catheter.

2. Bring each side of the tape up, folding it over the wings of the catheter, as shown at left. Press it down, parallel to the hub.

3. Next, apply tape to stabilize the catheter. Once a dressing is secured, apply a label. On the label, write the date and time of insertion, the type and gauge of the catheter, and your initials.

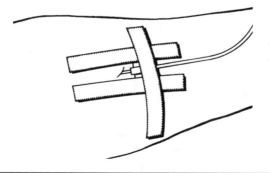

H method

1. Cut three strips of 1″ tape.

2. Place one strip of tape over each wing, keeping the tape parallel to the catheter.

3. Place the third strip of tape perpendicular to the first two, as shown. Put the tape directly on top of the wings. Make sure that the catheter is secure then apply a dressing and label. On the label, write the date and time of insertion, type and gauge of the catheter, and your initials.

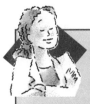

Peak technique

How to apply a transparent semipermeable dressing

Here's how to apply a transparent semipermeable dressing, which allows for visual assessment of the catheter insertion site:

• Make sure the insertion site is clean and dry.
• Remove the dressing from the package and, using
aseptic technique, remove the protective seal. Avoid
touching the sterile surface.
• Place the dressing directly over the insertion site and
the hub, as shown. Don't cover the tubing. Also, don't
stretch the dressing; doing so may cause itching.
• Tuck the dressing around and under the catheter hub to
make the site occlusive to microorganisms.

Grasp, lift, stretch
To remove the dressing, grasp one corner; then lift and
stretch.

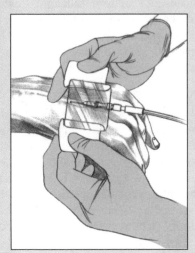

early signs of phlebitis and infiltration). The dressing is
waterproof, so it protects the site from contamination if it
gets wet. In addition, because the dressing adheres well to
the skin, there is less chance of accidentally dislodging
the venous access device.

Using a stretch net

You can make the venipuncture device more secure by applying a stretch net to the affected limb. (If you'll be using
the net on the patient's hand, cut a hole in the net sleeve
for his thumb.) The net reduces the risk of accidental dislodgment, especially with patients who are confused or
very active, and cuts down on the amount of tape needed
to prevent dislodgment.

Using an arm board

An arm board is an immobilization device that helps secure correct venous access device positioning and prevent
unnecessary motion that could cause infiltration or inflammation. This immobilization device is sometimes necessary when the insertion site is near a joint or in the dor-

sum of the hand. It's also used with a restraint for confused or disoriented patients.

The best arm board is no arm board

Because it's an immobilization device, the use of an arm board may be restricted by state or facility policies — so check first. Better yet, don't place the tip of the infusion device in a flexion area. Then you won't need an arm board.

The range-of-motion test

To determine whether an arm board is called for, move your patient's arm through its full range of motion (ROM) while watching the I.V. flow rate. If the flow stops during movement, you may need to use the arm board to prevent flexion of the extremity. Choose one that is long enough to prevent flexion and extension at the tip of the device. If necessary, cover it with a soft material before you secure it to the patient's arm. Be sure you can still observe the insertion site.

Additional arm board advice

Keep in mind that an arm board applied too tightly can cause nerve and tendon damage. If you need to use an arm board, remove it periodically so the patient can perform ROM activities and you can better observe for complications from restricted activity and infusion therapy.

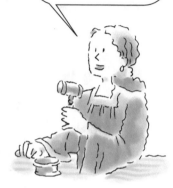

> Because an arm board is an immobilization device, its use may be restricted by state or facility policies.

Documenting the venipuncture

When you start an I.V. line, be sure to document the following:
- the date and time of the venipuncture
- the number of the solution container (if required by facility policy and procedures)
- the type and amount of solution
- the name and dosage of additives in the solution
- the type of venipuncture device used, including length and gauge
- the venipuncture site
- the number of insertion attempts, if more than one
- the flow rate
- any adverse reactions and the actions taken to correct them

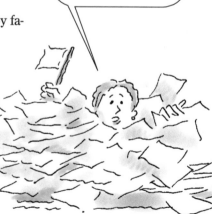

> Document the venipuncture? How could I forget?

• patient teaching and evidence of patient understanding
• the name of the person initiating the infusion.
Remember to document this information in all areas required by your facility's policy, such as the patient care Kardex, input and output flow sheets, the patient's chart, and medication sheets.

Maintaining peripheral I.V. therapy

After the I.V. infusion starts, focus on maintaining therapy and preventing complications. This involves routine and special care measures as well as discontinuing the infusion when therapy is completed. Also, you should be prepared to meet the special needs of pediatric, elderly, or home care patients who require I.V. therapy.

Routine care

Routine care measures help prevent complications. They also give you an opportunity to observe the I.V. site for signs of inflammation or infection — two of the most common complications. Perform these measures according to your facility's policy and procedures, wash your hands ahead of time, and wear gloves whenever you work near the venipuncture site.

Changing the dressing

Depending on your facility's policy, change the I.V. dressing every 3 to 7 days or whenever its integrity is compromised because it has become soiled, wet, or loose. As before, clean the insertion site with povidone-iodine, using a circular motion from the center outward. Allow the skin to dry before applying a new dressing. Of course, use aseptic technique.

Getting ready

Before performing a dressing change, gather this equipment:
• povidone-iodine or alcohol swab
• povidone-iodine ointment or another antimicrobial ointment (if your facility policy requires it)
• adhesive bandage, sterile 2″ × 2″ gauze pad, or transparent semipermeable dressing

Peak technique

Changing a peripheral I.V. dressing

To smoothly change a peripheral I.V. dressing, follow these steps:

Wash your hands and put on sterile gloves.

Hold the needle or catheter in place with your nondominant hand to prevent movement or dislodgment that could lead to infiltration; then gently remove the tape and the dressing.

Assess the venipuncture site for signs of infection (redness and tenderness), infiltration (coolness, blanching, edema), and thrombophlebitis (redness, firmness, pain along the path of the vein, edema).

If you detect these signs, apply pressure to the area with a sterile gauze pad and remove the catheter or needle. Maintain pressure on the area until the bleeding stops; then apply an ad-

hesive bandage. Using new equipment, insert the I.V. access device at another site.

If you don't detect complications, hold the needle or catheter at the hub and carefully clean around the site with a povidone-iodine or alcohol swab. Work from the site outward to avoid introducing pathogens into the cleaned area. Allow the area to dry completely.

If facility policy requires, apply povidone-iodine or another antimicrobial ointment.

Retape the device and apply a transparent semipermeable dressing, if available, or apply gauze and secure it.

- 1″ clean adhesive tape
- sterile gloves.

To change a dressing, follow the steps outlined in *Changing a peripheral I.V. dressing*.

Changing the I.V. solution

To avoid microbial growth, don't allow any I.V. container to hang for more than 24 hours. Before changing the I.V. container, check the new one for cracks, leaks, and other damage. Also check the solution for discoloration, turbidity, and particulates. Note the date and time the solution was mixed and the expiration date.

After washing your hands, clamp the line, remove the spike from the old container, and quickly insert the spike into the new one. Then hang the new container and adjust the flow rate as prescribed.

Changing the administration set

Change the administration set according to your facility's policy (usually every 48 to 72 hours if it's a primary infusion line) and whenever you note or suspect contamina-

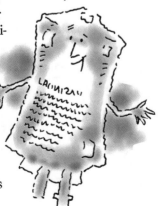

Can't stand those microbes. So please don't let me hang for more than 24 hours.

Peak technique

Changing the administration set

To quickly change the administration set for a peripheral infusion, follow these steps:

Wash your hands and put on gloves.

Reduce the I.V. flow rate. Then remove the old spike from the container, and place the cover of the new spike over it loosely.

Keeping the old spike upright and above the patient's heart level, insert the new spike into the I.V. container and prime the system.

Place a sterile gauze pad under the needle or hub of the plastic catheter to create a sterile field.

Disconnect the old tubing from the venipuncture device, being careful not to dislodge or move the I.V. device. If you have trouble disconnecting the old tubing, try one of these tech-niques: Use a pair of hemostats to hold the hub securely while twisting and removing the end of the tubing, or grasp the venipuncture device with one pair of hemostats and the hard plastic of the luer-lock end of the administration set with another pair and pull the hemostats in opposite directions. *Don't clamp the hemostats shut; this may crack the tubing adapter or the venipuncture device.*

Using aseptic technique, quickly attach the new primed tubing to the I.V. device.

Adjust the flow to the prescribed rate.

Label the new tubing with the date and time of the change.

tion. If possible, change the set when you start a new venous access device during routine site rotation.

Before changing the set, gather this equipment:
• an I.V. administration set
• a sterile 2″ × 2″ gauze pad
• adhesive tape for labeling or appropriate labeling tapes supplied by the hospital
• gloves.

Follow the guidelines set out in *Changing the administration set.*

Changing the I.V. site

As a standard of care, rotate the I.V. site every 48 to 72 hours, if possible. Sometimes, limited venous access will prevent you from changing sites this often. If that is the case, notify the doctor of the need to deviate from normal practice and be sure to document the reasons. Obtain an order to extend the dwell time of the current access site but remember to monitor more frequently for redness, pain, or swelling. Be prepared to change the entire sys-

tem, including the venipuncture device, if you detect signs
of thrombophlebitis, cellulitis, or I.V. therapy–related bac-
teremia.

Documentation

Record dressing, tubing, and solution changes, and note
the condition of the venipuncture site. If you obtain a
blood sample for culture and sensitivity testing, record the
date and time and the doctor's name.

Special care procedures

Besides your routine care procedures, be prepared to handle special situations such as administering additive infusions. Also, when peripheral venous access is no longer
possible, you may need to assist the doctor with other venous access interventions such as the insertion of a central line.

Additive infusions

To piggyback an I.V. drug into a primary line, use an add-
a-line administration set. To infuse two compatible solutions simultaneously, connect an administration set with
an attached needleless access catheter (or one with a needle) to the secondary solution container and prime the
tubing. (Using needles to apply a second infusion creates
increased risks associated with needle sticks, so exercise
extreme caution.) Hang the container at the same level as
the primary solution.

"Y" not?

Next, clean a Y-site in the lower part of the primary tubing, using a povidone-iodine or alcohol swab. Attach the
secondary infusion set to the Y-site and secure it. Adjust
each infusion rate independently. Remember that with this
setup, you don't have a backcheck valve above the Y-site,
so one solution may flow back into the other.

Vein dissection and hypodermoclysis

Though vein dissection and hypodermoclysis are seldom
performed anymore, you should be familiar with them.
Each provides a way of accessing a peripheral vein when

the usual venipuncture techniques become impossible due to obesity, venous collapse or sclerosis, or vasoconstriction from massive, rapid blood loss. The procedures are also performed on patients whose peripheral veins are exhausted.

A reflection on dissection

In vein dissection, also called venous cutdown, the doctor makes a small incision in the skin over the vein. He divides the subcutaneous tissues, then isolates the vein and temporarily ties a ligature around it. Next he makes a small incision in the vein, inserts a 3″ to 6″ (7.5- to 15-cm) plastic catheter into it, and anchors the catheter with a suture. The catheter can remain in place for several days.

Reserved for infants and the elderly

Hypodermoclysis is still performed in some long-term care facilities and at home. It's usually reserved for infants and elderly patients. It uses the subcutaneous route to achieve absorption of I.V. isotonic hydration fluids. This procedure is contraindicated for patients suffering from shock or severe electrolyte imbalance because the I.V. solution must be isotonic or tissue irritation will develop.

Identifying scalp veins

This illustration shows the scalp veins most frequently used for venipuncture.

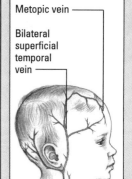

Metopic vein

Bilateral superficial temporal vein

Patients with special needs

I.V. therapy for pediatric and elderly patients poses special nursing challenges, especially regarding the effects of age-related differences in the skin and veins on I.V. line insertion and maintenance.

Pediatric patients

Inserting a venous access device in an infant or toddler can prove difficult because the veins are imbedded in fat, making them hard to isolate. (A premature infant has less subcutaneous fat, making the veins more prominent.)

Especially the scalp

In infants, the best sites for I.V. insertion include the hands, feet, antecubital fossa, dorsum of the hand and, especially, the scalp, which has an abundant supply of veins. (See *Identifying scalp veins*.) The head veins most frequently used are the bilateral superficial temporal veins

The scalp, with its abundant supply of veins, is one of the best sites for I.V. insertion in an infant.

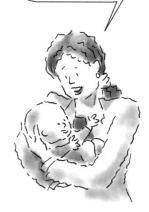

above the ear and the metopic vein running down the middle of the forehead.

Don't use after age 6 months

Scalp veins are extremely fragile and should be used only with infants under age 6 months; an older child is more likely to move his head and dislodge the venipuncture device. In toddlers, dorsal foot veins and saphenous veins in the leg can be used, but dorsal hand veins allow the greatest mobility.

Palpate first

Before performing a venipuncture on a scalp vein, palpate to ensure you have a vein — not an artery. In the scalp, arteries and veins may look similar. Remember, you'll feel a pulse with an artery.

Decreasing discomfort

Consider using a topical or transdermal anesthetic to decrease discomfort. If necessary, use clove-hitch and mummy restraints. Also seek to engage the parents to help keep the infant calm. If you need a tourniquet effect, tip the infant head down to facilitate filling of the superficial veins — don't use a tourniquet or rubber band. Insert the venous access device caudally to make stabilizing easier. When you see a blood return (usually it will be slight), tip the child back to a horizontal or vertical position.

Device advice

The preferred venous access device for infants and young children — no matter which vein you're using — is a small-diameter, winged over-the-needle catheter (commonly called a scalp vein catheter). This device is less likely to cause traumatic injury to the vein. Over-the-needle catheters are also recommended for long-term therapy and antibiotic therapy when venous access is poor.

Getting the site right

Stabilizing the I.V. site can be challenging with pediatric patients. Tape the site as you would for an adult so the skin over the access site is easily visible. Avoid overtaping the I.V. site; it makes inspecting the site and the surrounding tissues more difficult and practically guarantees trauma when the device is removed. Instead, cover the site

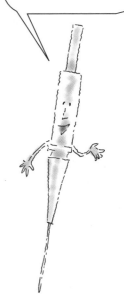

The preferred venous access device for infants and young children is a small-diameter, winged over-the-needle catheter.

with a stretch net, which can be rolled back easily for inspection. Some clinicians protect the insertion site by taping a plastic medicine cup over it.

Until a vein can be used

For children under age 6, an emergency procedure called intraosseous infusion has been successful in fluid resuscitation. An intraosseous needle — or, in emergencies, a 16G or 19G straight needle — is placed in the medullary cavity of a bone, usually in the distal end of the femur or the proximal or distal ends of the tibia. (With adults, the usual sites are the iliac crest or the sternum.) The I.V. solution is then infused directly into the cavity, which is rich in blood. Usually performed by emergency personnel, this procedure is indicated to provide resuscitative fluids, medication, and blood until a vein can be used for I.V. administration.

Elderly patients

Because an elderly person's veins are usually more prominent and his skin less resistant, you may find venipuncture easier than with pediatric patients. Even so, the normal aging process also presents drawbacks. Because the tissues are looser, you may have more difficulty stabilizing the vein. Also, because veins become more fragile, you'll need to perform the venipuncture quickly and efficiently to avoid excessive bruising. You'll also need to remove the tourniquet promptly to prevent increased vascular pressure from causing bleeding through the vein wall around the infusion device.

Less thrombogenic, easily manipulated, and flat

Typically, an elderly person's veins appear tortuous because of the skin's increased transparency and decreased elasticity. They'll also appear large if venous pressure is adequate. Winged steel needles may be used as I.V. insertion devices for elderly patients because they are less thrombogenic, can be easily manipulated, and lie flat against the skin to provide a stable site for the device. Be aware, however, that these needles increase the risk of infiltration.

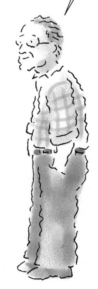

Now that I've gotten older, my veins are more fragile.

Be still, vein

To help stabilize the vein for insertion, stretch the skin proximal to the insertion site and anchor it firmly with your nondominant hand. Smaller, shorter access devices usually work best with elderly patients' fragile veins.

Complications of therapy

Complications of peripheral I.V. therapy can arise from the access device, the infusion, or the medication being administered and can be local or systemic.

Local, systemic, or a combination of the two

Local complications include:
• infiltration
• phlebitis
• catheter dislodgment
• occlusion
• vein irritation or pain at the I.V. site
• severed or fractured catheter
• hematoma
• venous spasm
• vasovagal reaction
• thrombosis
• thrombophlebitis
• nerve, tendon, or ligament damage.

Systemic complications include air embolism and allergic reaction. A complication may begin locally and become systemic — as when an infection at the venipuncture site progresses to septicemia. (For a complete description of local and systemic complications, see *Risks of peripheral I.V. therapy*, pages 89 to 93.)

The greatest threat (perhaps)

Perhaps the greatest threat to a patient receiving I.V. therapy is infiltration (infused fluid leaking into the surrounding tissues). Infiltration occurs when the access device punctures the vein wall or migrates out of the vein. The risk of infiltration may be as much as 70% greater with a steel needle than with a plastic catheter, depending on the skill of the person performing the venipuncture and the compliance of the patient.

(Text continues on page 94.)

Warning!

Risks of peripheral I.V. therapy

Complications of peripheral I.V. therapy may be local or systemic. This chart lists some common complications along with their signs and symptoms, possible causes, and nursing interventions, including preventive measures.

Signs and symptoms	Possible causes	Nursing interventions
Local complications		
Phlebitis • Tenderness at tip of device and above • Redness at tip of catheter and along vein • Puffy area over vein • Vein hard on palpation • Elevated temperature	• Poor blood flow around device • Friction from catheter movement in vein • Device left in vein too long • Clotting at catheter tip (thrombophlebitis) • Solution with high or low pH or high osmolarity	• Remove device. • Apply warm pack. • Notify doctor if patient has fever. • Document patient's condition and your interventions. *Prevention:* • Restart infusion using larger vein for irritating infusate, or restart with smaller-gauge device to ensure adequate blood flow. • Use filter to reduce risk of phlebitis. • Tape device securely to prevent motion.
Infiltration • Swelling at and above I.V. site (may extend along entire limb) • Discomfort, burning, or pain at site • Feeling of tightness at site • Decreased skin temperature around site • Blanching at site • Continuing fluid infusion even when vein is occluded, although rate may decrease • Absent backflow of blood • Slower flow rate	• Device dislodged from vein or perforated vein	• Remove device. • Apply ice (early) or warm soaks (later) to aid absorption. • Elevate limb. • Periodically assess circulation by checking for pulse and capillary refill. • Restart infusion above infiltration site or in another limb. • Document patient's condition and your interventions. *Prevention:* • Check I.V. site frequently (especially when using I.V. pump). • Don't obscure area above site with tape. • Teach patient to observe I.V. site and report discomfort, pain, or swelling.
Catheter dislodgment • Catheter partly backed out of vein • Infusate infiltrating	• Loosened tape or tubing snagged in bedclothes, resulting in partial retraction of catheter	• If no infiltration occurs, retape without pushing catheter back into vein. *Prevention:* • Tape device securely on insertion.

(continued)

Risks of peripheral I.V. therapy *(continued)*

Signs and symptoms	Possible causes	Nursing interventions
Local complications (continued)		
Occlusion • No increase in flow rate when I.V. container is raised • Blood backup in line • Discomfort at insertion site	• I.V. flow interrupted • Intermittent device not flushed • Blood backup in line when patient walks • Hypercoagulable patient • Line clamped too long	• Use mild flush pressure during injection. Don't force. If unsuccessful, reinsert I.V. device. *Prevention:* • Maintain I.V. flow rate. • Flush promptly after intermittent piggyback administration. • Have patient walk with his arm folded to chest to reduce risk of blood backup.
Vein irritation or pain at I.V. site • Pain during infusion • Possible blanching if vasospasm occurs • Red skin over vein during infusion • Rapidly developing signs of phlebitis	• Solution with high or low pH or high osmolarity, such as 40 mEq/L of potassium chloride, phenytoin, some antibiotics (vancomycin and nafcillin)	• Slow the flow rate. • Try using an electronic flow device to achieve a steady regulated flow. *Prevention:* • Dilute solutions before administration. For example, give antibiotics in 250-ml solution rather than 100 ml. If drug has low pH, ask pharmacist if drug can be buffered with sodium bicarbonate. (Refer to facility policy.) • If long-term therapy of irritating drug is planned, ask doctor to use central I.V. line.
Severed catheter • Leakage from catheter shaft	• Catheter inadvertently cut by scissors • Reinsertion of needle into catheter	• If broken part is visible, attempt to retrieve it. If unsuccessful, notify doctor. • If portion of catheter enters bloodstream, place tourniquet above I.V. site to prevent progression of broken portion. • Notify doctor and radiology department. • Document patient's condition and your interventions. *Prevention:* • Don't use scissors around I.V. site. • Never reinsert needle into catheter. • Remove unsuccessfully inserted catheter and needle together.

Risks of peripheral I.V. therapy *(continued)*

Signs and symptoms	Possible causes	Nursing interventions
Local complications (continued)		
Hematoma • Tenderness at venipuncture site • Bruising around site • Inability to advance or flush I.V. line	• Vein punctured through ventral wall at time of venipuncture • Leakage of blood from needle displacement	• Remove venipuncture device. • Apply pressure and warm soaks to affected area. • Recheck for bleeding. • Document patient's condition and your interventions. *Prevention:* • Choose a vein that can accommodate size of intended venous access device. • Release tourniquet as soon as successful insertion is achieved.
Venous spasm • Pain along vein • Sluggish flow rate when clamp is completely open • Blanched skin over vein	• Severe vein irritation from irritating drugs or fluids • Administration of cold fluids or blood • Very rapid flow rate (with fluids at room temperature)	• Apply warm soaks over vein and surrounding area. • Slow flow rate. *Prevention:* • Use blood warmer for blood or packed red blood cells when appropriate.
Thrombosis • Painful, reddened, and swollen vein • Sluggish or stopped I.V. flow	• Injury to endothelial cells of vein wall, allowing platelets to adhere and thrombus to form	• Remove device; restart infusion in opposite limb if possible. • Apply warm soaks. • Watch for I.V. therapy-related infection (thrombi provide an excellent environment for bacterial growth). *Prevention:* • Use proper venipuncture techniques to reduce injury to vein.
Thrombophlebitis • Severe discomfort • Reddened, swollen, and hardened vein	• Thrombosis and inflammation	• Remove device; restart infusion in opposite limb if possible. • Apply warm soaks. • Watch for I.V. therapy-related infection (thrombi provide an excellent environment for bacterial growth). *Prevention:* • Check site frequently. Remove device at first sign of redness and tenderness.

(continued)

Risks of peripheral I.V. therapy *(continued)*

Signs and symptoms	Possible causes	Nursing interventions
Local complications (continued)		
Nerve, tendon, or ligament damage • Extreme pain (similar to electric shock when nerve is punctured) • Numbness and muscle contraction • Delayed effects, including paralysis, numbness, and deformity	• Improper venipuncture technique, resulting in injury to surrounding nerves, tendons, or ligaments • Tight taping or improper splinting with arm board	• Stop procedure. *Prevention:* • Don't repeatedly penetrate tissues with venipuncture device. • Don't apply excessive pressure when taping or encircle the limb with tape. • Pad the arm board and, if possible, pad the tape securing the arm board.
Systemic complications		
Circulatory overload • Discomfort • Neck vein engorgement • Respiratory distress • Increased blood pressure • Crackles • Large positive fluid balance (intake is greater than output)	• Roller clamp loosened to allow run-on infusion • Flow rate too rapid • Miscalculation of fluid requirements	• Raise the head of the bed. • Administer oxygen as needed. • Notify doctor. • Administer medications (probably furosemide) as ordered. *Prevention:* • Use pump, controller, or rate minder for elderly or compromised patients. • Recheck calculations of fluid requirements. • Monitor infusion frequently.
Systemic infection (septicemia or bacteremia) • Fever, chills, and malaise for no apparent reason • Contaminated I.V. site, usually with no visible signs of infection at site	• Failure to maintain aseptic technique during insertion or site care • Severe phlebitis, which can set up ideal conditions for organism growth • Poor taping that permits access device to move, which can introduce organisms into bloodstream • Prolonged indwelling time of device • Immunocompromised patient	• Notify doctor. • Administer medications as prescribed. • Culture site and device. • Monitor vital signs. *Prevention:* • Use scrupulous aseptic technique when handling solutions and tubings, inserting venipuncture device, and discontinuing infusion. • Secure all connections. • Change I.V. solutions, tubing, and access device at recommended times. • Use I.V. filters.

Risks of peripheral I.V. therapy *(continued)*

Signs and symptoms	Possible causes	Nursing interventions
***Systemic complications** (continued)*		
Air embolism • Respiratory distress • Unequal breath sounds • Weak pulse • Increased central venous pressure • Decreased blood pressure • Loss of consciousness	• Empty solution container • Solution container empties; next container pushes air down line	• Discontinue infusion. • Place patient in Trendelenburg's position to allow air to enter right atrium and disperse through the pulmonary artery. • Administer oxygen. • Notify doctor. • Document patient's condition and your interventions. *Prevention:* • Purge tubing of air completely before infusion. • Use air-detection device on pump or air-eliminating filter proximal to I.V. site. • Secure connections.
Allergic reaction • Itching • Tearing eyes and runny nose • Bronchospasm • Wheezing • Urticarial rash • Edema at I.V. site • Anaphylactic reaction (within minutes or up to 1 hour after exposure), including flushing, chills, anxiety, agitation, generalized itching, palpitations, paresthesia, throbbing in ears, wheezing, coughing, seizures, and cardiac arrest	• Allergens such as medications	• If reaction occurs, stop infusion immediately. • Maintain patent airway. • Notify doctor. • Administer antihistaminic steroid, anti-inflammatory, and antipyretic drugs, as ordered. • Give 0.2 to 0.5 ml of 1:1,000 aqueous epinephrine subcutaneously. Repeat at 3-minute intervals and as needed, as ordered. • Administer cortisone if ordered. *Prevention:* • Obtain patient's allergy history. Be aware of cross-allergies. • Assist with test dosing. • Monitor patient carefully during first 15 minutes of administration of a new drug.

Of steel and plastic

Infiltration involving steel needles can occur any time after initiation of an infusion. With plastic catheters, infiltration is more likely to occur one or more days later, usually because the flexible tip of the catheter has penetrated the vein wall.

A joint risk

With either venipuncture device, the risk of infiltration increases whenever you insert it near a joint. If the tip of the venipuncture device isn't inserted far enough into the vein lumen, part of the tip remains outside the vein and infiltration develops quickly.

The fluid factor

The type of fluid being infused determines how much discomfort the patient feels during infiltration. Isotonic fluids usually don't cause much discomfort. Fluids with an acidic or alkaline pH, or those that are more than slightly hypertonic, are usually more irritating. Don't depend on the patient to complain of discomfort; large amounts of I.V. fluid — as much as 1 qt (1 L) — can escape into the surrounding tissues without the patient knowing it.

Looking on the bright side

Fortunately, you can minimize or prevent most complications by using proper insertion techniques and carefully monitoring the patient.

In case of complications

If complications do occur, document the signs and symptoms, patient complaints, name of the doctor notified, and treatment. If your patient develops a severe infusion-related problem — for instance, vesicant infiltration, circulatory compromise, a skin tear, fluid overload, or a severe allergic reaction — fill out an incident report according to your facility's policy and procedures. For legal purposes, document the details of the complication as well as medical and nursing interventions.

Discontinuing the infusion

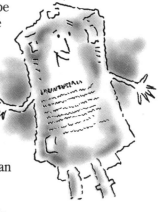

I need a break. Follow the steps below to finish up the infusion.

To discontinue the infusion, first clamp the infusion line; then remove the venipuncture device using aseptic technique. Here's how to proceed:
• After putting on gloves, lift the tape from the skin to expose the insertion site. You don't need to remove the tape or dressing as long as you can peel it back to expose the venipuncture device and skin.
• Be careful to avoid manipulating the device in the skin to prevent skin organisms from entering the bloodstream. Moving the device may also cause discomfort, especially if the insertion site has become phlebitic.
• Apply a sterile 2″ × 2″ dressing directly over the insertion site; then quickly remove the device. (Never use an alcohol pad to clean the site when discontinuing an infusion; this may cause bleeding and a burning sensation.)
• Maintain direct pressure on the I.V. site for several minutes, then tape a dressing over it, being careful not to encircle the limb. If possible, hold the limb upright for about 5 minutes to decrease venous pressure.
• Tell the patient to restrict his activity for about 10 minutes and to leave the site dressing in place for at least 8 hours. If he feels lingering tenderness at the I.V. site, apply warm, moist packs.
• Dispose of the used venipuncture equipment, tubing, and solution containers in a receptacle designated by your facility.
• Document the time of removal, the catheter length and integrity, and the condition of the site. Also, record how the patient tolerated the procedure and any nursing interventions.

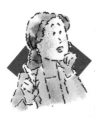

Quick quiz

1. The first step in performing a routine venipuncture is to:
    A.   prepare the venipuncture site.
    B.   dilate the vein.
    C.   use a local anesthetic.

Answer: B. The sequence in performing the venipuncture is to dilate the vein, then prepare the site. An anesthetic may or may not be used.

2. When applying a transparent dressing, it's important to:
   A. stretch the dressing as much as possible.
   B. cover the site and the tubing.
   C. tuck the dressing around and under the hub.
Answer: C. Tucking the dressing in this manner will make the site occlusive to microorganisms. Stretching the dressing will cause itching, and the tubing should never be covered.

3. The preferred and most accessible site for a venous access device in the infant under age 6 months is:
   A. the scalp.
   B. the hand.
   C. the antecubital fossa.
Answer: A. Although all of these sites are favorable, the veins of the scalp are the most accessible.

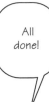

4. Your patient has swelling at the I.V. site, discomfort, burning, decreased skin temperature, and blanching around the site. These are signs of:
   A. phlebitis.
   B. infiltration.
   C. occlusion.

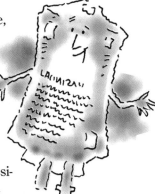

Answer: B. Signs of phlebitis include redness, possibly a hard vein on palpation, and possibly elevated temperature. Signs of occlusion include no forward movement of infusate into the vein, no blood return, and resistance to flushing.

Scoring

☆☆☆ If you answered all four items correctly, take a bow. At this juncture, fear no venipuncture.

☆☆ If you answered three correctly, congratulations. For the most part, you delivered the correct solutions.

☆ If you answered fewer than three correctly, don't get discouraged. Your quick quiz score is a peripheral matter. Review the chapter and try again.

3

Central venous therapy

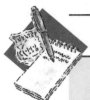

Just the facts

In this chapter you'll learn:

♦ the purpose of central venous (CV) therapy

♦ CV therapy equipment

♦ how to prepare a patient for catheter insertion

♦ how to assist with catheter insertion

♦ how to maintain and end CV therapy

♦ how to care for a patient with an implanted vascular access port.

Understanding central venous therapy

In CV therapy, drugs or fluids are infused directly into a major vein. CV therapy is used in emergencies or when a patient's peripheral veins are inaccessible. It may be ordered when a patient:
• needs infusion of a large volume of fluid
• requires multiple infusions
• requires long-term venous therapy.

At one time, only patients in intensive care and specialty units received CV therapy. Today, however, patients in any unit or even at home may receive CV therapy.

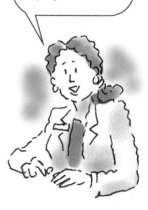

By reducing the need for repeated venipunctures, CV therapy preserves peripheral veins.

Benefits

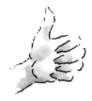

CV therapy offers many benefits, such as:
• access to the central veins
• rapid infusion of medications or large amounts of fluids
• way to draw blood samples and measure central venous pressure, an important indicator of circulatory function

• reduced need for repeated venipunctures, which decreases the patient's anxiety and preserves (or restores) the peripheral veins
• reduced risk of vein irritation from infusing irritating or caustic substances.

Risks

Like any other invasive procedure, CV therapy has its drawbacks. It increases the risk of life-threatening complications, such as:
• pneumothorax
• sepsis
• thrombus formation
• perforation of the vessel and adjacent organs.
   Using a CV catheter also has disadvantages:
• It requires more time and skill to insert than a peripheral I.V. catheter.
• It costs more to maintain than a peripheral I.V. catheter.
• It carries a risk of air embolism.

Venous circulation

The 5 quarts (L) of blood in an average adult body really gets around. After delivering oxygen and nutrients throughout the body, depleted blood flows from the capillaries to ever-widening veins, finally returning to the right side of the heart before collecting a fresh supply of oxygen from the lungs.
   CV circulation enters the right atrium through two major veins:

   the superior vena cava

   the inferior vena cava.

Going down

Before flowing into the right atrium, venous return from the head, neck, and arms enters the superior vena cava by three routes:
• through the subclavian vein
• through the internal and external jugular veins
• through the right and left innominate veins.

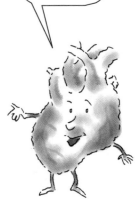

Venous blood enters my right atrium through the superior and inferior vena cava.

Going up

Venous return from the legs enters the inferior vena cava and returns blood to the right atrium by several routes:
- through the femoral venous system
- through multiple accessory venous pathways throughout the abdomen.

Getting to the point

In CV therapy, a catheter is inserted with its tip in one of three places (depending on venous accessibility and the prescribed infusion therapy):
- the superior vena cava
- the inferior vena cava
- the right atrium of the heart.

Blood flows unimpeded around the tip, allowing the rapid infusion of large amounts of fluid directly into the circulation. Because fluids are rapidly diluted by the venous circulation, highly concentrated or caustic fluids can be infused. (See *CV catheter pathways,* pages 100 and 101.)

Same destination, different route

In peripheral CV therapy, a variation of CV therapy, a catheter is inserted through a peripheral vein and the catheter tip is passed all the way to the superior vena cava. For instance, a catheter inserted in the arm (at the antecubital fossa) enters the basilic vein and is threaded through the subclavian vein and the innominate vein to the superior vena cava. To ease this procedure, newer catheters have longer introducers, smaller lumens, and variable lengths.

Types of catheters

Types of CV catheters include:
- nontunneled catheters
- tunneled catheters
- peripherally inserted central catheters (PICCs)
- implanted vascular access ports (VAPs).

Selecting the appropriate CV catheter for a patient depends on the type of therapy needed.

Nontunneled CV catheters

Nontunneled catheters, also called central catheters, are radiopaque, so placement can be checked by X-ray.

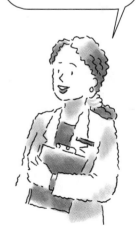

In peripheral CV therapy, a catheter is inserted through a peripheral vein and threaded to the superior vena cava.

Now I get it!

CV catheter pathways

Usually, a central venous (CV) catheter is inserted into the subclavian vein or the internal jugular vein. The catheter may terminate in the superior vena cava or the right atrium. The illustrations below show several common pathways of the CV catheter.

Inserted into the subclavian vein, this CV catheter terminates in the superior vena cava.

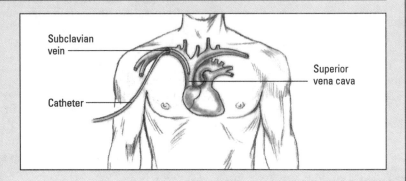

Inserted into the subclavian vein, this CV catheter extends to the right atrium.

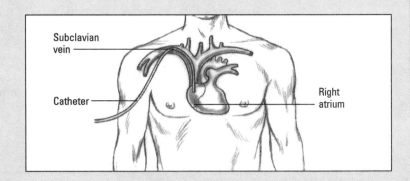

This CV catheter enters the internal jugular vein and terminates in the superior vena cava.

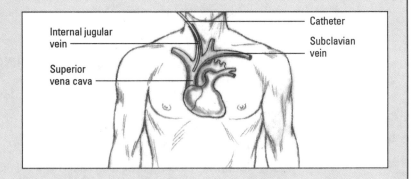

CV catheter pathways *(continued)*

This CV catheter, peripherally inserted into the basilic vein, terminates in the superior vena cava.

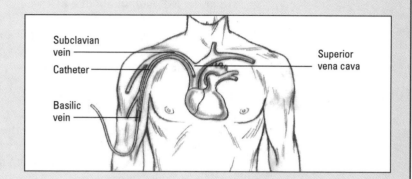

This CV catheter enters the subclavian vein and terminates in the superior vena cava. Note that the catheter tunnels (shown by broken line) from the insertion site, through the subcutaneous tissue, to an exit site on the skin. Also note how the position of the Dacron cuff helps hold the catheter in place.

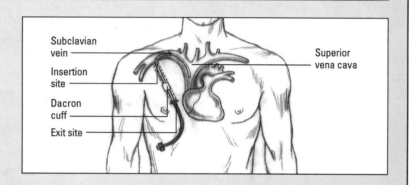

They're usually designed for short-term use, such as brief continuation of I.V. therapy following a patient's hospitalization. To avoid infection, nontunneled catheters are changed every 3 to 7 days. This type of catheter may not be appropriate for a patient starting long-term I.V. therapy.

Tunneled CV catheters

Tunneled CV catheters are designed for long-term use. They're also radiopaque and usually made of silicone. Silicone is much less likely to cause thrombosis than polyurethane or polyvinyl chloride because it's more physiologically compatible. This minimizes irritation or damage to the vein lining.

Cuff link

A tunneled CV catheter has a cuff that encourages tissue growth at the exit site. In about 2 to 4 weeks, the tissue anchors the catheter and keeps bacteria out of venous circulation. In most cases, the cuff is made of Dacron. An alternative, the Vitacuff, contains silver ions that provide antibacterial protection for about 3 months.

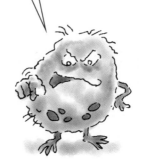

Tissue growth at the cuff of a tunneled catheter keeps bacteria out of venous circulation.

Tunnel tidbits

Tunneled catheters are better suited to the home care patient than nontunneled catheters because they're designed for long-term use. They're used in patients who have poor peripheral venous access or need long-term daily infusions, such as those with:
- cancer
- acquired immunodeficiency syndrome (AIDS)
- intestinal malabsorption
- anemia
- bone or organ infections
- other chronic diseases.
    Medications that are given by tunneled CV catheter include:
- antibiotics
- chemotherapy
- total parenteral nutrition (TPN)
- blood products.

Tunnel types

Common tunneled catheters for long-term use include the Broviac, Hickman, and Groshong catheters. The Groshong catheter has a pressure-sensitive valve in the catheter tip that keeps the lumen closed when not in use. The valve opens inward during blood aspiration and outward during blood or fluid administration. This valve eliminates the need to flush with heparin. (See *Guide to CV catheters.*)

Single, double, triple, or multi

Tunneled catheters can be single-lumen, double-lumen, triple-lumen, or multi-lumen and can vary in size. The Broviac tunneled CV catheter is a good choice for a patient — such as a child — with small central veins.

Running smoothly

Guide to CV catheters

Types of central venous (CV) catheters differ in their design, composition, and indications for use. This chart outlines the advantages, disadvantages, and nursing considerations for several commonly used catheters.

Catheter description and indications	Advantages and disadvantages	Nursing considerations
Short-term, single-lumen catheter *Description* • Polyvinyl chloride (PVC) or polyurethane • Approximately 8″ (20.3 cm) long • Variety of lumen gauges *Indications* • Short-term CV access • Emergency access • Patient who requires only a single lumen	*Advantages* • It can be inserted at bedside. • It's easily removed. • Stiffness aids central venous pressure (CVP) monitoring. *Disadvantages* • Catheter has limited functions. • PVC is thrombogenic. • PVC irritates inner lumen of vessel. • Catheter needs to be changed every 3 to 7 days.	• Minimize patient motion and activities. • Assess frequently for signs of infection and clot formation. 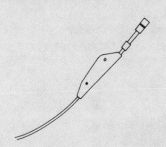
Short-term, multilumen catheter *Description* • PVC or polyurethane • Double, triple, or quadruple lumen at ¾″ (2-cm) intervals • Variety of lumen gauges *Indications* • Short-term CV access • Patient with limited insertion sites who requires multiple infusions	*Advantages* • It can be inserted at bedside. • It's easily removed. • Stiffness aids CVP monitoring. • It allows infusion of multiple solutions through the same catheter — even for the same task (for example, incompatible solutions). *Disadvantages* • Catheter has limited functions. • PVC is thrombogenic. • PVC irritates inner lumen of vessel. • Catheter needs to be changed every 3 to 7 days.	• Know gauge and purpose of each lumen. • Use the same lumen for the same task (for example, to administer TPN or to collect a blood sample). 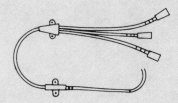

(continued)

Guide to CV catheters *(continued)*

Catheter description and indications	Advantages and disadvantages	Nursing considerations
Groshong catheter *Description* • Silicone rubber • Approximately 35″ (88.9 cm) long • Closed end with pressure-sensitive two-way valve • Dacron cuff • Available with single or double lumen *Indications* • Long-term CV access • Patient with heparin allergy	*Advantages* • It's less thrombogenic than catheters made with PVC. • Pressure-sensitive two-way valve eliminates heparin flushes. • Dacron cuff anchors catheter and prevents bacterial migration. *Disadvantages* • It requires surgical insertion. • It tears and kinks easily. • Blunt end makes it difficult to clear substances from its tip.	• Two surgical sites require dressing after insertion. • Handle catheter gently. • Check the external portion frequently for kinks or leaks. (Repair kit is available.) • Observe frequently for kinks or tears. • Remember to flush lumen with enough saline solution to clear catheter, especially after drawing or administering blood. 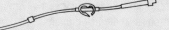
Hickman catheter *Description* • Silicone rubber • Approximately 35″ long • Open end with clamp • Dacron cuff 11¾″ (30 cm) from hub *Indications* • Long-term CV access • Home therapy	*Advantages* • It's less thrombogenic than catheters made with PVC. • Dacron cuff prevents excess motion and organism migration. • Clamps eliminate need for Valsalva's maneuver. *Disadvantages* • It requires surgical insertion. • Catheter has an open end. • It requires doctor for removal. • It tears and kinks easily.	• Two surgical sites require dressing after insertion. • Handle catheter gently. • Observe frequently for kinks or tears. (Repair kit is available.) • Clamp catheter whenever it becomes disconnected or open, using nonserrated clamp. 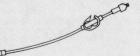
Broviac catheter *Description* • Identical to Hickman catheter except smaller inner lumen *Indications* • Long-term CV access • Patient with small central vessels (pediatric, elderly)	*Advantages* • Small lumen ensures better comfort. *Disadvantages* • Small lumen may limit its uses. • It has a single lumen, which limits its functions (cannot infuse multiple solutions at once).	• Check facility policy before drawing or administering blood products.

Guide to CV catheters *(continued)*

Catheter description and indications	Advantages and disadvantages	Nursing considerations
Hickman-Broviac catheter *Description* • Hickman and Broviac catheters combined in one catheter *Indications* • Long-term CV access • Patient who needs multiple infusions	*Advantages* • Double-lumen Hickman catheter allows sampling and administration of blood. • Broviac lumen delivers I.V. fluids, including total parenteral nutrition (TPN) fluids *Disadvantages* • It requires surgical insertion. • Catheter has an open end. • It requires doctor for removal. • It tears and kinks easily. 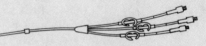	• Know purpose and function of each lumen. • Label lumens to prevent confusion.
Long-line catheter *Description* • Peripherally inserted central catheter • Silicone rubber • 20″ to 24″ (51 cm to 71 cm) long; available in 14G, 16G, 18G, 20G, and 22G *Indications* • Long-term CV access • Patient with poor central access • Patient at risk for fatal complications from insertion at central access sites • Patient who needs CV access but faces or has had head and neck surgery	*Advantages* • It's peripherally inserted. • It can be inserted at bedside with minimal complications. • It may be inserted by a trained, skilled, competent registered nurse in most states. • Single lumen or double lumen available. *Disadvantages* • Catheter may occlude smaller peripheral vessels. • It may be difficult to keep immobile. 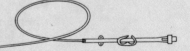	• Check frequently for signs of phlebitis and thrombus formation. • Insert catheter above the antecubital fossa. • Use arm board if necessary. • Catheter may alter CVP measurements.

Peripherally inserted central catheters

The most commonly used catheter for peripheral CV therapy is the PICC. A PICC, also known as a long-arm or long-line catheter, is inserted through a peripheral vein, with the tip ending in the superior vena cava or subclavian vein.

Generally, PICCs are used when patients need frequent blood transfusions or infusions of caustic drugs or solutions. PICCs are especially useful if the patient doesn't have reliable routes for short-term I.V. therapy.

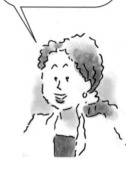

Generally, PICCs are used when patients need frequent blood transfusions or infusions of caustic drugs or solutions.

Why pick a PICC?

When a patient needs CV therapy for 5 days to several months or requires repeated venous access, a PICC may be the best choice. A PICC may also be ordered when a patient has the following conditions:
• chest injury due to trauma or burns
• respiratory problems due to chronic obstructive pulmonary disease (COPD), a mediastinal mass, cystic fibrosis, or pneumothorax.

Using a peripheral insertion site for a PICC helps prevent complications, such as pneumothorax, that may occur with a CV line.

PICCs are commonly used in patients with such conditions as:
• AIDS
• cancer
• recurrent infections (such as osteomyelitis and endocarditis)
• sickle cell anemia
• women who require I.V. therapy due to severe morning sickness.

Given by PICC

Infusions commonly given by PICC include:
• analgesics
• antibiotics
• blood products
• chemotherapy
• immunoglobulins
• narcotics
• TPN.

Take your PICC!

PICC specifics

PICCs are available in single- or double-lumen configurations and with or without guide wires. A guide wire stiffens the catheter to ease its advancement through the vein, but it can damage the vein if used incorrectly.

The patient receiving PICC therapy must have a peripheral vein large enough to accept an introducer needle.

Catheter gauge depends on the size of the patient's vein and the type of fluid or medication to be infused. PICCs range from 14G to 24G in diameter and from 7¾" to

23½″ (20 to 60 cm) in length. Other PICCs are configured for use in a neonate. If the patient is to receive blood or blood products through the PICC, you should use at least an 18G catheter. (See *Guide to PICCs*.)

Guide to PICCs

Below are some of the peripherally inserted central catheters (PICCs) from various manufacturers.

Per-Q-Cath

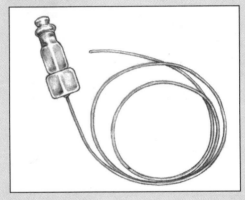

Dual-Lumen Per-Q-Cath

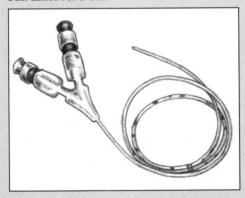

Per-Q-Cath and Dual Lumen Per-Q-Cath are manufactured by Bard Access Systems. Features include:
• single-lumen or double-lumen
• gauges from 16G to 23G
• catheter length of 23″ (60 cm)
• insertion tray available
• repair kit available.

OneCath

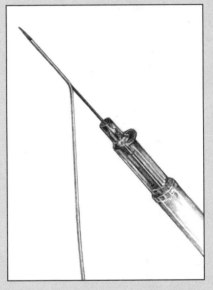

OneCath is manufactured by Luther Medical Products, Inc. Features include:
• introducer to prevent inadvertent needle sticks
• soft, biocompatible polyurethane catheter
• gauges from 16G to 20G
• catheter length of 23″
• protective sleeve to maintain catheter sterility during insertion
• 2″ (5-cm) increment markings on catheter for measurement during insertion.

(continued)

Guide to PICCs *(continued)*

Groshong

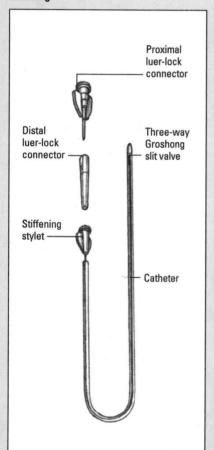

Proximal luer-lock connector

Distal luer-lock connector

Three-way Groshong slit valve

Stiffening stylet

Catheter

Arrow

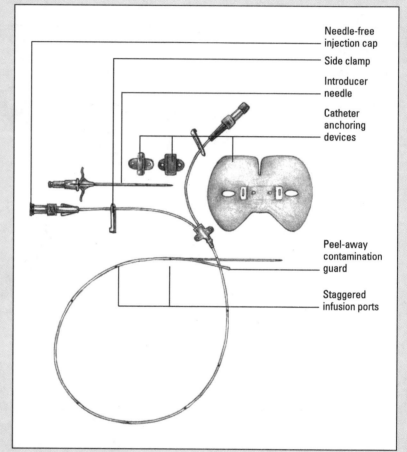

Needle-free injection cap

Side clamp

Introducer needle

Catheter anchoring devices

Peel-away contamination guard

Staggered infusion ports

Groshong is manufactured by Bard Access Systems. Features include:
• single lumen or double lumen
• gauges from 18G to 20G
• catheter lengths from 22½″ to 23″ (57 to 60 cm).

Arrow is manufactured by Arrow International. Features include:
• single lumen or double lumen
• gauges from 18G to 20G
• polyurethane catheter
• stylet-free insertion
• peel-away guard to maintain catheter sterility during insertion
• tip that deflects on contact with vessel walls to reduce intimal irritation during insertion
• anchoring device available.

Don't pressure a PICC

Don't use a tuberculin syringe or a 3-ml syringe with a PICC to administer a medication or flush the catheter. These syringes create too much pressure (measured in pounds per square inch) in the line. Such excessive pressure can cause the device to burst.

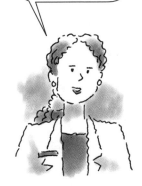

Widely used for home infusion therapy, PICCs may be inserted at bedside.

PICCs permitted by practice acts

In many states, nurse practice acts allow registered nurses who are trained and skilled in the proper technique to insert PICCs. PICCs are widely used for home infusion therapy because they may be inserted at bedside without a doctor in attendance.

PICC imposter

The term PICC may be incorrectly used to describe an extended peripheral catheter. This catheter is more correctly known as a midline device. Technically, the midline device isn't a CV catheter because its tip doesn't rest in the CV circulation but in the axillary vein. A true PICC tip terminates in the superior or inferior vena cava. When caring for a home care patient with a PICC, make sure you know where the catheter terminates and the entire length of the catheter, both indwelling and external.

PICC ups

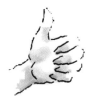

PICCs have a definite up side:
• PICCs provide long-term access to central veins. A PICC can be left in place for up to 1 year because the catheter is made of soft, physiologically compatible silicone or polyurethane. A single catheter may be used for an entire course of therapy.
• A PICC provides a safe, reliable route for infusion therapy and occasional blood sampling.
• PICCs have antithrombogenic properties that minimize the risk of blood clots and phlebitis associated with other types of CV catheters.
• PICCs are extremely cost-effective compared with other long-term and short-term CV catheters.

PICC downs

A PICC may be unsuitable for a patient with bruises, scarring, or sclerosis from earlier multiple venipunctures at the intended PICC site. PICC therapy works best when it's introduced early in treatment; it shouldn't be considered a

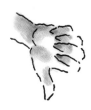

last resort for patients with sclerosed or repeatedly punctured veins.

Implanted vascular access ports

As the number of chronically ill patients increases, so does the need for long-term I.V. therapy. When an external catheter isn't suitable, an implanted device may be used.

An implanted VAP functions much like a long-term CV catheter except that it has no external parts; it's implanted in a pocket under the skin. (See *Comparing VAPs and long-term CV catheters.*)

The indwelling catheter that is attached to a VAP is surgically tunneled under the skin until the catheter tip lies in the superior vena cava. The catheter may be threaded through the subclavian vein, for example. A VAP is also suitable for epidural, intra-arterial, or intraperitoneal placement.

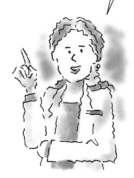

An implanted VAP functions much like a long-term CV catheter except that it's implanted in a pocket under the skin.

VAP advantages

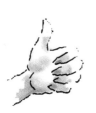

Implanted devices are easier to maintain than external devices. They require heparinization only once a month to maintain patency. VAPs also pose less risk of infection because they have no exit site through which microorganisms can invade. VAPs offer several other advantages for patients, including:
• minimal activity restrictions
• few self-care measures for the patient to learn and perform
• few dressing changes (except when accessed and used to maintain continuous infusions or intermittent infusion devices).

Finally, because VAPs create only a slight protrusion under the skin, many patients find them easier to accept than external venous access devices. A patient with a VAP may shower, swim, and exercise without worrying about the device, as long as the device isn't accessed. The doctor decides how soon after insertion the patient may undertake these activities.

VAP disadvantages

Because it's implanted, a VAP may be more difficult for the patient to manage, especially for daily or frequent infusions. Accessing the device requires insertion of a special-

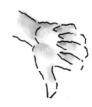

Comparing VAPs and long-term CV catheters

A vascular access port (VAP) offers patients many of the advantages of a long-term central venous (CV) catheter, along with an unobtrusive design that many patients find easier to accept. Both devices are indicated when poor venous access prohibits peripheral I.V. therapy. Deciding which device to use depends on the type and duration of treatment, the frequency of access, and the patient's condition. The following chart shows how the two devices compare.

Type of treatment	VAP	Long-term catheter
Continuous infusion of drugs or fluids	Yes, but maintaining continuous needle access eliminates the benefits of implantation	Yes
Self-administration of drugs or fluids	Yes, but it may be more difficult for patient or family member to manage	Yes
Bolus injections of vesicant or irritant drugs by health care professionals	Yes	Yes
Duration of treatment		
Less than 3 months	No, because the high cost of implanting and removing the device precludes it	Yes
More than 3 months	Yes, but cost of implantation and removal may exceed cost benefit if treatment lasts less than 6 months	Yes
Frequency of access		
Three or more times a week	Yes, but it may minimize the advantage of having an implanted device	Yes
Less than once a week	Yes	No, because the high cost of maintaining the catheter precludes it
Patient concerns		
Negative effect on body image	No	Possibly
Negative reaction to needle punctures	Possibly	No
Ability to care for external catheter	Not needed	Needed
Cost of dressing changes and heparinization	Minimal	Considerable

ized needle through subcutaneous tissue, which may be uncomfortable for patients who fear or dislike needle punctures.

Also, implanting and removing the VAP requires surgery and possible hospitalization, which can be costly. The comparatively high cost of a VAP makes it worthwhile only for patients who require infusion therapy for at least 6 months. Another type of implantable vascular access device — an implantable pump — may be used for patients who require continuous low-volume infusions. (See *Understanding implantable pumps.*)

For more information about VAP implantation and infusions, turn to pages 144 to 164.

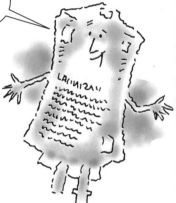

Preparing for central venous therapy

The first step in preparing for CV therapy is selecting an insertion site for the CV catheter. You also need to prepare the patient both physically and mentally. Depending on which procedure is to be used, you may then gather and prepare the appropriate equipment.

Selecting the insertion site

With the exception of PICC insertions, CV devices are usually inserted by a doctor. If inserting a central line is an elective rather than an emergency procedure, you may collaborate with the patient and the doctor in selecting a site.

In CV therapy, the insertion site varies, depending on:
• type of catheter
• patient's anatomy and age
• duration of therapy
• vessel integrity and accessibility
• history of previous neck or chest surgery such as mastectomy
• presence of chest trauma
• possible complications.

Veins commonly used as CV insertion sites include the subclavian, internal and external jugular, and brachiocephalic. Rarely, the femoral and brachial veins may be used. (See *Comparing CV insertion sites,* page 115.)

Now I get it!

Understanding implantable pumps

An implantable pump is usually placed in a subcutaneous pocket made in the abdomen below the umbilicus. An implantable pump has two chambers separated by a bellows. One chamber contains the I.V. solution, and the other contains a charging fluid. The charging fluid chamber exerts continuous pressure on the bellows, forcing the infusion solution through the silicone outlet catheter into a central vein. The pump also has an auxiliary septum that can be used to deliver bolus injections of medication. Generally, the pump is indicated for patients who require continuous low-volume infusions.

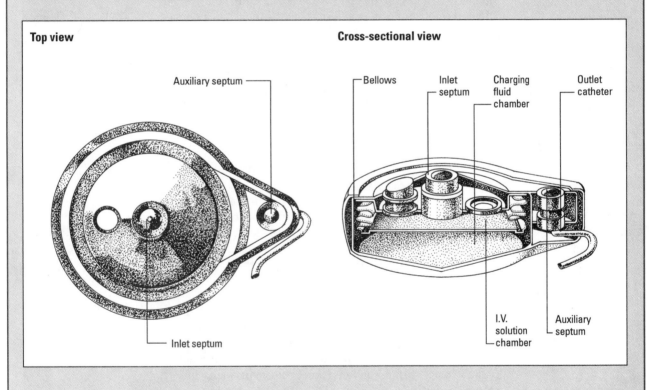

Top view

Auxiliary septum

Inlet septum

Cross-sectional view

Bellows   Inlet septum   Charging fluid chamber   Outlet catheter

I.V. solution chamber   Auxiliary septum

Subclavian vein

The subclavian vein is the most common insertion site for CV therapy. It affords easy access and a short, direct route to the superior vena cava and the CV circulation.

The subclavian vein is a large vein with high-volume blood flow, making clot formation and vessel irritation less likely. The subclavian site also allows the greatest patient mobility after insertion.

Through the skin and to the angle of Louis

When using the subclavian site, the doctor inserts the catheter into the vein percutaneously (through the skin and into the vessel with one puncture), threading it into the superior vena cava. This technique requires a venipuncture close to the apex of the lung and major vessels of the thorax.

As the catheter enters the skin between the clavicle and first rib, the doctor directs the needle toward the angle of Louis, under the clavicle. The procedure may be difficult if the patient moves during insertion or has a chest deformity or poor posture.

Internal jugular vein

The internal jugular vein provides easy access in small patients. This insertion site is commonly used in children but not infants.

Dangerously close

The right internal jugular vein provides a more direct route to the superior vena cava than the left internal jugular vein. However, its proximity to the common carotid artery can lead to serious complications, such as uncontrolled hemorrhage, emboli, or impeded flow, especially if the carotid artery is punctured during catheter insertion (which can cause irreversible brain damage).

Other drawbacks

Using the internal jugular vein has other drawbacks. For example, it limits the patient's movement and may be a poor choice for home therapy because of cosmetic considerations. Because of the location of the internal jugular vein, it's also difficult to keep an occlusive dressing in place.

Femoral veins

Femoral veins may be used if other sites aren't suitable. Although the femoral veins are large vessels, using them for catheter insertion entails some complications, such as the following:
• Insertion may be difficult, especially in larger individuals.
• Local lymph nodes may be punctured during insertion.

> Using the subclavian vein provides a direct route to the superior vena cava...

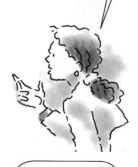

> ....it also reduces the risk of clot formation and vessel irritation.

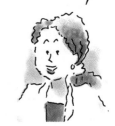

Advice from the experts

Comparing CV insertion sites

The chart below lists the most common insertion sites for a central venous (CV) catheter and the advantages and disadvantages of each.

Site	Advantages	Disadvantages
Subclavian vein	• Easy access • Easy to keep dressing in place • High flow rate, which reduces risk of thrombus	• Proximity to subclavian artery (if artery is punctured during catheter insertion, hemorrhage can occur) • Difficulty controlling bleeding • Increased risk of pneumothorax
Internal jugular vein	• Short, direct route to right atrium • Catheter stability, resulting in less movement with respiration • Decreased risk of pneumothorax	• Proximity to the common carotid artery (if artery is punctured during catheter insertion, uncontrolled hemorrhage, emboli, or impedance to flow can result) • Difficulty keeping dressing in place • Proximity to the trachea
External jugular vein	• Easy access, especially in children • Decreased risk of pneumothorax or arterial puncture	• Less direct route • Lower flow rate, which increases risk of thrombus • Difficulty keeping dressing in place • Tortuous vein, especially in elderly patients
Cephalic, basilic veins	• Least risk of major complications • Easy to keep dressing in place	• Possible cutdown required • Possible difficulty locating antecubital fossa in obese patients • Difficulty keeping elbow immobile, especially in children

• The femoral site inherently carries a greater risk of local infection, and keeping a dressing clean and intact in the groin area is a challenge. (Dressing adherence is a big concern when selecting an insertion site.)

Straighten up

When a femoral vein is used in CV therapy, the patient's leg needs to be kept straight and movement limited. This prevents bleeding and keeps the catheter from becoming kinked internally or dislodged. Infection can also occur at the insertion site from catheter movement into and out of the incision.

Peripheral veins

The peripheral veins most commonly used as insertion sites are the following:
- cephalic
- basilic
- median cubital of the antecubital fossa
- external jugular.

Far from internal organs

Because they're located far from major internal organs and vessels, peripheral veins cause fewer traumatic complications on insertion. However, accessing peripheral veins may cause phlebitis. The tight fit of the catheter in the smaller vessel allows only minimal blood flow around the catheter. Catheter movement may irritate the inner lumen or block it, causing blood pooling (stasis) and thrombus formation.

At the bend of the elbow

Accessing peripheral sites in the antecubital space may limit the patient's mobility because the device exits the skin at the bend of the elbow. Inserting the catheter above the antecubital space increases patient mobility and prevents kinking but makes it difficult to palpate the veins.

Cephalic and basilic veins

Although the cephalic vein is more accessible than the basilic vein, its sharp angle makes it more difficult to thread a catheter through it. The larger, straighter basilic vein is usually the preferred insertion site.

External jugular vein

The external jugular vein may provide a CV insertion site. Using the external jugular vein this way presents few complications. However, threading a catheter into the superior vena cava may be difficult because of the sharp angle encountered on entering the subclavian vein from the external jugular vein. For this reason, the catheter tip may remain in the external jugular vein. This position allows high-volume infusions but makes CV pressure measurements inaccurate.

Dilution dilemma

External jugular veins shouldn't be used to administer highly caustic medications because blood flow around the tip of the catheter may not be strong enough to sufficiently dilute the solutions as they enter the vein.

Insertion site concerns

There are notable concerns in choosing an insertion site for a CV catheter. Examples of these include:
- presence of scar tissue
- interference with surgical site or other therapy
- configuration of the lung apices
- patient's lifestyle or daily activities.

Scar wars

In some patients, scar tissue from previous surgery or trauma may prohibit access to major blood vessels or make insertion of a catheter difficult. Alternatively, if the patient is facing surgery in the area of a central vein, another site may need to be chosen. A peripheral site, such as the basilic vein, or a central site on the side of the body unaffected by surgery is a likely alternative site.

Tracheostomy treachery

An alternative site may be necessary if the patient is receiving other therapy that interferes with the insertion site. For example, if the patient has a tracheostomy, the internal or external jugular site should be avoided because the tracheostomy tapes come too close to these insertion sites. This predisposes the patient to infection and may cause the catheter to dislodge.

Look out for the lungs

Another site consideration is the location of the lung apices. In patients on mechanical ventilation, especially those receiving positive end-expiratory pressure therapy, intrathoracic pressures increase, which may elevate the lung apices and increase the chance of lung puncture and

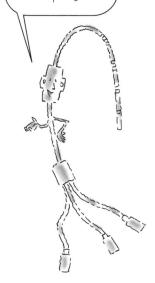

Upon entering the subclavian vein, I encounter a sharp angle.

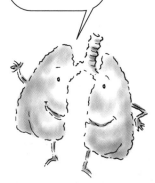

When selecting a CV insertion site, consider the location of my apices.

pneumothorax. Patients with COPD also have displaced lung apices, so consideration should be given to venous access sites outside the thorax in these patients.

Practically done

Practical considerations play a role in site selection. For example, a home therapy patient with a PICC may have only one hand with which to work. A woman with a long-term tunneled catheter that exits near her brassiere straps would have a limited choice of clothing.

Aware and alert

Be aware of the catheter's insertion site and the location of the catheter tip. That way, you can be alert for potential problems, such as thrombosis, catheter displacement, and infection.

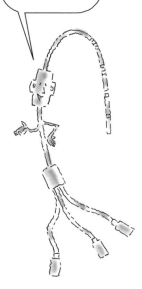

Be aware of the insertion site and where my tip is located.

Preparing the patient

Accurate and thorough patient teaching increases the success of CV therapy. Before therapy begins, make sure the patient understands:
- the procedure
- its benefits
- what to expect during and after catheter insertion.

The primary responsibility for explaining the procedure and its goals rests with the doctor. Your role may include allaying the patient's fears and answering questions about the following:
- movement restrictions
- cosmetic concerns
- management regimens.

Explaining the procedure

Ask the patient if he has ever received I.V. therapy before, particularly CV therapy. Evaluate the patient's learning capabilities and adjust your teaching technique accordingly. For example, use appropriate language when describing the procedure to a child. Also, ask the parents to help you phrase the procedure in terms their child understands. If time and resources permit, use pictures and physical models to enhance your teaching.

Dress code

If catheter insertion is to take place at the bedside, explain that sterile procedures require the staff to wear gowns, masks, and gloves. Tell your patient he may need to wear a mask as well. If time allows, let your patient, especially a child, try on the mask.

An important position

To minimize the patient's anxiety, explain how he'll be positioned during the procedure. If the subclavian or jugular vein will be used, he'll be in Trendelenburg's position for at least a short period, and a towel may be placed under his back between the scapulae. (In Trendelenburg's position, the head is low and the body and legs are on an inclined plane.)

Reassure the patient that he won't be in this position longer than necessary. Stress the position's importance for dilating the veins, which aids insertion and helps prevent insertion-related complications.

This may sting

Warn the patient to expect a stinging sensation from the local anesthetic and a feeling of pressure during catheter insertion.

Testing, testing

Explain any other tests that may be done. For example, the doctor may obtain a venogram before the catheter insertion to check the status of the vessels, especially if the catheter is intended for long-term use. After CV catheter insertion, blood samples are often drawn to establish baseline coagulation profiles, and a chest X-ray is always done to confirm catheter placement.

Explaining self-care measures

In explaining care measures to your patient, make sure you cover the following topics:
• Teach the patient Valsalva's maneuver, and have him demonstrate it to you at least twice. This maneuver helps prevent air embolism. The patient may need to perform it in the future whenever the catheter is open to the air. This training is especially important when the patient is taking care of his catheter at home.
• If the catheter is to be in place long-term or will be managed at home, explain thoroughly all care procedures, such as how to change the dressing and how to flush the device. Ask the patient to return demonstrate the various

techniques and procedures, and include other family members, as appropriate. A home-therapy coordinator or discharge planner should coordinate teaching and follow-up assessments before and after catheter insertion.

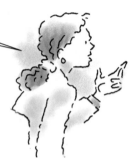

Ask the patient to return demonstrate Valsalva's maneuver...

...as well as techniques and procedures for catheter care.

Preparing the equipment

Besides the I.V. solution, infusion equipment typically includes an administration set with tubing containing an air-eliminating in-line filter. Expect to use an infusion pump when positive pressure is required, for example, when solutions are administered through a CV line at low flow rates or during intra-arterial infusion.

A drip controller permits infusion at a lower pressure.

Some facilities use drip controllers for CV therapy, which permit infusion at a lower pressure. Drip controllers are used most often with infants and children, who could suffer serious complications from high-pressure infusion.

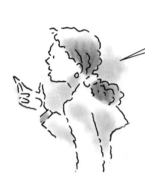

Getting equipped

When you're assisting with an insertion at the patient's bedside, first collect the necessary equipment. Most facilities use preassembled disposable trays that include the CV catheter. Although most trays include the necessary equipment, be sure to check. If you don't have a preassembled tray, gather the following items:
• linen-saver pad
• scissors
• povidone-iodine solution
• sterile gauze pads
• solution of 70% alcohol

- local anesthetic
- 3-ml syringe with 25G needle for introduction of anesthetic
- sterile syringe for blood samples
- sterile towels or drapes
- suture material
- sterile dressing
- CV catheter.

   You also need to obtain extra syringes and blood sample containers if the doctor wants venous blood samples to be drawn during the procedure.

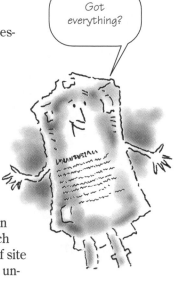

Got everything?

Mask, gown, and gloves required

Make sure that everyone participating in the insertion has a mask, gown, and gloves. You may also need such protection for the patient, especially if there's a risk of site contamination from oral secretions or if the patient is unable to cooperate.

It's a setup

To set up the equipment, follow these steps:
- Attach the tubing to the solution container.
- Prime the tubing with the solution.
- Fill the syringes with saline or heparin flush solutions, based on policy and procedures at your facility.
- Prime and calibrate any pressure monitoring setups.

Aseptic, air-free, secure, and sealed

In addition, take the following precautions:
- All priming must be done using strict aseptic technique.
- All tubing must be free from air.
- After you've primed the tubing, recheck all the connections to make sure they're secure.
- Make sure all open ends are covered with sealed caps.

Performing central venous therapy

The same basic procedure is used whether catheter insertion is done at the bedside or in the operating room. Specific steps may vary. Before the doctor inserts the catheter, you need to do the following:

 Position the patient.

Prepare the insertion site.

Monitoring, administering, applying, and documenting

After the catheter is inserted, your primary responsibilities include:
- monitoring the patient
- administering therapy.
     You also need to:
- apply a dressing to the insertion site
- document your interventions and all information related to the catheter insertion.

Positioning the patient

After you've assembled the equipment, position the patient and make him as comfortable as possible.

Visible and accessible

Position the patient in Trendelenburg's position (for insertion in the subclavian or internal jugular veins). This position distends neck and thoracic veins, making them more visible and accessible. Filling the veins also lessens the chance of air emboli because the venous pressure is higher than atmospheric pressure.

Trendelenburg's position makes neck and thoracic veins more visible.

Between the scapulae

If the subclavian vein is to be used, you may need to place a rolled towel or blanket between the patient's scapulae. This allows for more direct access and may prevent puncture of the lung apex or adjacent vessels.

Under the opposite shoulder

If a jugular vein is to be used, place a rolled blanket under the opposite shoulder to extend the neck and make anatomic landmarks more visible.

Preparing the insertion site

Prepare the insertion site by taking these steps:
- Place a linen-saver pad under the site to prevent soiling the bed.

• Make sure the skin is free from hair, because the follicles can harbor microorganisms. (See *Removing hair from a CV insertion site*.)

• Prepare the intended venipuncture site with 70% alcohol, then with povidone-iodine solution, using sterile gauze pads. If the patient is allergic to iodine, you may use only 70% alcohol, taking care to vigorously prepare the site. Use a circular motion to prepare the skin, starting at the insertion site and gradually making wider circles with each motion. Don't wipe the same area twice, and be sure to discard each gauze pad after each complete cycle.

Sterile drape style

After the site is prepared, the doctor places sterile drapes around it and, possibly, around the patient's face as well. (This makes the patient's mask unnecessary.) If the patient's face is draped, you can help ease anxiety by uncovering his eyes. The drapes should provide a work area at least as large as the length of the catheter or guide wire.

Inserting the catheter

During catheter insertion, you may be responsible for monitoring the patient's tolerance of the procedure and providing emotional support. The doctor usually prepares the equipment, which comes with a central venous access kit and requires aseptic technique.

Blood samples

You may obtain venous blood samples after the catheter is inserted. You'll need a sterile syringe that is large enough to hold all of the needed blood. Place the blood in the proper sample container or, using a needle or needleless system, access a saline lock at the end of the port with a Vacutainer. This device draws blood directly into the appropriate tube.

Patient participation

Each time the catheter hub is open to air — such as when the syringe is changed — tell the patient to perform Valsalva's maneuver and clamp the port to decrease the risk of air embolism.

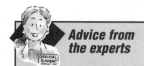

Advice from the experts

Removing hair from a CV insertion site

Infection-control practitioners and the Intravenous Nurses Society recommend clipping the hair close to the skin rather than shaving.

Irritation, open wounds, infection
Shaving may cause skin irritation and create multiple, small, open wounds, increasing the risk of infection. (If the doctor orders the area to be shaved, try to shave it the evening before; this allows minor skin irritations to partially heal before irritating cleaning substances are applied.)

Rinse, wash, and remove
After you remove the hair, rinse the skin with saline solution to remove hair clippings. You may also need to wash the skin with soap and water before the actual skin prep to remove surface dirt and body oils.

Monitoring the patient

After the catheter has been inserted, monitor the patient for complications. Make sure you tailor your assessment and interventions to the particular catheter insertion site. For example, if the site is close to major thoracic organs, as is a subclavian or internal jugular site, you should closely monitor the patient's respiratory status, watching for dyspnea, shortness of breath, and sudden chest pain.

Arrhythmia alert

Inserting the catheter can cause arrhythmias if the catheter enters the right ventricle and irritates the cardiac muscle. For this reason, make sure you monitor the patient's cardiac status. (Arrhythmias usually abate as the catheter is withdrawn.) If the patient isn't attached to a cardiac monitor, palpate the radial artery to detect any rhythm irregularities.

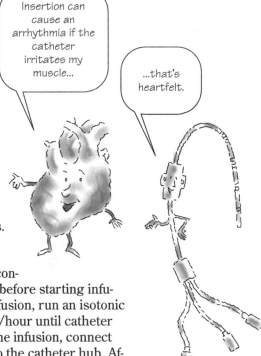

Insertion can cause an arrhythmia if the catheter irritates my muscle...

...that's heartfelt.

A stitch in time

When the proximal end of the catheter rests on the sterile drape, the doctor will use one or two sutures to secure the catheter to the skin. Most short-term catheters have preset tabs to hold the sutures.

Look inside

Finally, a chest X-ray is ordered to confirm the location of the catheter tip before starting infusions. If the line is to be used for infusion, run an isotonic fluid at a rate no greater than 20 ml/hour until catheter placement is confirmed. To begin the infusion, connect the I.V. tubing or intermittent cap to the catheter hub. After the X-ray confirmation, adjust the flow rate as prescribed.

Poor positioning poses problems

A catheter may be positioned poorly, especially if it's inserted into the internal or external jugular veins. This may cause several problems. It can:
• make dressing changes difficult
• make maintaining an occlusive dressing impossible
• cause the catheter to kink.

Applying a dressing

Maintain sterile technique and place a sterile dressing over the insertion site of a short-term catheter or exit site of the catheter. To apply the dressing, follow these steps:
• Clean the site with 70% alcohol followed by povidone-iodine solution, using the same method as the initial skin preparation.
• Place a drop of antibiotic ointment at the site, if facility policy directs, and cover the site with a dry, sterile gauze pad or transparent, semipermeable dressing.
• Seal the dressing with nonporous tape, checking that all edges are well secured. Label the dressing with the date, the time, your initials, and the catheter length.

Comfortable and elevated, clean and dry

After you apply the dressing, place the patient in a comfortable position and reassess his status. Elevate the head of the bed 45 degrees to help the patient breathe more easily. Remember to keep the site clean and dry to prevent infection. Also remember to keep the dressing occlusive to prevent air embolism and contamination.

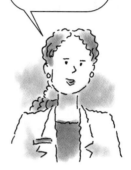

To prevent infection, keep the catheter insertion site clean and dry.

Documenting catheter insertion

Record all pertinent information in the nurses' notes and on the I.V. flow sheet, if your facility uses one. Make sure your documentation includes the following:
• type of catheter used
• location of insertion
• catheter tip position as confirmed by an X-ray
• patient's tolerance of the procedure
• blood samples taken.

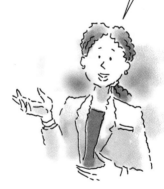

To prevent air embolism, keep the dressing occlusive.

A measure of migration

Some facilities recommend documenting the length of catheter remaining outside the body so other nurses can compare the measurements, checking for catheter migration.

Maintaining central venous infusions

One of your primary responsibilities is maintaining CV infusions. This includes meticulous care of the CV catheter insertion site as well as the catheter and tubing.

Routine care

Expect to perform the following care measures:
• Change the dressing every 48 to 72 hours or whenever it becomes moist, loose, or soiled.
• Care for the catheter by changing the I.V. tubing, solution container, and cap and flushing the catheter.
• If needed and requested, administer a secondary infusion or obtain blood samples.

Changing dressings

To reduce the risk of infection, always wear gloves and a mask when changing the dressing. Anyone within 10′ (3 m) of the patient should also wear a mask, including the patient. If he's unable to tolerate a facial mask, have him turn his head away from the catheter during the dressing change.

Getting equipped

Many facilities use a preassembled dressing-change tray that contains all the necessary equipment. If your facility doesn't use this type of tray, gather the following equipment:
• povidone-iodine swabs and ointment
• alcohol swabs
• sterile 2″ × 2″ gauze pads
• 1″ adhesive tape or transparent, semipermeable dressing
• sterile drape
• sterile gloves and masks
• clean gloves
• bag to dispose of old dressing.
   CV dressings are usually changed every 48 hours, but new brands of dressing can remain in place for as long as 7 days, depending on the type of dressing and the facility's policy and procedures. (See *Changing a CV dressing,* page 128.)

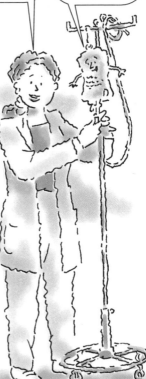

Change the dressing every 48 to 72 hours...

...or whenever it becomes moist, loose, or soiled.

Changing solutions and tubing

Change the I.V. solution and tubing every 24 hours or as directed by your facility's policy, maintaining strict aseptic technique. You don't need to wear a mask while performing this procedure, unless there is a contamination risk; for example, if you have an upper respiratory tract infection.

> If possible, change the solution and tubing at the same time.

Patient participation

To prevent air embolism, have the patient perform Valsalva's maneuver and clamp the port each time the catheter hub is open to air. Many facilities eliminate the need for this by using a connecting tubing with a slide clamp between the catheter hub and the I.V. tubing, which allows the I.V. tubing to be clamped during changes.

Two at once

If possible, change the solution and tubing at the same time. You may not be able to do this if, for example, the tubing is damaged or the solution runs out before it's time to change the tubing.

Switching solutions

To change the solution, follow these steps:
• Gather a solution container and an alcohol swab.
• Wash your hands.
• Put on gloves.
• Remove the cap and seal from the solution container.
• Clamp the CV line.
• Remove the spike quickly from the solution container, and reinsert it into the new container.
• Hang the new bottle and adjust the flow rate.

Turning over the tubing

To change the tubing, gather an I.V. administration set, a sterile 2″ × 2″ gauze pad, an extension set, an alcohol wipe, and gloves. For instructions on what to do next, see *Changing CV tubing,* page 129.)

Peak technique

Changing a CV dressing

After you assemble all needed equipment, follow the step-by-step technique below to safely change a central venous (CV) dressing.

Getting ready
• Wash your hands. Then, place the patient in a comfortable position.
• Prepare a sterile field. Open the bag, placing it away from the sterile field but still within reach.

Out with the old
• Put on clean gloves and remove the old dressing.
• Inspect the old dressing for signs of infection. You may want to culture any discharge at the site or on the old dressing. If not, discard the dressing and gloves in the bag. Be sure to report an infection to the doctor immediately and to document it in the nurses' notes.
• Check the position of the catheter and the insertion site for signs of infiltration or infection, such as redness, swelling, tenderness, or drainage.

In with the new
• Put on sterile gloves and clean the skin around the catheter with alcohol, wiping outward from the insertion site in a circular manner. Clean the site with alcohol three times.
• Clean the skin around the site with povidone-iodine, moving outward from the insertion site. Do this three times also. Don't use solutions containing acetone; they may cause some catheters to disintegrate. Also, make sure the alcohol is completely dry before cleaning with povidone-iodine; otherwise, the combination may form a tincture of iodine solution, which can cause skin irritation and breakdown.
• Re-dress the site with sterile 4″ × 4″ gauze pads, and tape the dressing in place. A transparent semipermeable dressing may also be used. If your facility's policy directs, apply povidone-iodine ointment to the insertion site; then cover the site with a sterile 2″ × 2″ gauze pad, followed by a sterile 4″ × 4″ gauze pad. Tape all edges completely.
• If the catheter is taped (not sutured) to the skin, carefully replace the soiled tape with sterile tape, using the chevron method. To do so, first cut a strip of tape about ½″ (1.27 cm) wide and slide it under the catheter, sticky side up. Then crisscross the tape over the top of the catheter. Finally, place a second strip of tape over the first strip. Be sure the catheter is secure.

Write it down
• Label the dressing with the date, time, and your initials.
• Discard all used items properly; reposition the patient comfortably.

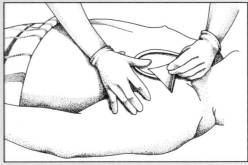

Remove the old dressing.

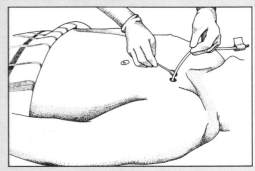

Clean the insertion site.

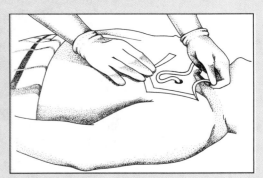

Re-dress the site.

Flushing the catheter

Flush the CV catheter routinely, according to your facility's policy, to maintain patency. The Intravenous Nurses Society recommends flushing with a heparin solution (100 units/ml). When the system is maintained as an intermittent infusion device, the flushing procedure varies depending on the following:

- facility policy
- medication administration schedule
- type of catheter used.

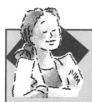

Peak technique

Changing CV tubing

After assembling the needed equipment, follow these guidelines to safely and quickly change central venous (CV) tubing:

- Wash your hands.

- Place a 2″ × 2″ sterile gauze pad under the needle or catheter hub to create a sterile field.

- Reduce the I.V. flow rate and remove the old spike from the bag. Loosely spread the cover from the new spike over the old spike.

- Keep the old spike in an upright position above the patient's heart, and insert the new spike into the I.V. container. Prime the system.

- Instruct the patient to perform Valsalva's maneuver. Quickly disconnect the old tubing from the needle or catheter hub, being careful not to dislodge the venipuncture device. If it's difficult to disconnect, use a hemostat to hold the hub securely while the end of the tubing is twisted and removed. Don't clamp the hemostat shut because the tubing adapter, needle, or catheter hub may crack, requiring a change of equipment and I.V. site.

- Quickly attach the new primed tubing to the venipuncture device, using aseptic technique.

- Adjust the flow to the prescribed rate.

- Label the new tubing with the date and time of change.

Two things at once

To change the tubing and solution simultaneously, follow these steps:

- Wash your hands.

- Hang the new I.V. bag and primed tubing on the I.V. pole.

- Stop the flow in the old tubing.

- Quickly disconnect the old tubing and connect the new tubing, as described above.

When

Generally, a CV catheter with a two-way valve (Groshong catheter) is flushed with saline solution once a day when not in use. All lumens of a multilumen catheter (unless it's a Groshong catheter) must be flushed regularly with a heparin saline solution, depending on your facility's policy and practice. (No flushing is needed with a continuous infusion through a single-lumen catheter.)

How

Most facilities use a heparinized saline flush solution, available in premixed, 10-ml multidose vials. Recommended concentration strengths vary from 10 units of heparin/ml to 1,000 units of heparin/ml. For CV line heparinization, always use 100 units/ml concentration unless contraindicated by the patient's condition. Remember that the heparin solution used to flush shouldn't affect the patient's clotting factors. Be extremely careful when selecting a heparin solution to make sure to choose the correct concentration.

Some facilities use saline solution instead of heparinized saline solution to flush catheters. Research shows that heparin isn't always necessary to keep the line open.

How often? How much?

Flushing recommendations vary from once every 8 hours to once per day. The recommended amount of flushing solution also varies. Most practitioners and facility policies recommend using 3 to 5 ml of solution to flush the catheter, although some policies call for as much as 10 ml of solution. Different catheters require different amounts of solution.

Most facilities' policies recommend using 3 to 5 ml of solution to flush the catheter...

...some call for as much as 10 ml of solution.

Six (count 'em) steps

To flush the catheter, follow these steps:

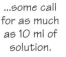 Clean the cap with an alcohol swab (using a 70% alcohol solution).

Allow the cap to dry.

 Inject the recommended or prescribed type and amount of flush solution.

After flushing, follow these steps to prevent blood backflow and possible clotting in the line:

 Maintain positive pressure by keeping your thumb on the plunger of the syringe.

 Engage the clamping mechanism in the central line.

  Withdraw the syringe.

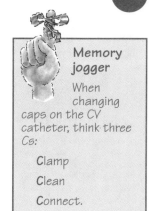

> **Memory jogger**
>
> When changing caps on the CV catheter, think three Cs:
>
> Clamp
>
> Clean
>
> Connect.

Changing caps

CV catheters used for infrequent infusions have intermittent injection caps similar to heparin lock adapters used for peripheral I.V. infusion therapy. The frequency of cap changes varies according to facility policy and the number of times that the cap is used.

A couple of warnings

Use strict aseptic technique when changing the cap; repeated puncturing of the injection port increases the risk of infection. Also, pieces of the rubber stopper may break off after repeated punctures, placing the patient at risk for embolism.

Clamp, clean, and connect

To change the cap, follow these steps:
• Close the clamping mechanism on the line.
• Clean the connection site with an alcohol or povidone-iodine swab.
• Instruct the patient to perform Valsalva's maneuver while you quickly disconnect the old cap and connect the new cap, using aseptic technique. If the patient can't perform Valsalva's maneuver, time the disconnect maneuver with the patient's respiratory cycle, and remove the cap during the expiratory phase. Make sure the new cap is purged of air and ready to be applied.

Infusing secondary fluids

To add other fluids to the patient's CV infusion, first make sure:

☝ solutions running in the same line are compatible

✌ connections are well secured with tape.

Piggyback ride

Secondary I.V. lines may be piggybacked into a side port or Y-port of a primary infusion line, instead of being connected directly to the catheter lumen. However, if there is no primary infusion prescribed, the medication may be infused through the CV line.

Drawing blood

You may use the CV catheter to obtain ordered blood samples, especially if the patient has poor peripheral veins. (See *Drawing blood from a CV catheter.*)

Documentation

Record your assessment findings and interventions according to your facility's policy. Include the following information:
• the type, amount, and rate of infusion
• dressing changes, including the appearance and location of the catheter and the site
• how the patient tolerated the procedure
• tubing and solution changes
• cap changes
• flushing procedures, including any problems encountered, and the amount and type of solution used
• blood samples collected, including the type and amount.

Special care

Besides performing routine care measures during CV infusions, be prepared to:
• handle common problems that may arise during infusion such as replacing a fractured, dislodged, or disconnected catheter
• prevent problems, such as catheter tears and kinks, fluid leaks, and clot formation at the catheter's tip

• tailor your interventions to meet the special infusion requirements of pediatric, elderly, and home therapy patients
• manage potential traumatic complications, such as a

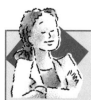

Peak technique

Drawing blood from a CV catheter

After assembling your equipment, use these step-by-step instructions to safely draw blood from a central venous (CV) catheter.

Collecting with an evacuated tube
To draw blood using an evacuated tube, follow the steps listed below.

Get ready
• Wash your hands and put on sterile gloves.
• Stop the I.V. infusion and place an injection cap on the lumen of the catheter.
• If multiple infusions are running, stop them and wait 1 minute before drawing blood from the catheter. This allows I.V. fluids and medications to be carried away from the catheter, preventing them from becoming mixed with the blood sample you'll be drawing.
• Clean the end of the injection cap with antiseptic swabs (povidone-iodine and alcohol).

Draw the blood
• Place a 5-ml lavender-top evacuated tube into its plastic sleeve. Use this tube to collect and discard the filling volume of the catheter, plus an extra 2 to 3 ml. Most studies indicate that about 5 ml is enough blood to discard. (At some health care facilities, the first 5 ml of blood isn't discarded if the patient is scheduled for multiple blood studies. Instead, the blood is infused back into the patient after the sample is drawn.)
• Insert the needle into the injection cap of the catheter. The first milliliter may be clear until the blood flows through the catheter.
• When blood stops flowing into the tube, remove and discard the tube, if appropriate.
• Use the appropriate evacuated tubes for the ordered blood tests. After you've drawn the necessary blood, flush the catheter with saline solution and resume the infusion. If you're not going to use the lumen immediately, heparinize the catheter.

• If you can't get blood flowing from the catheter, the tip of the catheter could be against the vessel wall. To correct this, ask the patient to raise his arms over his head, turn on his side, cough, or perform Valsalva's maneuver. You can also try flushing the catheter with saline solution before making another attempt to draw blood.

Collecting with a syringe
If evacuated tubes for collecting blood aren't available, obtain the blood sample with a syringe. To do so, collect syringes, evacuated tubes for the sample, gloves, and saline or heparin flush solution. Then follow the steps listed below.

Get ready
• First stop all infusions.
• Select the port from which to withdraw the blood; it should be at least 20G and preferably 16G or 18G.
• Put on gloves.
• Using aseptic technique, disconnect the tubing or heparin lock cap. (If the catheter has a clamp, use it before disconnecting; if the catheter doesn't have a clamp, have the patient perform Valsalva's maneuver.)

Draw the blood
• Insert the syringe and draw back 5 ml of blood.
• Discard the syringe.
• Connect a second syringe and draw the amount of blood you need.
• Flush the catheter with the recommended amount of saline solution or heparin. (The amount depends on the type of catheter and the frequency and type of infusions. Check the manufacturer's recommendations and your facility's policy.)
• Place the blood in the evacuated tubes.
• Label the evacuated tubes and send them to the laboratory.

pneumothorax, and systemic complications such as sepsis. (See *Managing common problems in CV therapy.*)

Repairing or replacing a catheter

A serrated hemostat will eventually break down silicone rubber and tear the catheter, causing blood to back up and fluid to leak from the device. If air enters the catheter through the tear, an air embolism could result. Prevent catheter tears by using nonserrated clamps. If the catheter or part of the catheter breaks, cracks, or becomes nonfunctional, the doctor usually replaces the entire CV line with a new one.

Twisted

The catheter can become kinked or pinched either above or beneath the skin. Kinks beneath the skin are detected by X-ray and can sometimes be corrected by simply repositioning the patient. If repositioning the patient doesn't resolve the situation, the catheter may need to be unsutured and repositioned or replaced.

Thinking of unkinking?

Never attempt to straighten kinks in stiff catheters, such as those made from polyvinyl chloride. These catheters fracture easily. Fractured particles may enter the circulation and act as an embolus. The doctor may try to unkink a long-term catheter; this is possible because it's made of pliable silicone rubber. The unkinking is done under guided fluoroscopy using aseptic technique.

An ounce of prevention

You may be able to prevent catheter kinks by taping and positioning the catheter properly. For example, looping the extension tubing once and securing it with tape adjacent to the dressing prevents the catheter from being pulled if the tubing gets entangled. This also helps prevent the catheter from moving or telescoping at the insertion site, a major cause of catheter-related infections and site irritations.

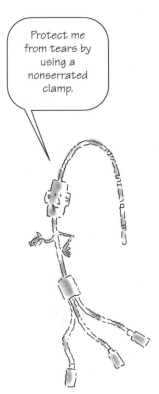

Protect me from tears by using a nonserrated clamp.

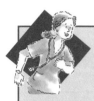

Running smoothly

Managing common problems in CV therapy

Maintaining central venous (CV) therapy requires being prepared to handle potential problems. The following chart tells you how to recognize and manage some common problems.

Problem	Possible causes	Nursing interventions
Fluid won't infuse	• Closed clamp • Displaced or kinked catheter • Thrombus	• Check the infusion system and clamps. • Change the patient's position. • Have the patient cough, breathe deeply, or perform Valsalva's maneuver. • Remove dressing and examine external portion of catheter. • If a kink isn't apparent, obtain an X-ray order. • Try to withdraw blood. • Try a gentle flush with saline solution. (Doctor may order a thrombolytic flush.)
Unable to draw blood	• Closed clamp • Displaced or kinked catheter • Thrombus • Catheter movement against vessel wall with negative pressure	• Check the infusion system and clamps. • Change the patient's position. • Have the patient cough, breathe deeply, or perform Valsalva's maneuver. • Remove dressing and examine external portion of catheter. • Obtain an X-ray order.
Fluid leaking at the site	• Displaced catheter • Lymph fluid leaking from tract • Tear in catheter	• Check patient for signs of distress. • Change dressing and observe site for redness. • Notify the doctor. • Obtain an X-ray order. • Prepare for a catheter change, if necessary. • If tear occurred in a Hickman, Groshong, or Broviac catheter, obtain a repair kit.
Disconnected catheter	• Patient moved • Not securely connected to tubing	• Apply catheter clamp, if available. • Place sterile syringe or catheter plug in the catheter hub. • Change the I.V. extension set. Don't reconnect the contaminated tubing. • Clean the catheter hub with alcohol or povidone-iodine. Don't soak the hub. • Connect clean I.V. tubing or a heparin lock plug to the site. • Restart the infusion.

Managing clot formation

If you have difficulty withdrawing blood or infusing fluid, there may be a clot at the tip of the catheter. Two points about such a clot:

- It impedes the flow of blood.
- It provides a protein-rich environment for bacterial growth.

Salvaging a catheter

Occasionally, the clot forms so that fluids infuse easily while blood aspiration is difficult or impossible. The fibrin clot may be dissolved by instilling urokinase, a thrombolytic agent. The agent may be instilled by a doctor or registered nurse trained in this procedure.

This procedure is usually recommended for long-term CV catheters because they're difficult to replace and costly. However, this attempt to salvage a device is not always appropriate or possible.

A clot at the catheter tip provides a protein-rich environment for bacterial growth.

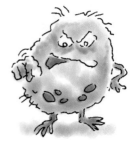

Patients with special needs

There are a few additional considerations involved in caring for pediatric, elderly, and home therapy patients.

Pediatric and elderly patients

Essentially the same catheters are used in both pediatric and elderly patients, with four possible differences:

 catheter length

 lumen size

 insertion sites

 amount of fluid infused.

In infants, for example, the jugular vein is the preferred insertion site, even though it's much more difficult to maintain than other sites. Usually, the doctor and the patient's family select a mutually acceptable site if the catheter will be used for long-term therapy.

Home therapy patients

Long-term CV catheters allow patients to receive fluids, medications, and blood infusions at home. These catheters have a much longer life because they're less thrombogenic and less prone to infection than short-term devices.

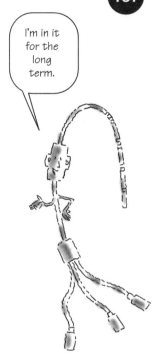

I'm in it for the long term.

A candidate for home care?

The care procedures used in the home are the same as those used in the hospital, including the use of aseptic technique. A candidate for home CV therapy must have the following:
• family member or friend who can assist in safe and competent administration of I.V. fluids
• backup helper
• suitable home environment
• telephone
• transportation
• adequate reading skills
• ability to prepare, handle, store, and dispose of the equipment.

Before discharge, after discharge

To ensure your patient's safety, patient teaching begins well before the patient is discharged. After discharge, a home-therapy coordinator provides follow-up care. This helps ensure compliance until the patient or caregiver can independently provide catheter care and infusion therapy at home. Many home therapy patients learn to care for the catheter themselves and to infuse their own medications and solutions.

Many home therapy patients learn to perform catheter care and to infuse their own medications and solutions.

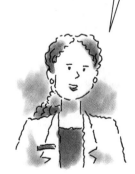

Complications of central venous therapy

Complications can occur at any time during CV therapy.

Traumatic complications

Traumatic complications, such as pneumothorax, typically occur on insertion but may not be noticed until after the procedure is completed. (See *Risks of CV therapy,* pages 138 to 140.)

Pneumothorax

The most common traumatic complication, pneumothorax is associated with insertions of a CV catheter into the subclavian or internal jugular veins. It's usually discovered on the chest X-ray that confirms catheter placement if the patient doesn't have symptoms immediately.

(Text continues on page 140.)

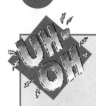

Risks of CV therapy

As with any invasive procedure, central venous (CV) therapy poses risks, including pneumothorax, air embolism, thrombosis, and infection. The following chart outlines how to recognize, manage, and prevent these complications.

Pneumothorax, hemothorax, chylothorax, or hydrothorax

Signs and symptoms	*Possible causes*	*Nursing interventions*	*Prevention*
• Chest pain • Dyspnea • Cyanosis • Decreased breath sounds on affected side • With hemothorax, decreased hemoglobin because of blood pooling • Abnormal chest X-ray	• Lung puncture by catheter during insertion or exchange over a guide wire • Large blood vessel puncture with bleeding inside or outside of lung • Lymph node puncture with leakage of lymph fluid • Infusion of solution into chest area through infiltrated catheter	• Notify doctor. • Remove catheter or assist with removal. • Administer oxygen as ordered. • Set up and assist with chest tube insertion. • Document interventions.	• Position patient's head down with a towel roll between the scapulae to dilate and expose the internal jugular or subclavian vein as much as possible during catheter insertion. • Assess for early signs of fluid infiltration, such as swelling in shoulder, neck, chest, and arm area. • Ensure immobilization of patient with adequate preparation for procedure and restraint during procedure; active patients may need to be sedated or taken to the operating room for CV catheter insertion. • Minimize patient activity after insertion, especially if peripheral CV catheter is used.

Air embolism

Signs and symptoms	*Possible causes*	*Nursing interventions*	*Prevention*
• Respiratory distress • Unequal breath sounds • Weak pulse • Increased central venous pressure (CVP) • Decreased blood pressure • Churning murmur over precordium • Change in or loss of consciousness	• Intake of air into CV system during catheter insertion or tubing changes; inadvertent opening, cutting, or breaking of catheter	• Clamp catheter immediately. • Turn patient on his left side, head down, so air can enter right atrium and be dispersed via pulmonary artery. Maintain position for 20 to 30 minutes. • Don't have the patient perform Valsalva's maneuver. (A large intake of air would worsen the situation.) • Administer oxygen. • Notify doctor. • Document interventions.	• Purge all air from tubing before hookup. • Teach patient to perform Valsalva's maneuver during catheter insertion and tubing changes (bear down or strain and hold breath to increase CVP). • Use air-eliminating filters proximal to patient. • Use infusion-control device with air detection capability. • Use luer-lock tubing, tape connections, or use locking devices for all connections.

Risks of CV therapy *(continued)*

Thrombosis

Signs and symptoms	Possible causes	Nursing interventions	Prevention
• Edema at puncture site • Erythema • Ipsilateral swelling of arm, neck, and face • Pain along vein • Fever, malaise • Tachycardia	• Sluggish flow rate • Composition of catheter material (some materials such as polyvinyl chloride are more thrombogenic) • Hematopoietic status of patient • Preexisting limb edema • Infusion of irritating solutions • Repeated use of same vein or long-term use • Preexisting cardiovascular disease	• Notify doctor. • Possibly, remove catheter. • Possibly, infuse anticoagulant doses of heparin. • Verify thrombosis with diagnostic studies. • Apply warm wet compresses locally. • Don't use limb on affected side for subsequent venipuncture. • Document interventions.	• Maintain flow through catheter at steady rate with infusion pump, or flush at regular intervals. • Use catheters made of less thrombogenic materials or catheters coated to prevent thrombosis. • Dilute irritating solutions. • Use 0.22-micron filter for infusions.

Local infection

Signs and symptoms	Possible causes	Nursing interventions	Prevention
• Redness, warmth, tenderness, and swelling at insertion or exit site • Possible exudate of purulent material • Local rash or pustules • Fever, chills, malaise	• Failure to maintain aseptic technique during catheter insertion or care • Failure to comply with dressing change protocol • Wet or soiled dressing remaining on site • Immunosuppression • Irritated suture line	• Monitor temperature frequently. • Culture site. • Re-dress aseptically. • Possibly, use antibiotic ointment locally. • Treat systemically with antibiotics or antifungals, depending on culture results and doctor's order. • Catheter may be removed. • Document interventions.	• Maintain strict aseptic technique. Use gloves, masks, and gowns when appropriate. • Adhere to dressing change protocols. • Teach patient about restrictions on swimming, bathing, and so on. (Patients with adequate white blood cell counts can do these activities if doctor allows.) • Change wet or soiled dressing immediately. • Change dressing more frequently if catheter is located in femoral area or near tracheostomy. • Complete tracheostomy care after catheter care.

(continued)

Risks of CV therapy *(continued)*

Systemic infection

Signs and symptoms	Possible causes	Nursing interventions	Prevention
• Fever, chills without other apparent reason • Leukocytosis • Nausea, vomiting • Malaise • Elevated urine glucose level	• Contaminated catheter or infusate • Failure to maintain aseptic technique during solution hookup • Frequent opening of catheter or long-term use of single I.V. access • Immunosuppression	• Draw central and peripheral blood cultures; if same organism, catheter is primary source of sepsis and should be removed. • If cultures don't match but are positive, catheter may be removed or the infection may be treated through the catheter. • Treat patient with antibiotic regimen, as ordered. • Culture tip of catheter if removed. • Assess for other sources of infection. • Monitor vital signs closely. • Document interventions.	• Examine infusate for cloudiness and turbidity before infusing, and check fluid container for leaks. • Monitor urine glucose level in patients receiving total parenteral nutrition; if greater than 2+, suspect early sepsis. • Use strict sterile technique for hookup and disconnection of fluids. • Use 0.22-micron filter. • Catheter may be changed frequently to decrease chance of infection. • Keep the system closed as much as possible. • Teach patient aseptic technique.

A pneumothorax may be minimal and may not require intervention (unless the patient is on positive-pressure ventilation). A thoracotomy is performed and a chest tube inserted if the pneumothorax is large enough to cause signs and symptoms, such as:
- chest pain
- dyspnea
- cyanosis
- decreased or absent breath sounds on the affected side.

Sneaky signs and symptoms

Initially, the patient may be asymptomatic; signs of distress gradually show up as the pneumothorax gets larger. For this reason, you need to monitor the patient closely and auscultate for breath sounds for at least 8 hours after catheter insertion.

If unchecked, pneumothorax may progress to tension pneumothorax, a medical emergency. The patient exhibits such signs as:
- acute respiratory distress
- asymmetrical chest wall movement
- possibly, a tracheal shift away from the affected side.

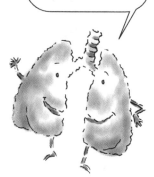

Yikes! Insertion of a catheter into subclavian or internal jugular veins may cause pneumothorax.

A chest tube must be inserted immediately before respiratory and cardiac decompensation occur.

Arterial puncture

The second most common life-threatening complication is arterial puncture. Arterial puncture may lead to hemothorax and internal bleeding, which may not be detected immediately. A hemothorax is treated like pneumothorax, except that the chest tube is inserted lower in the chest to help evacuate the blood.

Yikes! Internal bleeding

Left untreated, internal bleeding caused by arterial puncture leads to hypovolemic shock. Signs and symptoms include:
• increased heart rate
• decreased blood pressure
• cool, clammy skin
• obvious swelling in the neck or chest
• mental confusion (especially if the common carotid arteries are involved)
• formation of a hematoma (a large, blood-filled sac), which causes pressure on the trachea and adjacent vessels.

Rare but risky

There are a few additional, but rare, complications of CV therapy:
• Tracheal puncture is associated with insertion of a catheter into the subclavian vein.
• Development of a fistula between the innominate vein and the subclavian artery may result from perforation by the guide wire on insertion into the vessel.
• Chylothorax results when a lymph node is punctured and lymph fluid leaks into the pleural cavity.
• Hydrothorax (or infusion of solution into the chest), thrombosis, and local infection are also potential complications of CV therapy.

Systemic complications

Systemic complications such as sepsis typically occur later in therapy.

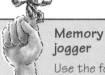

Memory jogger

Use the following mnemonic to remember the signs and symptoms of tension pneumothorax so that you can "ACT fast" to protect your patient.

Acute respiratory distress

Chest wall motion is asymmetrical

Tracheal shifting.

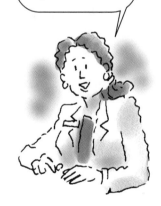

Left untreated, internal bleeding caused by arterial puncture leads to hypovolemic shock.

Sepsis

Catheter-related sepsis is the most serious systemic complication. It may lead to:
• septic shock
• multisystem organ failure
• death.

Most sepsis attributed to CV catheters is caused by skin surface organisms, such as *Staphylococcus epidermidis, S. aureus,* and *Candida albicans.*

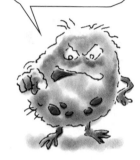

Most sepsis attributed to CV catheters is caused by skin surface organisms.

Observe closely

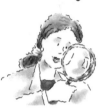

Strict aseptic technique and close observation are the best defense against sepsis. Regularly check the catheter insertion site for signs of localized infection, such as redness, drainage, or tenderness along the catheter path. If the patient shows signs of generalized infection such as unexplained fever, draw blood cultures from a peripheral site as well as from the device itself.

Out with the old, in with the new

If catheter-related sepsis is suspected, the catheter may be removed and a new one inserted in a different site. Culture the catheter tip after removal. Administer antibiotics, as ordered, and draw blood for repeat cultures after the antibiotic course is complete.

PICC-specific complications

PICC therapy causes fewer and less severe complications than other CV lines. Pneumothorax is extremely rare because the insertion site is peripheral. Catheter-related sepsis is usually related to site contamination.

Phlebitis — mechanical or bacterial

Mechanical phlebitis — painful inflammation of a vein — may be the most common PICC complication. It may occur during the first 72 hours after PICC insertion and is more common in left-sided insertions and when a large-gauge catheter is used.

If the patient develops mechanical phlebitis, apply warm moist compresses to his upper arm, elevate the extremity, and restrict activity to mild exercise. If the phlebitis continues or worsens, remove the catheter, as ordered.

Bacterial phlebitis can occur with PICCs; however, this usually occurs later in the infusion therapy. If drainage

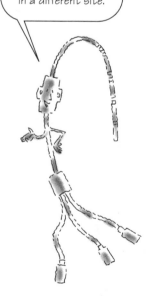

If sepsis is suspected, I may need to be replaced by a new catheter in a different site.

occurs at the insertion site and the patient's temperature increases, notify the doctor. The catheter may have to be removed.

Bleeding

Expect minimal bleeding from the PICC insertion site for the first 24 hours. Bleeding that persists needs additional evaluation. A pressure dressing should be left in place over the insertion site for at least 24 hours. After that, if there's no bleeding, the dressing can be changed and a new transparent dressing applied without a gauze pressure dressing.

Air embolism

Air embolism in PICC therapy is less common than in traditional CV lines, because the line is inserted below heart level.

Pain

Some patients complain of pain at the PICC insertion site, usually because the device is located in an area of frequent flexion. Pain may be treated two ways:

☝ applying warm compresses

✌ restricting activities until the patient becomes adjusted to the presence of the PICC.

Discontinuing central venous therapy

You or the doctor may remove the catheter, depending on your state's nurse practice act, your facility's policy, and the type of catheter. Long-term catheters and implanted devices are always removed by the doctor. But PICC lines may be removed by a qualified nurse.

Discontinue continuous, begin intermittent

You may receive an order to discontinue continuous infusion therapy and begin intermittent infusion therapy. If so, follow the same procedure used for peripheral I.V. therapy (see chapter 2, page 75).

Removing the catheter

Begin catheter removal with a couple of precautions:

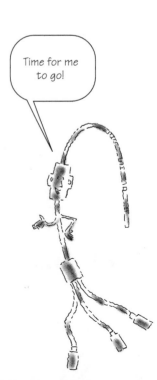

Time for me to go!

☝ First, check the patient's record for the most recent placement confirmed by an X-ray to trace the catheter's path as it exits the body.

✌ Then make sure that backup assistance is available if a complication such as uncontrolled bleeding occurs during catheter removal. This complication is common in patients with coagulopathies.

Patient preparation

Before you remove the catheter, explain the procedure to the patient. Tell him that he'll need to turn his face away from the site and perform Valsalva's maneuver when the catheter is withdrawn. If necessary, review the maneuver with him.

Getting equipped

Before removing the catheter, gather the following equipment:
• sterile gauze
• clean gloves
• sterile gloves
• forceps
• sterile scissors
• povidone-iodine solution
• alcohol swabs
• transparent, semipermeable dressing
• tape.
    If you're sending the tip of the catheter for culture, you also need a sterile specimen container and an extra pair of sterile scissors. (See *Removing a CV catheter.*)

Note this

After removing the catheter, be sure to document:
• patient tolerance
• condition of the catheter, including the length
• time of discontinuation of therapy
• cultures ordered and sent
• other pertinent information.

VAP implantation and infusion

Implanted under the skin, a VAP consists of a silicone catheter attached to a reservoir covered by a self-sealing

Peak technique

Removing a CV catheter

After assembling your equipment, follow the step-by-step guidelines listed below to safely remove a central venous (CV) catheter.

Getting ready
- Place the patient in a supine position to prevent emboli.
- Wash your hands and put on clean gloves.
- Turn off all infusions and prepare a sterile field.
- Remove the old dressing and change to sterile gloves.
- Prepare the site first with alcohol, then with povidone-iodine solution. Inspect the site for signs of drainage or inflammation.

Removing the catheter
- Clip the sutures and remove the catheter in a slow, even motion. Have the patient perform Valsalva's maneuver as the catheter is withdrawn to prevent air emboli.
- Apply povidone-iodine ointment to the insertion site to seal it.
- Inspect the catheter to see if any portions broke off during the removal. If so, notify the doctor immediately and monitor the patient closely for signs of distress. If a culture is to be obtained, clip approximately 1″ (2.5 cm) off the distal end of the catheter, letting it drop into the sterile specimen container.
- Place a transparent semipermeable dressing over the site. Label the dressing with the date and time of the removal and your initials.
- Properly dispose of the I.V. tubing and equipment you used.

Monitoring the patient
Insidious bleeding may develop after removing the catheter. Remember that some vessels such as the subclavian vein aren't easily compressed. By 72 hours, the site should be sealed and the risk of air emboli should be past; however, you may still need to apply a dry dressing to the site.

Make a notation on the nursing care plan to recheck the patient and insertion site frequently for the next few hours. Check for signs of respiratory decompensation, possibly indicating air emboli, and for signs of bleeding, such as blood on the dressing, decreased blood pressure, increased heart rate, paleness, or diaphoresis.

Noteworthy
Document the time and date of the catheter removal and any complications that occurred, such as catheter shearing, bleeding, or respiratory distress. Also be sure to record signs of blood, drainage, redness, or swelling of the site.

---

silicone rubber septum. Implanting a VAP requires surgery. The device may be placed in the arm, chest, abdomen, flank of the chest, or thigh.

Through the VAP

Usually, you'll use a VAP to deliver intermittent infusions. For example, you may use one to deliver:
- chemotherapy
- I.V. fluids
- pain control
- medications
- blood products.

VAPs may also be used to deliver TPN. When administering TPN, you'll need to closely monitor the access site

Do you know what a VAP is?

Sure do. It's a silicone catheter attached to a reservoir covered by a self-sealing silicone rubber septum.

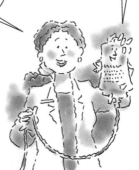

to assess skin integrity. VAPs may be used for long-term antibiotic therapy or to obtain blood samples.

Punctilious about punctures

To reduce the number of punctures to a VAP, an intermittent infusion device or lock may be used.

Proceed with caution

VAPs should be used cautiously in patients with a high risk of developing an allergic reaction or infection.

Selecting the equipment

The VAP selected for a patient depends on two things:

✌ the type of therapy needed

✌ how often the port needs to be accessed. (Typically, VAPs are used for intermittent infusions and only require access during the prescribed therapy.)

The selection of infusion equipment will depend partly on the type of VAP selected and the implantation site. Generally, you will use the same infusion equipment as in peripheral I.V. and CV therapy, including an infusion solution and an administration set with tubing.

VAP selection

Depending on the patient's size and the type of therapy, a VAP catheter with one or two large or small lumens may be chosen. For example, blood sampling or transfusion therapy requires a larger-size lumen than does I.V. fluid administration.

VAP variations

VAPs come in two basic types:

✌ top entry

✌ side entry.

In a top-entry VAP (such as the Med-I-Port, Port-A-Cath, Passport, and Infuse-A-Port), the needle is inserted perpendicular to the reservoir. In a side-entry VAP (such as the S.E.A. Port), the needle is inserted almost parallel to the reservoir. (See *Comparing top-entry and side-entry VAPs.*)

Material concerns

The VAP reservoir may be made of the following materials:
- titanium (Port-A-Cath)
- stainless steel (Q-Port)
- molded plastic (Infuse-A-Port).

The type of VAP reservoir used depends on the patient's therapeutic needs. For example, a patient undergoing magnetic resonance imaging should have a device made of titanium or plastic, instead of stainless steel, to avoid distorting test results.

Noncoring needles needed

To avoid damaging the port's silicone rubber septum, use only noncoring needles. A noncoring needle has an angled or deflected point that slices the septum on entry, rather than coring it as a conventional needle does. When the noncoring needle is removed, the septum reseals itself. (See *A close look at noncoring needles,* page 148.)

Comparing top-entry and side-entry VAPs

Vascular access ports (VAPs) come in two basic designs: top entry and side entry. In a top-entry port, the needle is inserted perpendicular to the reservoir. In a side-entry port, the needle is inserted into the septum nearly parallel to the reservoir. (A needle stop prevents the needle from coming out of the other side of the port.)

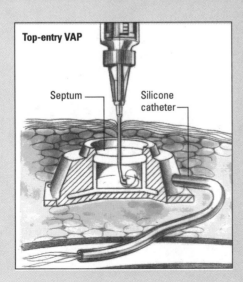

Top-entry VAP

Septum — Silicone catheter

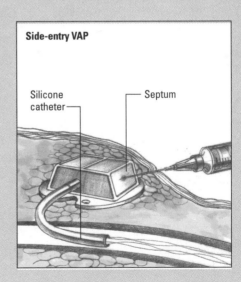

Side-entry VAP

Silicone catheter — Septum

Noncoring needles come with metal or plastic hubs in straight or right-angle configurations, with or without an extension set. Each configuration comes in various lengths (depending on the depth of septum implantation) and gauges (depending on the rate of infusion). (See *Choosing the right VAP needle.*)

Over the needle and to the port...

An over-the-needle catheter, such as the Surecath, allows continuous access to the port. This style of catheter is more comfortable for the patient and there's less risk of the device migrating out of the septum.

In an over-the-needle catheter, a solid-spike introducer and flexible catheter are passed through the silicone septum. Then the introducer is removed and the flexible Teflon catheter is positioned along the contour of the patient's chest wall. (See *Using an over-the-needle catheter.*)

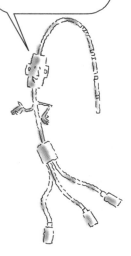

> Want continuous access to the port? Try an over-the-needle catheter.

A close look at noncoring needles

Unlike a conventional hypodermic needle, a noncoring needle has a deflected point, which slices the port's septum instead of coring it. Noncoring needles come in two types: straight and right angle.

Generally, expect to use a right-angle needle with a top-entry port and a straight needle with a side-entry port. When administering a bolus injection or continuous infusion, you'll also use an extension set.

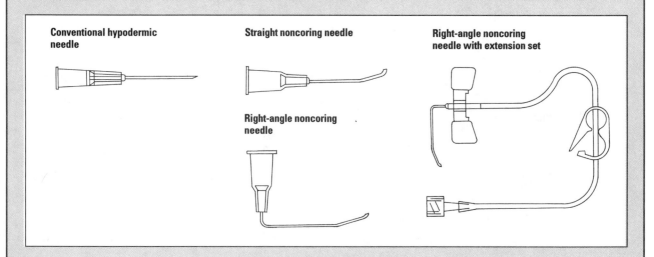

Conventional hypodermic needle

Straight noncoring needle

Right-angle noncoring needle

Right-angle noncoring needle with extension set

VAP implantation

A doctor surgically implants the VAP, usually using local anesthesia with conscious sedation. Occasionally, general anesthesia may be used.

It begins with an incision

Implanting the VAP involves the following steps:
• The doctor makes a small incision and introduces the catheter into the superior vena cava through either the subclavian, jugular, or cephalic vein. Fluoroscopy is used to verify placement of the catheter tip.

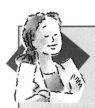

Peak technique

Using an over-the-needle catheter

An over-the-needle catheter, such as the Surecath device shown below, provides continuous access to an implanted port. The Surecath consists of a solid-spike introducer and a flexible catheter, which you pass through the portal septum and into the chamber. You then withdraw the introducer, leaving the catheter in place.

Inserting the device

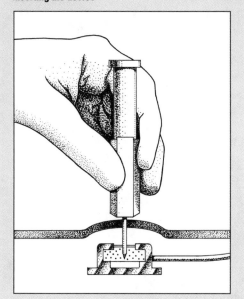

Catheter in place

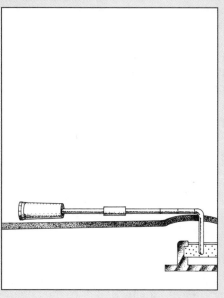

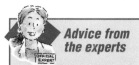

Advice from the experts

Choosing the right VAP needle

When choosing a vascular access port (VAP) needle, consider the following. Remember that you should use only noncoring needles with a VAP.

Experts recommend:
• a 19G needle for blood infusion or withdrawal
• a 20G needle for most infusions (other than blood infusion or withdrawal), including total parenteral nutrition
• a 22G needle for flushing.

Right angle vs. straight
Most often, a right-angle noncoring needle is used; rarely, a longer needle such as a straight 2" noncoring needle is used to access a deeply implanted port.

You can use either a straight needle or a right-angle needle to inject a bolus into a top-entry port. For continuous infusions, however, experts recommend using a right-angle needle because it's easily secured to the patient. Side-entry ports are designed for use with straight noncoring needles only.

• The doctor then creates a subcutaneous pocket over a bony prominence on the chest wall and tunnels the catheter to the pocket.
• Next, the doctor connects the catheter to the reservoir, places the reservoir in the pocket, and flushes it with heparinized saline solution.
• Finally, the doctor sutures the reservoir to the underlying fascia and closes the incision.

You may then apply a dressing to the wound site, according to your facility's policy and procedures. Once the implantation site is healed, use routine dressing practices when the VAP is in use.

Preparing the patient

Because VAP implantation is an operating room procedure, teaching should cover preoperative and postoperative considerations.

Pre-op pointers

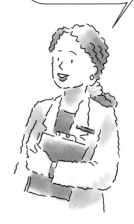

Make sure the patient understands what's expected of him after implantation.

Use the following pointers to guide your teaching before VAP implantation:
• Make sure the patient understands the procedure, its benefits, and what is expected of him after the implantation. Be prepared to supplement information provided by the doctor. You'll also need to allay the patient's fears and answer questions about movement restrictions, cosmetic concerns, and maintenance regimens. Clear explanations help ensure the patient's cooperation.
• Explain to the patient the purpose of a venogram, which may be ordered to determine the best vessel to use. The venogram is performed while the patient is under anesthesia and before postoperative swelling occurs, allowing immediate use of the device.
• Make sure you describe how the patient will be positioned during the procedure.

Obtaining consent

Most hospitals require a signed informed consent form before any invasive procedure. Tell the patient he'll be asked to sign a consent form and explain what this means.

Sign on the dotted line

The doctor obtains consent; occasionally, you may witness the patient's signature. Before the patient signs, make sure he understands the procedure. If not, delay signing until you or the doctor clarifies the procedure and the patient demonstrates understanding.

Rarely, a patient requires emergency VAP implantation. The consent form can be signed by the next of kin or legal guardian. In this case, your teaching may be deferred until after the device is in place.

Post-op pointers

Discuss the following postoperative care topics:
• Remind the patient that once the device is in place, he will have to keep scheduled appointments to have the port heparinized. Another option is to teach him or his family how to heparinize the port.
• Tell the patient to report signs and symptoms of systemic infection (fever, malaise, and flulike symptoms) and local infection (redness, tenderness, and drainage at the port or tunnel track site).
• The patient will need to receive prophylactic antibiotics before undergoing any dental or surgical procedures to prevent contamination and colonization of the VAP. Tell him to inform his dentist or doctor that he has an implanted device. Tell the patient to carry identification material pertaining to specific care protocols, serial number, and model of the VAP.
• Teach the patient to recognize and report signs and symptoms of infiltration, such as pain or swelling at the site, especially if he'll be receiving continuous infusions. Stress the need for immediate intervention to avoid damaging the tissue surrounding the port.

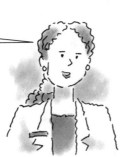

Remind the patient to keep appointments to have the port heparinized...

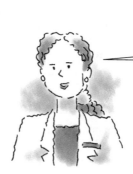

...and teach him the signs and symptoms of infection and infiltration.

Monitoring the patient

After the VAP is implanted, observe the patient for several hours. The device can be used immediately after placement. Some swelling and tenderness may persist for about 72 hours, making the device initially difficult to palpate and slightly uncomfortable for the patient.

The incision requires routine postoperative care for 7 to 10 days. Assess the implantation site for signs of the following:
- infection
- clotting
- redness
- device rotation
- skin irritation.

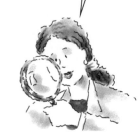

After the VAP is implanted, observe the patient for several hours.

Infusion by VAP

To administer an infusion using a VAP, the doctor first accesses the port with the appropriate needle in the operating room. When you're ready to initiate infusion therapy, you'll need to set up the equipment and prepare the site.

Preparing the equipment

To set up infusion equipment, follow these steps:
- Attach the tubing to the solution container.
- Prime the tubing with fluid.
- Fill two syringes, one with 5 ml of normal saline and the other with 5 ml of heparin solution (100 units/ml), if setting up an intermittent system.
- Prime the noncoring needle and extension set with the saline from the syringe. (Prime the tubing and purge it of air using strict aseptic technique.)
- After priming the tubing, recheck all the connections for tightness. Make sure that all open ends are covered with sealed caps.

Preparing the site

To prepare the insertion site, obtain an implantable port access kit, if your facility uses them. If a kit isn't available, gather the following equipment:
- sterile gloves
- three alcohol swabs
- three povidone-iodine swabs

- sterile 3″ × 3″ gauze pad
- sterile 1″ × 1″ gauze pad
- transparent dressing
- tape
- mask
- sterile drape.

Clear the field

When you're ready to prepare the access site, take the following precautions:
- Establish a sterile field for the sterile supplies, and inspect the area around the port for signs of infection or skin breakdown.
- An ice pack may be placed over the area for several minutes to numb the site.
- Apply a thick layer of the anesthetic cream over the injection port, and cover with a transparent dressing. Be sure to remove this cream completely before putting on sterile gloves and preparing the access site.

Preparing the access site

To prepare the access site, follow these steps:
- Wash your hands thoroughly and put on sterile gloves.
- Clean the area with an alcohol swab, starting at the center of the port and working outward with a firm circular motion over a 4″ to 5″ (10- to 12.5-cm) area. Repeat this procedure twice more, allowing the alcohol to dry thoroughly.
- Clean the area with a povidone-iodine swab in the same manner described above. Repeat this procedure twice. Most importantly, allow the povidone-iodine to dry.
- If facility policy calls for a local anesthetic, check the patient's record for possible allergies. As indicated, anesthetize the insertion site by injecting 0.1 ml of lidocaine (Xylocaine), without epinephrine, intradermally. Transdermal analgesia may also be used but must be applied approximately 1 hour before the access procedure.

If using transdermal analgesia, apply it about 1 hour before the access procedure.

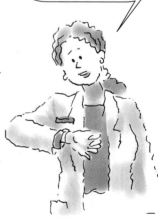

Accessing the site

When accessing a top-entry VAP, you'll usually use a right-angle noncoring needle and a 5-ml syringe filled with saline solution. Follow the instructions in *How to access a top-entry VAP,* page 154.

Side entrance

To gain access to a side-entry port, follow the same procedure used to access a top-entry port. However, insert the needle parallel to the reservoir instead of perpendicular to it.

Save time, decrease discomfort, prolong port life

While the patient is hospitalized, an intermittent infusion cap or lock may be attached to the end of the extension set. The cap contains a clamping mechanism to provide ready access for intermittent infusions.

Besides saving valuable nursing time, an accessed VAP reduces the discomfort of reaccessing the port. It also prolongs the life of the port septum by decreasing the number of needle punctures.

Giving a bolus injection

To give a bolus injection, you need:

Peak technique

How to access a top-entry VAP

After assembling your equipment , use the following step-by-step guidelines to safely and securely access a top-entry VAP:

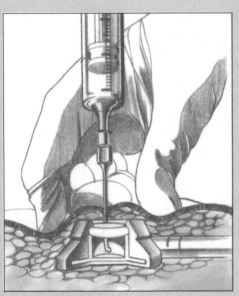

• Palpate the area over the port to locate the port septum.

• Anchor the port between your thumb and the first two fingers of your non-dominant hand. Then using your dominant hand, aim the needle at the center of the device.

• Insert the needle perpendicular to the port septum, as shown. Push the needle through the skin and septum until you reach the bottom of the reservoir.

• Check needle placement by aspirating for a blood return.

• If you're unable to obtain blood, remove the needle and repeat the procedure. Inability to obtain blood might indicate that the catheter is against the vessel wall. Ask the patient to raise his arms, perform Valsalva's maneuver, or change position to free the catheter. If you still can't obtain a blood return, notify the doctor: A fibrin sleeve on the distal end of the catheter may be blocking the opening.

• Flush the device with normal saline solution. If you detect swelling or if the patient reports pain at the site, remove the needle and notify the doctor.

• a 10-ml syringe filled with saline solution
• a syringe containing the prescribed medication
• a syringe filled with the appropriate heparin flush solution (optional). (See *How to administer a bolus injection by VAP.*)

Starting continuous infusion

To prepare for a continuous infusion with a VAP, gather the following equipment:
• prescribed I.V. solution or medication
• I.V. administration set with an air-eliminating filter, if ordered
• 10-ml syringe filled with saline solution
• antibacterial ointment (such as povidone-iodine ointment), as ordered
• adhesive tape
• sterile 2″ × 2″ gauze pad
• sterile tape or adhesive skin closures
• transparent semipermeable dressing.

Make sure the access needle is attached with an extension set that has a clamp, and you're ready to administer the infusion. (See *How to administer a continuous VAP infusion,* page 156.)

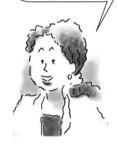

Get ready to start a continuous infusion via a VAP. First, gather the equipment you need.

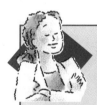

Peak technique

How to administer a bolus injection by VAP

Follow the step-by-step instructions below to safely and accurately give a bolus injection via a vascular access port (VAP).

Attach, check, clamp, connect
• Attach a 10-ml syringe filled with saline solution to the end of the extension set, and remove all the air. Then attach the extension set to a noncoring needle.
• Check for a blood return. Then flush the port with saline solution, according to your facility's policy. (Some facilities require flushing the port with heparin solution first.)
• Clamp the extension set and remove the saline syringe.
• Connect the medication syringe to the extension set. Open the clamp and inject the drug, as ordered.

Examine, clamp, flush
• Examine the skin surrounding the needle for signs of infiltration, such as swelling or tenderness. If you note these signs,

stop the injection and intervene appropriately.
• When the injection is complete, clamp the extension set and remove the medication syringe.
• Open the clamp and flush with 5 ml of saline solution after each drug injection to minimize drug incompatibility reactions.
• Flush with heparin solution, as your facility's policy directs.

Write it down
Document the injection according to your facility's policy. Include the following information: the type and amount of medication injected, the time of the injection, the appearance of the site, the patient's tolerance of the procedure, and any pertinent nursing interventions.

Maintaining VAP infusions

To maintain infusion therapy with a VAP, perform such care measures as:
- flushing the VAP with the appropriate heparin solution if the VAP is used intermittently
- assessing the site at established intervals

Peak technique

How to administer a continuous VAP infusion

Follow the step-by-step instructions below to administer a continuous vascular access port (VAP) infusion safely and accurately.

Assemble, remove, flush, connect, and begin
- Assemble the equipment.
- Remove all air from the extension set by priming it with an attached syringe of saline solution. Now attach the extension set to a noncoring needle.
- Flush the port system with saline solution. Clamp the extension set and remove the syringe.
- Connect the administration set, and secure the connections with tape, if necessary.
- Unclamp the extension set and begin the infusion.

Apply, place under, examine
- Apply a small amount of antibacterial ointment to the insertion site.
- Place a gauze pad under the needle hub if it doesn't lie flush with the skin.
- To help prevent needle dislodgment, secure the needle to the skin with sterile tape or adhesive skin closures, as shown below.

- Apply a transparent semipermeable dressing over the needle insertion site.
- Examine the site carefully for infiltration. If the patient complains of burning, stinging, or pain at the site, discontinue the infusion and intervene appropriately.

Obtain, clamp, attach
- When the solution container is empty, obtain a new I.V. solution container, as ordered, with primed I.V. tubing.
- Clamp the extension set and remove the old I.V. tubing.
- Attach the new I.V. tubing with the solution container to the extension set. Open the clamps, and adjust the infusion rate.

Write it down
Document the infusion according to your facility's policy, including the following information: the type, amount, rate, and time of infusion; the patient's tolerance of the procedure; the appearance of the site; and any pertinent nursing interventions.

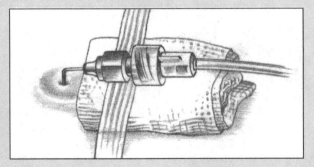
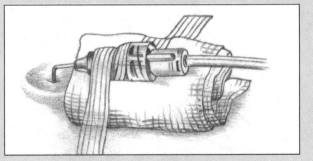

• changing the dressing per the facility's protocol or whenever the dressing's integrity is compromised.
• managing common equipment problems and patient complications
• discontinuing therapy when ordered, or converting the VAP to an intermittent system to keep the device patent until it's needed again.

Flushing a VAP

Follow these guidelines to determine when to flush a VAP:
• If your patient is receiving a continuous or prolonged infusion, flush the port after infusions and change the dressing and needle or needleless device every 5 to 7 days. Change the tubing and solution according to your facility's protocols.
• If your patient is receiving an intermittent infusion, flush the port periodically with saline and heparin solutions. Keep in mind that the Groshong-type VAP doesn't require heparinization.
• To help prevent clot formation in the device, flush the VAP with heparin solution after each saline flush. When the VAP isn't accessed, flush it once every 4 weeks.

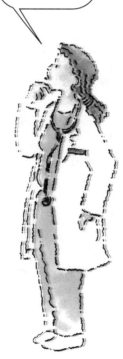

When you're ready to flush the VAP, follow these steps.

Getting equipped

To flush the VAP, first gather the following equipment:
• 22G noncoring needle with an extension set
• 10-ml syringe filled with 5 ml of sterile normal saline
• 10-ml syringe filled with 5 ml of heparin flush solution (100 units/ml)

Ready, set, flush

Prepare the injection site, as described above. Then follow these steps:
• Attach the 10-ml syringe with 5 ml of normal saline solution to the extension set and noncoring needle, applying gentle pressure to the plunger to expel all air from the set.
• Palpate the area over the port to locate it, and then access the port.
• Aspirate a blood return and flush the VAP with normal saline to confirm patency. Then flush with the heparin solution.
• While stabilizing the VAP with two fingers, withdraw the noncoring needle.

Obtaining blood samples

You can obtain blood samples from an implanted VAP in two ways:

 with a syringe

with an evacuated tube. (See *How to obtain a blood sample from a VAP.*)

Clearing the VAP

If clotting threatens to block the VAP, making flushing and infusions sluggish, the doctor may order a fibrinolytic agent such as urokinase to clear the port and catheter.

To clear the VAP, gather the following equipment:
• 20G or 22G noncoring needle with an extension set
• 1-ml syringe filled with urokinase (5,000 I.U. in 1 ml sterile water is the usual dosage for clotted catheters)
• empty 10-ml syringe
• 5-ml syringe and 10-ml syringe, both filled with saline solution
• sterile syringe filled with heparin flush solution.

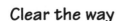
Clear the way

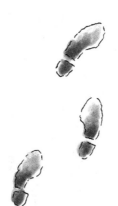

Follow these steps to clear the port and catheter:
• Palpate the area over the port and access the VAP as described.
• Check for blood return.
• Flush the VAP with 5 ml of saline solution, and clamp the extension tubing.
• Attach the 1-ml syringe, and unclamp the extension tubing.
• Instill the urokinase solution using a gentle pull-push motion on the syringe plunger to mix the solution in the access equipment, VAP, and catheter.
• Clamp the extension set, and leave the solution in place for 15 minutes.
• Then attach an empty 10-ml syringe, unclamp the extension set, and aspirate the urokinase and clot with the 10-ml syringe. Discard this syringe. This will prevent the accidental injection of the urokinase into the systemic circulation.
• If the clot can't be aspirated, wait 15 minutes and try again. You can safely instill urokinase solution as many as three times in a 4-hour period if the patient's platelet count

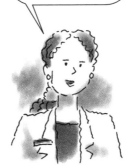

If clotting threatens to block the VAP, a fibrinolytic agent may be used to clear the port and catheter.

Peak technique

How to obtain a blood sample from a VAP

After assembling your equipment, follow the step-by-step guidelines below to safely obtain a blood sample from a vascular access port (VAP).

Syringe technique

To obtain a blood sample with a syringe, first gather the following equipment: a 19G or 20G noncoring needle with an extension set, a 10-ml syringe filled with 5 ml of saline solution, a 20-ml sterile syringe, a 20-ml sterile syringe filled with saline solution, blood sample tubes, and a sterile syringe filled with heparin flush solution.

Prepare the site, then follow these steps:
• Attach the 10-ml syringe with 5 ml of saline solution to the noncoring needle and extension set. Remove all air from the set.
• Palpate the area over the port to locate it. Then access the port.
• Flush the VAP with 5 ml of saline solution.
• Withdraw at least 5 ml of blood; then clamp the extension set and discard the syringe.
• Connect a 20-ml sterile syringe to the extension set; unclamp the set.
• Aspirate the desired amount of blood into the 20-ml syringe.
• After obtaining the sample, clamp the extension set, remove the syringe, and attach a 20-ml syringe filled with saline solution. Unclamp the extension set.
• Immediately flush the VAP with 20 ml of saline solution. (Solution concentrations and amounts may vary according to facility policy.)
• Clamp the extension set, remove the saline syringe, and attach a sterile heparin-filled syringe. Perform the heparin flush procedure.
• Transfer the blood into appropriate blood sample tubes.

Evacuated tube technique

To obtain a blood sample using an evacuated tube, first gather the following equipment: a 19G or 20G noncoring needle with an extension set, a luer-lock injection cap, a 10-ml syringe of saline solution, alcohol or povidone-iodine swabs, an evacuated tube needle and holder (disposable tubes come with the needle or needleless device already attached), blood sample tubes (label one "Discard"), a 20-ml sterile syringe filled with saline solution, and a sterile syringe filled with heparin flush solution. Prepare the site; then follow these steps:

• Apply the evacuated tube needle to the tube's holder.
• Attach the luer-lock injection cap to the noncoring needle extension set, using sterile technique. Remove all air from the set with the saline-filled syringe.
• Palpate the area over the port to locate it. Then access the port.
• Flush the VAP with 5 ml of saline solution to ensure correct noncoring needle placement. Remove the saline syringe.
• Wipe the injection cap with an alcohol or povidone-iodine swab.
• Insert the evacuated tube needle or needleless device into the injection cap.
• Insert the blood sample tube labeled "Discard" into the evacuated tube holder.
• Allow the tube to fill with blood; remove the tube and discard.
• Insert another tube and allow it to fill with blood. Repeat this procedure until you obtain the necessary amount of blood.
• Remove the evacuated tube needle or needleless device from the injection cap.
• Insert the 20-ml saline-filled syringe and immediately flush the VAP with 20 ml of saline solution; then remove the syringe.
• Next, attach the heparin-filled syringe and needle and perform the heparin flush procedure.
• After you've flushed the VAP with saline solution and heparin, clamp the extension set.

Obtaining blood samples during therapy

You may be ordered to obtain blood samples either before administering a bolus injection or during a continuous infusion. If you'll be administering a bolus injection, use the syringe method to obtain the blood sample, but don't flush with heparin solution.

If the patient is already receiving a continuous infusion, shut off the infusion and clamp the extension set. Then disconnect the extension set, maintaining aseptic technique. Follow the procedure for obtaining a blood sample with a syringe, up to and including the saline flush procedure. After the catheter is flushed with saline solution, clamp the extension set and remove the syringe. Reconnect the I.V. extension set. Then unclamp it and adjust the flow rate.

is greater than 20,000/µl. Repeat the procedure only once in a 4-hour period if the patient's platelet count is less than 20,000/µl.

• After the blockage is cleared, flush the catheter with at least 10 ml of saline solution, then flush with heparin solution, as described above.

Fibrinolytics aren't for everyone

Treatment with a fibrinolytic agent is contraindicated in patients with the following conditions:

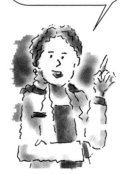

Careful! Fibrinolytic agents shouldn't be used in patients with these conditions.

• active bleeding
• intracranial neoplasms
• hypersensitivity to urokinase
• liver disease
• subacute bacterial endocarditis or visceral tumors
• stroke in the past 2 months. (See *Fibrinolytics may be forbidden*.)

Documenting VAP infusions

Record your assessment findings and interventions according to your facility's policy. Include the following information:
• type, amount, rate, and duration of the infusion
• appearance of the site
• development of problems and steps taken to resolve them
• needle gauge and length and dressing changes for continuous infusions
• blood samples obtained, including the type and amount
• patient-teaching topics covered and the patient's response to the procedure.

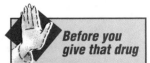

Before you give that drug

Fibrinolytics may be forbidden

Because fibrinolytic agents increase the risk of bleeding, urokinase may be contraindicated in patients who've had surgery within the past 10 days; who have active internal bleeding such as GI bleeding; or who've experienced central nervous system damage, such as infarction, hemorrhage, trauma, surgery, or primary or metastatic disease within the past 2 months.

Special precautions

Routine care measures are subject to a few glitches. Be prepared to handle common problems that may arise during an infusion with a VAP. Problems may include inability to:
• flush the VAP
• withdraw blood from the VAP
• palpate and access the VAP. (See *Managing common VAP problems.*)

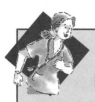

Running smoothly

Managing common VAP problems

To maintain a vascular access port (VAP), you must be able to handle common problems. This chart outlines problems you may encounter, their possible causes, and the appropriate nursing interventions.

Problem and possible causes	Nursing interventions
Inability to flush or withdraw blood	
• Kinked tubing or closed clamp	• Check tubing or clamp.
• Catheter lodged against vessel wall	• Reposition patient. • Teach patient to change position to free catheter from the vessel wall. • Raise the arm that is on the same side as catheter. • Roll patient to the opposite side. • Have patient cough, sit up, or take a deep breath. • Infuse 10 ml of saline solution into catheter. • Regain access to catheter or VAP, using a new sterile needle.
• Incorrect needle placement • Needle not advanced through septum	• Regain access to device. • Teach home care patient to push down firmly on noncoring needle device in septum and to verify needle position by aspirating for a blood return.
• Clot formation	• Assess patency by trying to flush VAP while the patient changes position. • Notify doctor; obtain order for urokinase instillation. • Teach patient to recognize clot formation, to notify the doctor if it occurs, and to avoid forcibly flushing VAP.
• Kinked catheter, catheter migration, port rotation	• Notify doctor immediately. • Tell patient to notify doctor if he has difficulty using VAP.
Inability to palpate VAP	
• Deeply implanted port	• Note portal chamber scar. • Use deep palpation technique. • Ask another nurse to try locating VAP. • Use a 1½" to 2" noncoring needle to gain access to VAP.

A big exception for small patients

Generally, the procedures for implanting and maintaining a VAP are the same for pediatric and elderly patients as for adult patients, with one big exception: For pediatric patients, general anesthesia is typically used during implantation.

Home VAP

A home care patient requires thorough teaching about procedures and follow-up visits from a home care nurse to ensure compliance, safety, and successful treatment.

If the patient is to access the port himself, explain that the most uncomfortable part of the procedure is inserting the needle into the skin. Once the needle has penetrated the skin, the patient will feel some pressure but little pain. Eventually, the skin over the port becomes desensitized from frequent needle punctures. Until then, the patient may want to use a topical anesthetic.

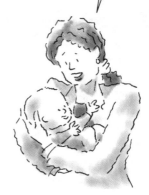

Usually, when a child undergoes VAP implantation, general anesthesia is used.

To the back of the port

Stress the importance of pushing the needle into the port until the needle bevel touches the back of the port. Many patients tend to stop short of the back of the port, leaving the needle bevel in the rubber septum. This can cause blockage or slow the infusion rate.

Recognizing risks

A patient with a VAP faces risks similar to those associated with a traditional CV catheter, such as infection and infiltration. Teach the patient or caregiver how to recognize signs and symptoms of these complications. Make sure they know how to intervene or how to reach the home health agency. (See *Complications of VAP therapy.*)

Instruct your patient to push the needle into the port until the needle bevel touches the back of the port.

Interrupting VAP therapy

When interrupting VAP therapy, remove the access needle from a VAP only after it has been flushed for maintenance. Although there is usually little or no bloody drainage when the access needle is removed, observe these precautions:
• Wear gloves.
• Dispose of the needle properly.
• Place a small dressing temporarily over the VAP site.

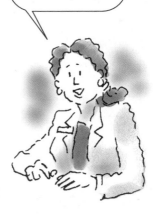

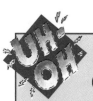

Warning!

Complications of VAP therapy

The following chart lists common complications of vascular access port (VAP) therapy as well as their signs and symptoms, causes, nursing interventions, and preventive measures.

Signs and symptoms	Possible causes	Nursing interventions	Prevention
Site infection or skin breakdown			
• Erythema and warmth at the port site • Oozing or purulent drainage at port site or VAP pocket • Fever	• Infected incision or VAP pocket • Poor postoperative healing	• Assess site daily for redness; note any drainage. • Notify doctor. • Administer antibiotics, as prescribed. • Apply warm soaks for 20 minutes four times a day.	• Teach patient to inspect for and report any redness, swelling, drainage, or skin breakdown at the port site.
Extravasation			
• Burning sensation or swelling in subcutaneous tissue	• Needle dislodged into subcutaneous tissue • Needle incorrectly placed in VAP • Needle position not confirmed; needle pulled out of septum	• Don't remove needle. • Stop infusion. • Notify doctor; prepare to administer antidote, if prescribed.	• Teach patient how to gain access to the device, verify placement of the device, and secure the needle before initiating the infusion.
Thrombosis			
• Inability to flush port or administer infusion	• Frequent blood sampling • Infusion of packed red blood cells (RBCs)	• Notify doctor; obtain order to administer urokinase.	• Flush VAP thoroughly right after obtaining blood sample. • Administer packed RBCs as a piggyback with saline solution and use an infusion pump; flush with saline solution between units.
Fibrin sheath formation			
• Blocked port and catheter lumen • Inability to flush port or administer infusion	• Adherence of platelets to catheter	• Notify doctor; prepare to administer urokinase.	• Use port only to infuse fluids and medications; don't use to obtain blood samples. • Administer only compatible substances through port.

Discontinuing a VAP

To prepare to discontinue therapy, first gather the following equipment:
• 10-ml syringe filled with 5 ml of normal saline solution
• 20G needle or needleless device
• 10-ml syringe filled with 5 ml of sterile heparin flush solution (100 units/ml)
• sterile gloves
• sterile 2″ × 2″ gauze pad and tape.
   Then, follow these steps:
• After shutting off the infusion, clamp the extension set and remove the I.V. tubing.
• Attach the syringe filled with saline solution using aseptic technique.
• Unclamp the extension set, flush the device with the saline solution, and remove the saline syringe.
• Attach the heparin syringe, flush the VAP with the heparin solution, and clamp the extension set.

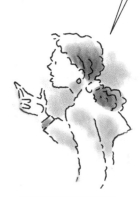

After flushing the port with heparin solution, remove the noncoring needle by following these steps.

Removing the noncoring needle

After flushing the port with heparin solution, remove the noncoring needle by following these steps:
• First, put on gloves.
• Place the gloved index and middle fingers from the nondominant hand on either side of the port septum.
• Stabilize the port by pressing down with these two fingers, maintaining pressure until the needle is removed.
• Using your gloved (dominant) hand, grasp the noncoring needle and pull it straight out of the port.
• Apply a dressing as indicated.
• If no more infusions are scheduled, remind the patient that he'll need a heparin flush in 4 weeks.

Almost done. I just need to document a few things.

Don't forget to document

After removing the noncoring needle, document the following:
• removal of the infusion needle
• status of the site
• use of the heparin flush
• patient's tolerance of the procedure
• your teaching efforts
• problems you encountered and resolved.

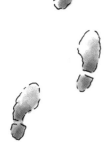
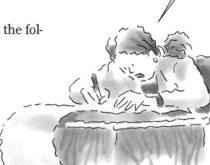

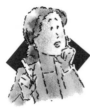

Quick quiz

1. CV therapy is indicated in all of the following instances except:
    A. infusion of a large volume of fluid.
    B. short-term venous access.
    C. an emergency.
Answer: B. CV therapy isn't indicated in short-term venous access.

2. The advantages of CV therapy include:
    A. ability to rapidly infuse fluids, draw blood specimens, and measure central venous pressure.
    B. minimal or no complications on insertion.
    C. increased patient mobility.
Answer: A. There are several potentially life-threatening complications from inserting a CV line, including pneumothorax, sepsis, and vessel and organ perforation. It also decreases patient mobility.

3. The veins commonly used as CV insertion sites include:
    A. femoral.
    B. brachial.
    C. subclavian.
Answer: C. The subclavian veins are commonly used as CV insertion sites, as are the internal and external jugular and the cephalic. Although femoral and brachial veins may be used, this is rare.

4. Nursing responsibilities when preparing a patient for CV therapy include all of the following except:
    A. explaining the procedure and care measures of the therapy.
    B. selecting the equipment.
    C. obtaining consent.
Answer: C. The doctor is responsible for obtaining consent, but the nurse may be responsible for witnessing the patient's signature.

5. The catheter more appropriate for pediatric patients would be a:
    A. Broviac tunneled CV catheter.
    B. Hickman-Broviac tunneled CV catheter.
    C. PICC.

Answer: A. The Broviac tunneled CV catheter is more appropriate for use in individuals with small central veins, such as pediatric patients.

6. When drawing a specimen, the amount of blood discarded from a VAP is:
   A. 1 ml
   B. 3 ml
   C. 5 ml
Answer: C. You should discard 5 ml of blood before drawing the specimen.

Scoring

☆☆☆   If you answered six questions correctly, right on! You took a central route to understanding this chapter.

☆☆   If you answered three to five questions correctly, good job. You followed the text right to the heart of the matter.

☆   If you answered fewer than three questions correctly, don't fret. Instead, center yourself and reaccess the material.

I.V. medications

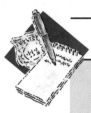

Just the facts

In this chapter you'll learn:

♦ the purpose, advantages, and disadvantages of I.V. medications

♦ how to calculate dosages and administration rates

♦ how to prepare I.V. medications

♦ how to select the proper equipment

♦ how to administer direct injection, intermittent infusion, and continuous infusion

♦ about patient-controlled analgesia devices

♦ how to monitor patients for common complications of I.V. medication therapy

♦ how to care for pediatric and elderly patients receiving I.V. medications.

Understanding I.V. medications

Hospital patients receive about 40% of their medications by the I.V. route. I.V. medications may be given by:
• direct injection
• intermittent infusion
• continuous infusion.

Think I.V. when...

An I.V. medication may be ordered when:
• a patient needs a rapid therapeutic effect
• the medication can't be absorbed by the GI tract, either because it has a high molecular weight or is unstable in gastric juices

• the patient may receive nothing by mouth and an irritating drug would cause pain or tissue damage if given I.M. or subcutaneously (S.C.)
• a controlled administration rate is needed.

Benefits

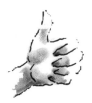

Compared with the oral, S.C., and I.M. routes, the I.V. route has many advantages:
• It effects immediate drug action by directly introducing a drug into the circulation. Therapeutic blood levels can be achieved rapidly, which makes I.V. delivery the preferred route in emergencies.
• It circumvents gastric absorption problems.
• It allows for accurate titration.
• It causes less discomfort for the patient.

Rapid response

I.V. medications go directly into the patient's circulation, rapidly achieving therapeutic blood levels. This difference in absorption explains why, for drugs such as propranolol, I.V. doses are much smaller than oral doses.

Effective absorption

Absorption of S.C., I.M., and orally administered drugs may be problematic for two reasons:
• Absorption may be erratic with S.C. and I.M. drugs.
• Some oral medications are unstable in gastric juices and digestive enzymes.
Giving drugs I.V. avoids these problems.

Bypass the first pass

Many oral medications are absorbed slowly, and absorption may be erratic or incomplete. In part, these absorption problems occur because oral medications are metabolized by the liver.
    In the liver, significant amounts of the drug are processed and eliminated before they reach the bloodstream. This process, known as first-pass metabolism, may be so rapid and extensive (in the case of lidocaine, for example) that it precludes oral administration.

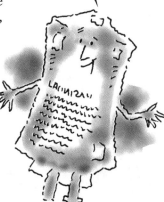

With all due modesty, I allow a rapid therapeutic response.

Accurate titration

Because gastric absorption isn't a factor with I.V. therapy, you can accurately titrate doses by adjusting the concentration of the infusate and the administration rate.

Less discomfort

I.V. administration prevents the pain and discomfort of I.M. and S.C. injections. However, rapid delivery of some I.V. medications can cause venous irritation. You may sometimes reduce venous irritation by further diluting an I.V. medication in a larger volume of solute.

Other benefits

The I.V. route provides an alternative when the oral route must be bypassed, such as when your patient is unconscious or uncooperative or can take nothing by mouth.

In addition, if an adverse reaction occurs, I.V. drug delivery can be stopped immediately. With other routes, absorption would continue until the drug was physically removed by vomiting, gastric suctioning, or dialysis.

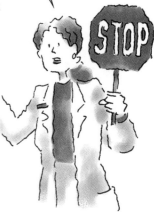

If an adverse reaction occurs, I.V. drug delivery can be stopped immediately.

Risks

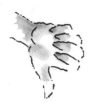

Like all administration routes, the I.V. route has certain risks. These include:
• solution and drug incompatibilities
• poor vascular access in some patients
• immediate adverse reactions.

Incompatibility

To successfully mix medication in a solution for infusion, two things need to be compatible:
• drug
• diluent.

If you're not sure about the compatibility of a mixture, ask the pharmacist or check an up-to-date compatibility chart.

Not a good mix

Incompatibility can occur when drugs are mixed in a syringe or solution container or during delivery of an I.V.

drug through an existing infusion line. For example, incompatibility can occur in the following situations:
- Several drugs are added to a large volume of fluid to produce an admixture.
- Drugs in separate solutions are administered concurrently or in close succession through the same I.V. line.
- A drug is reconstituted or diluted with the wrong solution.
- One drug reacts with another drug's preservatives.

Complexity can cause incompatibility

Most I.V. drugs are compatible with commonly used I.V. solutions. But the more complex the solution, the greater the risk of incompatibility.

An I.V. solution containing divalent cations (such as calcium) also has a higher incidence of incompatibility. For example, lactated Ringer's solution and Ringer's injection can present mixing problems because they contain potassium, calcium, chloride, and lactate. Incompatibility problems are also common in mixtures containing:

> Give me the simple life. The more complex a solution, the greater the risk of incompatibility.

- other electrolytes
- mannitol
- bicarbonate
- nutritional solutions.

Influences on incompatibility

The major factors that affect incompatibility include:
- the order in which drugs are mixed
- drug concentrations
- the amount of time the drugs are in contact with each other
- temperature
- exposure to light
- pH.

Also, when a drug loses more than 10% of its potency, it's considered incompatible with whatever caused the loss of potency. (See *Factors affecting drug compatibility*.)

Specific incompatibilities fall into three categories:

 physical

 chemical

 therapeutic.

Now I get it!

Factors affecting drug compatibility

Incompatibility is an undesirable chemical or physical reaction between a drug and a solution or between two or more drugs. The following factors can affect the compatibility of an I.V. drug or solution.

Order of mixing

Mixing order is a concern when you're adding more than one drug to an I.V. solution. Chemical changes occur after you add each drug. A drug that is compatible with the I.V. solution alone may be incompatible with the mixture of the I.V. solution and another drug. Changing the order in which you mix the drugs may prevent incompatibility.

Drug concentration

The higher the drug concentration, the more likely an incompatibility will develop. Gently invert the container after adding each drug to evenly disperse it throughout the solution, preventing a high-concentration buildup. Do this before starting an infusion and before adding another drug to the container.

Contact time

The longer two or more drugs are together, the more likely an incompatibility will occur. You should know if two drugs are incompatible before deciding how to give them. Suppose, for example, your patient is receiving a continuous heparin infusion, and gentamicin sulfate is ordered. Because these two drugs have an im-

mediate incompatibility, you should not piggyback the gentamicin into the heparin solution. If you do, your patient won't receive a therapeutic dose of gentamicin.

Temperature

Higher temperatures promote chemical reactions. The higher the temperature of an admixture, the greater the risk of incompatibility. For this reason, prepare the admixture immediately before administering it, or refrigerate it until needed.

Light

Prolonged exposure to light can affect the stability of certain drugs. Nitrofurantoin and amphotericin B, for example, must be protected from light during administration to maintain their stability.

pH

Generally, drugs and solutions that are to be mixed should have similar pH values to avoid incompatibility. The pH of each I.V. solution is listed on the manufacturer's label. You'll find the pH of each drug on the package insert.

Physical incompatibility

A physical incompatibility (also called a pharmaceutical incompatibility) occurs more often with multiple additives. Signs of physical incompatibility can be seen in the solution and include:
• precipitation
• haze
• gas bubbles
• cloudiness.

> Study I.V. solutions for signs of physical incompatibility — precipitates, haze, bubbles, and cloudiness.

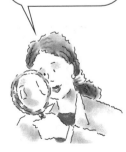

The presence of calcium in a solution (such as Ringer's solution) often increases the likelihood that a precipitate might form if the solution is mixed with another drug.

Other physical incompatibilities occur as a result of drug degradation such as the degradation of norepinephrine when added to sodium bicarbonate.

Chemical incompatibility

With chemical incompatibility, mixing two drugs alters the integrity and potency of active ingredients. Decomposition of a drug indicates a chemical incompatibility. Factors commonly associated with chemical incompatibility include:

• drug concentration
• pH of the solution
• volume of solution used to mix medications
• length of time that the medications are in contact with each other
• temperature
• light.

The most common chemical incompatibility involves the reaction between acidic and alkaline drugs and solutions. For example, mixing heparin solutions with intermittent aminoglycoside infusions commonly creates a chemical incompatibility, leading to such reactions as precipitate formation, color change, or gas bubbles.

> Better keep me out of the sun. Bright light may provide the energy for a chemical reaction to occur.

Bright light, such as sunlight, may provide the energy needed for a chemical reaction. To avoid such a reaction, certain drugs must be protected from light. Examples of drugs that need protection from light when they're diluted are amphotericin B and sodium nitroprusside (Nipride).

Therapeutic incompatibility

Therapeutic incompatibilities may occur when two or more drugs are administered concurrently. This may happen when a patient is prescribed two antibiotics — for example, chloramphenicol and penicillin. Chloramphenicol reportedly antagonizes the antibacterial effects of penicillin. Therefore, penicillin should be infused at least 1 hour before chloramphenicol.

Poor vascular access

In an emergency, you may find that normally accessible veins have collapsed from vasoconstriction or hypovolemia. Venipuncture may also be difficult in patients who require frequent or prolonged I.V. therapy. You may find that they've developed small, scarred, inaccessible veins from repeated venipunctures or infusions of irritating drugs.

If peripheral venous access isn't possible, the doctor may use a central vein, frequently by the subclavian route. If venipuncture isn't possible, drugs may be given I.M. or S.C. However, these routes can be used only if the volume to be infused is small and the drugs cause little or no tissue irritation.

If venipuncture isn't possible, drugs may be given I.M. or S.C...

...but only if the volume is small and the drugs cause little or no tissue irritation.

Adverse reactions

Because I.V. drugs quickly produce high blood levels, severe adverse reactions may occur immediately. The type of adverse reaction depends largely on the type of drug that's infused.

Consider cross-sensitivity

Hypersensitivity to I.V. drugs, although uncommon, can occur immediately or any time after administration. Keep cross-sensitivity in mind; if a patient is hypersensitive to a particular drug, he may be hypersensitive to chemically similar drugs. The most severe hypersensitivity reaction is anaphylaxis. Penicillin and its synthetic derivatives make up one of the drug families most likely to produce anaphylaxis.

Perilous preservatives

Your patient may suffer an adverse reaction from the preservative in a drug or I.V. solution. Large amounts of benzyl alcohol, for example, may cause seizures in neonates. Sulfites, another type of preservative, can cause sensitivity reactions, particularly in persons with asthma.

Intolerance turned topsy-turvy

You may encounter patients who have an inherent inability to tolerate certain chemicals. They can experience another kind of adverse reaction, called an idiosyncratic reaction. For example, in a particular patient, a tranquilizer may cause excitation rather than sedation.

Calculating I.V. drug dosages

Often, you must calculate an ordered dosage and verify that the dosage is within the recommended range.

Weight or body surface area

With some drugs (I.V. immune globulin, for instance), dosage is based on the patient's weight in kilograms. To convert a patient's weight from pounds to kilograms, simply divide the number of pounds by 2.2. (Remember, 2.2 lb equals 1 kg.)

With other drugs (such as chemotherapeutic agents), the dosage may be based on the patient's body surface area. One method for determining body surface area is to use a nomogram. (See *Using a nomogram for children,* page 175, and *Using a nomogram for adults*, page 176.)

Calculating administration rates

Typically, an order for I.V. medication prescribes the number of milliliters to infuse over a period of time. For instance, an order may call for 1,000 ml of dextrose 5% in half-normal saline solution every 8 hours.

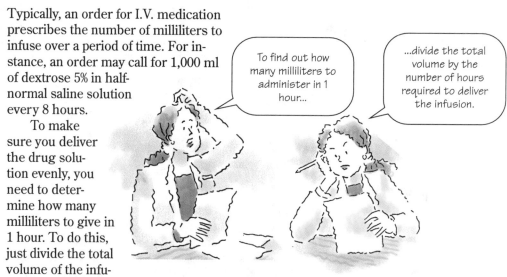

To find out how many milliliters to administer in 1 hour...

...divide the total volume by the number of hours required to deliver the infusion.

To make sure you deliver the drug solution evenly, you need to determine how many milliliters to give in 1 hour. To do this, just divide the total volume of the infusion by the number of hours the infusion is to take. In this case, divide 1,000 ml by 8 hours to determine that you must give 125 ml/hour.

Additional orders

Additional I.V. orders affect your calculations. Suppose the patient who's receiving 1,000 ml of dextrose 5% in half-normal saline solution every 8 hours also needs to receive gentamicin 80 mg once every 8 hours by intermittent infusion. There are two possible ways to handle this:

☝ After determining that the patient is able to tolerate the extra volume, you may simply incorporate the antibiotic fluid into the total daily intake.

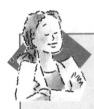

Peak technique

Using a nomogram for children

To estimate a child's body surface area with a nomogram, find the child's weight in the right column and his height in the left column. Mark these two points, then draw a line between them. The point where the line intersects the surface area column in the middle gives you the body surface area in square meters (m²).

On this nomogram, the child's height is 36″ and his weight is 55 lb. A straight line drawn between the two columns intersects the center column at 0.8. That tells you this patient's body surface area is 0.8 m².

If the child is of average size you can determine body surface area from weight alone by using the shaded area.

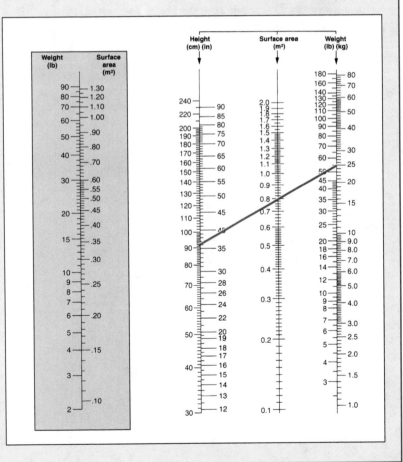

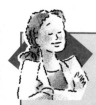

After determining that gentamicin and the primary infusate (dextrose 5% in half-normal saline solution) are compatible, you may recalculate the infusion rate for the

Peak technique

Using a nomogram for adults

To estimate an adult's body surface area with a nomogram, find your patient's weight in the right column and his height in the left column. Mark these two points; then draw a line between them. The point where the line intersects the middle column gives you the body surface area in square meters (m²).

On this nomogram, the patient's height is 5′ 3″ and her weight is 110 lb. A straight line drawn between the two columns intersects the center column at 1.50. That tells you this patient's body surface area is 1.5 m².

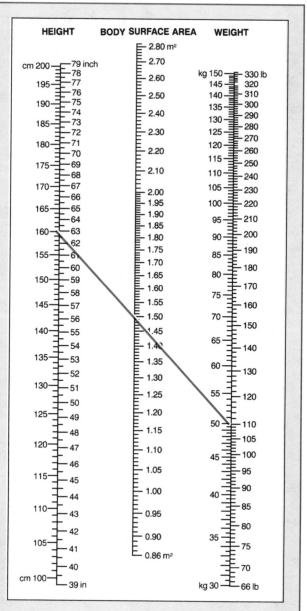

primary infusion after the antibiotic has been administered.

Ready, set, recalculate

If you need to recalculate the infusion rate, some simple subtraction and division are needed. To recalculate the infusion rate for the example above, use these two steps:

✍ Subtract the time needed to give the gentamicin from the total time period. For example, if you administer the gentamicin over 1 hour, there are 7 hours left to give the primary solution.

✌ Divide 1,000 by 7 to find that you must deliver the primary solution at a rate of 143 ml/hour.

I take life one minute at a time...

...so be prepared to convert milliliters per hour to drops per minute.

Equipment considerations

Your calculations may also depend on the delivery equipment. If you're using an infusion pump, simply set the dial for the desired milliliters per hour rate. But if you're using a controller that doesn't automatically convert milliliters per hour to drops per minute, or if you're using an administration set, you have to convert milliliters per hour to drops per minute (gtt/minute).

To do this, you must know the number of drops per milliliter that the particular I.V. tubing delivers. Microdrip tubings deliver 60 gtt/ml, but macrodrip tubings vary. To find drops per milliliter information, check the product wrapper or box; then use this formula:

$$\text{Drip rate in drops/minute} = \frac{\text{Total milliliters}}{\text{Total minutes}} \times \text{Drip factor in drops/ml}$$

Administering I.V. medications

Before you give an I.V. medication to your patient, you need to prepare the medication for delivery and select the right equipment.

Preparing medications

Most I.V. drug solutions are prepared in the pharmacy by pharmacists or pharmacy technicians. Occasionally, however, you have to prepare I.V. drug solutions yourself.

Safety first

When you're preparing a medication for I.V. administration, be sure to take some basic safety measures, such as the following:

• Maintain aseptic technique. Always wash your hands before mixing, and avoid contaminating any part of the vial, ampule, syringe, needle, or container that must remain sterile. When you're inserting the needle into and withdrawing it from the vial, make sure the needle tip doesn't touch any part of the vial that isn't sterile. Also, make sure you don't inadvertently puncture your finger; to keep your hands steady, brace one against the other while you're inserting and withdrawing the needle.

• When drawing up the drug before adding it to the primary solution, make sure you use a syringe that's large enough to hold the entire dose. The needle should be at least 1″ long to penetrate the inner seal of the port on an I.V. bag. In many facilities, practitioners use a 5-micron filter needle for mixing drug powder or withdrawing drugs from glass ampules. This needle is then removed, a sterile 1″ needle is reapplied to the syringe, and the drug is then admixed. (See *Keep it safe.*)

Play it safe. Maintain aseptic technique.

Reconstituting powdered drugs

Many I.V. drugs are supplied in powder form and have to be reconstituted with liquid diluents.

Choose a fluid

Common diluents include:
• normal saline solution
• sterile water for injection
• dextrose 5% in water.

Note the manufacturer's instructions about the appropriate type or amount of diluent. Some drugs should be reconstituted with diluents that contain preservatives. (See *Reconstituting powdered drugs,* page 180.)

Before you give that drug!

Keep it safe

Make sure you follow a few basic tips for ensuring safety when you administer I.V. medications.

Check it out
Check the expiration date on the drug and the diluent, and look for any special diluent requirements. Note whether the drug requires filtration. Also inspect the drug, diluent, and solution for particles and cloudiness. After reconstitution, again check for any visible signs of incompatibility in the admixture. Remember, incompatibility is more likely with drugs or I.V. solutions that have a high or low pH. Most drugs are moderately acidic, but some are alkaline, including heparin, aminophylline, ampicillin sodium, and sodium bicarbonate.

Mixing in a minibag
If you're mixing a drug in a minibag or minibottle of normal saline solution or dextrose 5% in water, you may be able to use the solution in the minicontainer as the diluent. But be sure to inspect it and discard any solution that appears cloudy or contains particles. Some solutions change color after several hours. If you're not sure whether to use a discolored solution, ask the pharmacist.

Two chambers

Some drugs come in double-chambered vials that contain powder in the lower chamber and a diluent in the upper one. To combine the contents, press the rubber stopper on top of the vial to dislodge the rubber plug separating the compartments. The diluent then mixes with the drug in the bottom chamber.

Diluting liquid drugs
Liquid medication may be packed in:
• single-dose ampules or vials
• multidose vials
• prefilled syringes
• disposable cartridges.
Liquid drugs don't need reconstitution, but they often require further dilution.

Liquid drugs don't require reconstitution...

...but they may require further dilution.

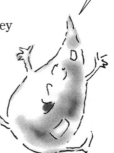

180

Add-a-drug

There are several methods you can use to add a drug to an I.V. container. Additive vials of a drug can be attached directly to administration tubing. If the vial contains a drug powder, first reconstitute it. Then you can infuse the drug solution directly from the vial, using dedicated vented tubing. (See *Adding a drug to an I.V. container.*)

Labeling solution containers

A container prepared in the pharmacy has a label showing the following information:
- patient's full name
- patient's room number

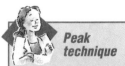

Peak technique

Reconstituting powdered drugs

To safely reconstitute powdered drugs, gather your equipment; then follow these step-by-step guidelines.

Draw up and clean
- Draw up the amount and type of diluent specified by the manufacturer.
- Clean the rubber stopper of the drug vial with an alcohol swab, using aseptic technique.

Insert, inject, and mix
- Insert the needle connected to the syringe of diluent into the stopper at a 45- to 60-degree angle. This minimizes coring or breaking off rubber pieces, which would then float inside the vial.
- Inject the diluent.
- Mix thoroughly by gently inverting the vial. If the drug doesn't dissolve within a few seconds, let it stand for 10 to 30 minutes. If necessary, invert the vial several times to dissolve the drug. Don't shake vigorously (unless directed) because some drugs may froth.

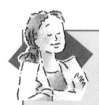

Peak technique

Adding a drug to an I.V. container

To add a drug to an I.V. container, use the following step-by-step techniques to ensure safe mixing.

Adding to an I.V. bottle
To add a drug to an I.V. bottle, first clean the rubber stopper or latex diaphragm with alcohol. Then insert the needle (either 19G or 20G) of the medication-filled syringe into the center of the stopper or diaphragm and inject the drug. Next, invert the bottle at least twice to ensure thorough mixing. Now remove the latex diaphragm and insert the administration spike.

Adding to an I.V. bag
To add a drug to a plastic I.V. bag, insert the needle of the medication-filled syringe into the clean latex medication port and inject the drug. (The needle should be 19G or 20G and 1" long; a short needle won't pierce the inner port seal, and a small-volume additive such as insulin will remain in the port.) After injecting the drug, grasp the top and bottom of the bag and quickly invert it twice. Don't squeeze or shake the bag.

Adding to an infusing solution
- If you have a choice, don't add a drug to an I.V. solution that's already infusing because of the risk of altering the drug concentration. However, if you must add a drug, make sure the primary solution container contains enough solution to provide adequate dilution. To add the drug, clamp the I.V. tubing and take down the container. Then, with the container upright, add the drug.
- If you're adding the drug to a bottle, clean the rubber stopper with an alcohol swab, insert the needle through the stopper, and inject the drug. If you're adding the drug to an I.V. bag, clean the rubber injection port with an alcohol swab before you inject the drug.
- After injecting the drug into the container, invert it several times to ensure thorough mixing and prevent a bolus effect.

- date
- name and amount of the I.V. solution and drugs
- other vital information.

Look to the label

If you prepare the drug solution, be sure to label the container with the same information provided by a pharmacy. Also, note the date and time you mixed the drug solution, and sign or initial the label. Make sure your label doesn't cover the manufacturer's label. If you use a time strip, label it with the patient's name and room number and the infusion rate (in milliliters per hour, drops per minute, or both).

Selecting the equipment

The type of equipment you choose depends on how the drug is administered. There are several questions to consider. (See *Choosing the right equipment,* page 182.)

Preparing for drug delivery

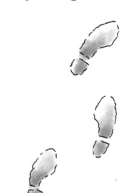

Before you administer I.V. medication by any method, take time to properly prepare the patient and the medication. Follow these steps:

- Confirm the patient's identity by checking his full name and facility identification number on his wristband. Also, ask him to identify himself, verbally if possible. If the patient is unable to identify himself, ask another nurse to corroborate his identity. Check his history for allergies and explain the procedure to him. (See *Remember the five rights.*)
- Make sure you know some key information about the drug you're giving. For instance, you should know the normal dosage, expected effects, adverse reactions, contraindications, and drug interactions. If you're unfamiliar with the drug and don't have access to the drug package insert or a drug reference book, ask your pharmacist any drug-related questions.
- Follow the Centers for Disease Control and Prevention (CDC) guidelines to protect yourself and your patient from blood-borne pathogens and infection. This means wearing gloves (and possibly a gown and mask) when exposed to body fluids.

Before you give that drug

Remember the five rights

Before you administer an I.V. drug to a patient, make sure you check the five rights:

- right drug
- right patient
- right time
- right dosage
- right route.

There's actually a 6th right
At the same time, make sure the patient understands the medication he's to receive and knows he has the right to refuse to take the medication.

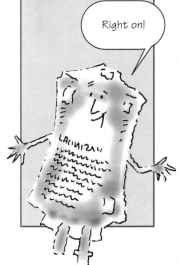

Right on!

Choosing the right equipment

Consider the following questions to help you choose equipment that's appropriate for administering any drug.

Pump or controller

Do you need a pump or controller to deliver a particular drug? Health care facilities usually have policies regarding the use of these devices. Pumps and controllers, most of which still require specific administration sets, are frequently used when you need a precise or very low infusion rate. They're also used when you're administering fluids or admixtures through a central venous catheter.

Drip rate

What is the ordered drip rate and what is your facility's policy on using macrodrip and microdrip tubing? Many policies require microdrip tubing when the infusion rate is less than 63 ml/hour.

Intermittent infusions

Is your patient going to receive intermittent drug infusions as well as the primary drug solution? If so, you may need a primary tubing that has an injection port close to the drip chamber and a backcheck valve that will automatically shut off the primary solution when the secondary solution is infusing.

Simultaneous infusions

Is your patient going to receive a simultaneous infusion of a secondary drug solution? If so, choose tubing that has an injection port close to the venipuncture device so you don't have to stop the primary infusion.

Special tubing

Does the drug solution require special tubing? Tubing without polyvinyl chloride is recommended for certain drugs such as nitroglycerin.

Glass or plastic

Is the solution container made of glass or plastic? If you're using a glass container, you need vented I.V. tubing. Use nonvented tubing for a collapsible plastic bag.

Infant or small child

Is your patient an infant or a small child? Many facilities have policies that permit only volume-control sets for such patients. These devices limit the volume available to the patient and decrease the risk of inadvertent fluid overload.

Needle-free

Consider using a needleless system, if available. You can piggyback drugs or additional I.V. solutions into a primary line without using a needle. Instead, a system is used that consists of a blunt-tipped device and a rubber injection port, as shown below. These items are called access devices or adaptation devices. The port may be part of a special administration set or an adapter for existing administration sets. This rubber injection port has a preestablished slit that can open and reseal immediately.

A needleless system can greatly reduce the risk of accidental needle-stick injuries, but it can't eliminate all such injuries because this system can't be used to perform venipunctures. Needleless systems can be used to obtain blood for blood gas analysis and other laboratory tests; indwelling lines such as A-lines or central lines can be adapted for use with the needleless system. It's possible to adapt a line for use with needleless systems with replaceable injection ports.

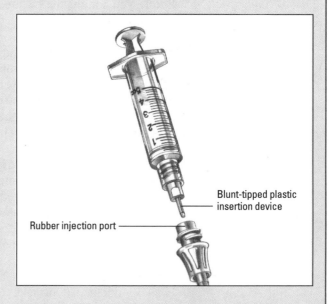

Blunt-tipped plastic insertion device

Rubber injection port

Infusion methods

You can give I.V. medications by three methods:
• direct injection
• intermittent infusion
• continuous infusion.
    You may also administer an I.V. medication using a specialized device, such as a patient-controlled analgesia (PCA) electronic infusion device. (See *Comparing administration methods,* pages 184 and 185.)

Direct injection

Direct injection can be used to deliver a single dose (bolus) or intermittent multiple doses. Commonly called an I.V. push, a direct injection can be administered two ways:

 directly into a vein

 through an existing infusion line.

Uh-oh

Direct injection may cause localized site complications. This method exerts more pressure on the vein than other methods, posing a greater risk of infiltration in patients with fragile veins.

Slow down

Most drugs must be given over a specific period of time when using direct injection. To avoid speed shock, don't administer any drug in less than 1 minute, unless the order directs you to do so or the patient is in cardiac or respiratory arrest.
    If your patient has any of the following conditions, slower injection times or greater drug dilution may be required to avoid decreased drug tolerance:
• systemic edema
• pulmonary congestion
• decreased cardiac output
• reduced urine output, renal flow, or glomerular filtration rate.

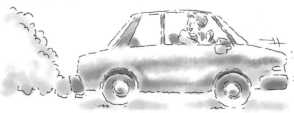

My motto: Slow down. Avoid speed shock.

Comparing administration methods

This chart gives you the indications, advantages, and disadvantages of common I.V. administration methods.

Methods and indications	Advantages	Disadvantages
Direct injection		
Into a vein (no infusion line) • When a nonvesicant drug with low risk of immediate adverse reaction is required for a patient with no other I.V. needs (for example, outpatients requiring I.V. contrast injections for radiologic examinations or cancer patients receiving chemotherapeutic agents)	• Eliminates risk of complications from indwelling venipuncture device • Eliminates inconvenience of indwelling venipuncture device	• Can only be given by doctor or specially certified nurse • Requires venipuncture, which can cause patient anxiety • Requires two syringes—one to administer medication and one to flush the vein after administration • Risk of infiltration from steel needle • Drug can't be diluted and delivery can't be interrupted if irritation occurs • Carries risk of clotting with the administration of a drug over a long period and with a small volume
Through existing infusion line • When drug is incompatible with I.V. solution and must be given as bolus injection • When patient requires immediate high blood levels (for example, regular insulin, dextrose 50%, atropine, and antihistamines) • In emergencies, for immediate drug effect	• Doesn't require time or authorization to perform venipuncture because the vein is already accessed • Doesn't require needle puncture, which can cause patient anxiety • Allows use of I.V. solution to test patency of venipuncture device before drug administration • Allows continued venous access in case of adverse reactions • Reduces risk of infiltration with vesicant drugs because most continuous infusions are started with an over-the-needle catheter	• Carries the same inconveniences and risk of complications associated with indwelling venipuncture device
Intermittent infusion		
Piggyback method • Often used with drugs given over short periods at varying intervals (for example, antibiotics and gastric-secretion inhibitors)	• Avoids multiple needle injections required by I.M. route • Permits repeated administration of drugs through single I.V. site • Provides high drug blood levels for short periods without causing drug toxicity	• May cause periods when drug blood level becomes too low to be clinically effective (for example, when peak and trough times aren't considered in the medication order)

Comparing administration methods *(continued)*

Methods and indications	Advantages	Disadvantages
Intermittent infusion *(continued)*		
Heparin lock • When patient requires constant venous access but not a continuous infusion	• Provides venous access for patients with fluid restrictions • Provides better patient mobility between doses • Preserves veins by reducing venipunctures • Lowers cost if used with limited number of drugs	• Requires close monitoring during administration so device can be flushed on completion • Heparin flush can't be used if patient has heparin sensitivity • Cost can rise rapidly when using device for several drugs because of equipment required
Volume-control set • When patient requires low volume of fluid	• Requires only one large-volume container • Prevents fluid overload from a runaway infusion • Allows chamber to be reused	• High cost • Carries high risk of contamination • If set doesn't contain membrane to block air passage when empty, you must close flow clamp when the set empties
Continuous infusion		
Through primary line • To maintain continuous serum levels, if infusion is not likely to be stopped abruptly	• Maintains steady serum levels • Presents less risk of rapid shock and vein irritation because of large volume of fluid diluting the drug	• Risk of incompatibility increases with drug contact time • Restricts patient mobility • Carries increased risk of undetected infiltration
Through secondary line • When patient requires continuous infusion of two or more compatible admixtures administered at different rates • When there's a significant chance of abruptly stopping one admixture without infusing remaining drug in I.V. tubing	• Allows primary infusion and each secondary infusion to be given at different rates • Allows primary line to be totally shut off and kept on stand-by to maintain venous access in case secondary line must be abruptly stopped • Short contact time before infusion may allow the administration of incompatible admixtures — something not possible with long contact time	• Can't be used for drugs with immediate incompatibility • Carries increased risk of vein irritation or phlebitis from increased number of drugs • Use of multiple I.V. systems (for example, primary lines with secondary lines attached), especially with electronic pumps or controllers, can create physical barriers to patient care and limit patient mobility

Speed up

Certain drugs metabolize quickly and must be administered quickly to achieve the desired effect. One such drug is adenosine, used for the treatment of supraventricular tachycardia.

Injection into a vein

To inject a drug directly into a vein, you need the following supplies:
- winged small-vein needle
- syringe with medication
- 3-ml syringe filled with saline solution
- povidone-iodine
- alcohol swab
- tourniquet
- gloves
- tape
- sterile pressure dressing.

Use the winged needle for I.V. push because it can be inserted quickly and easily. You also need dressing materials to apply to the venipuncture site after administration and a nonpermeable container in which to discard contaminated equipment. (See *Injecting a drug directly into a vein.*)

Injection into an existing line

To give an injection directly into the injection port of an existing line, you need the following supplies:
- the medication
- syringe with a 20G to 22G 1″ needle or a needleless system (preferred)
- alcohol swab.

You may also need a saline-filled syringe for flushing. (See *Injecting a drug into an existing line,* page 188.)

Intermittent infusion

The most common and flexible method of administering I.V. drugs is intermittent infusion. In this method, drugs are administered over a specified period at varying intervals. This helps to maintain and monitor therapeutic blood levels. You may deliver a small volume (1 to 250 ml) over several minutes or a few hours.

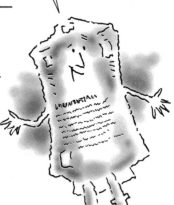

My main gig: intermittent infusion. It's the most common and flexible method of administering I.V. drugs.

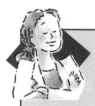

Peak technique

Injecting a drug directly into a vein

After assembling your equipment, follow the steps outlined below to inject a drug directly into a vein safely and accurately.

Apply, connect, select, withdraw
• Apply the tourniquet and clean the I.V. site with a povidone-iodine or alcohol swab.
• Connect the syringe with medication to the small-vein needle and push the plunger to expel the air.
• Select the largest suitable vein to allow for rapid dilution. Put on gloves and insert the needle in the vein with the bevel up.
• Withdraw a small amount of blood to confirm needle placement.

Release, secure, inject, aspirate
• Release the tourniquet.
• Place a short narrow strip of tape or a transparent dressing over each needle wing to secure the device during administration.
• Inject the drug at an even rate, as ordered.
• Gently aspirate the plunger at frequent intervals to reconfirm needle placement and ensure the delivery of all medication.

Observe, disconnect, remove, dispose
• Observe your patient for any signs of adverse reactions during and after the injection.
• Disconnect the medication syringe from the small-vein needle. Attach the syringe filled with saline to the needle and flush the device to ensure the complete delivery of all medication.
• Remove the venipuncture device and immediately place a sterile pressure dressing over the I.V. site.
• Dispose of contaminated hazardous equipment where appropriate.

Something to consider
If your patient needs further I.V. therapy — or if the drug can cause immediate adverse reactions — consider getting an order for an indwelling access device.

Secondary line

To infuse a drug through a secondary line, you need the following:
• medication in the unit-dose container
• secondary infusion tubing
• needleless device or 22G 1″ needle
• alcohol swab
• 1″ adhesive tape
• extension hook for the primary container.

Piggyback ride

You can deliver an intermittent infusion through a piggyback line that is connected to the primary line through a port, a saline or heparin lock, or a volume-control set.

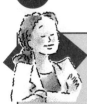

Peak technique

Injecting a drug into an existing line

After assembling your equipment, follow the step-by-step technique described below to inject a drug into an existing line safely.

Check, flush, invert, clean
• Check the I.V. site for redness, tenderness, edema, or leakage. If you detect any of these signs of complications, change the site before you administer the drug.
• If the new drug and the existing infusate are compatible, keep the infusion running. If the drug isn't compatible with the infusate but is compatible with saline solution, use a saline-filled syringe to flush the line before injecting the drug.
• Invert the syringe and gently push the plunger to remove all air.
• Using an alcohol swab, clean the rubber cap of the injection port closest to the venous access device.

Stabilize, inject, observe, withdraw
• Stabilize the injection port with one hand and insert the needle or needleless device through the center of the rubber cap. Don't force the insertion. If you meet resistance, position the needle or needleless device at a different angle.
• Inject the drug at an even rate, as ordered. Never inject so fast that you stop the primary infusion or allow the drug to flow back into the tubing.
• Observe the patient for any signs of a reaction during and after the injection.
• Withdraw the needle or needleless device and reestablish the desired flow rate.

Check the backcheck

The primary line should have a side Y-port with a backcheck valve that stops the flow from the primary line during drug infusion and resumes the primary flow after infusion. (See *Setting up a piggyback set.*)

Do it!

To perform the procedure, follow these steps:
• Check the I.V. site for infiltration, phlebitis, or infection.
• Check the primary infusion line for patency.
• Ensure that the drug to be piggybacked is compatible with the primary infusion.
• Hang the medication container on the I.V. pole.
• Close the flow clamp on the secondary tubing, remove the covers to the medication container and tubing spike, and insert the spike firmly into the medication container port.

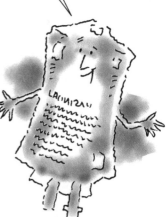

Let's do it! Let's deliver an intermittent infusion!

Setting up a piggyback set

Used only for intermittent drug infusions, a piggyback set includes a secondary container (a small I.V. bag or bottle) and short tubing with a drip chamber. To use it, connect the piggyback set to a primary line with a Y-port (or piggyback port), as shown. You must use an extension hook to position the primary I.V. container below the secondary container.

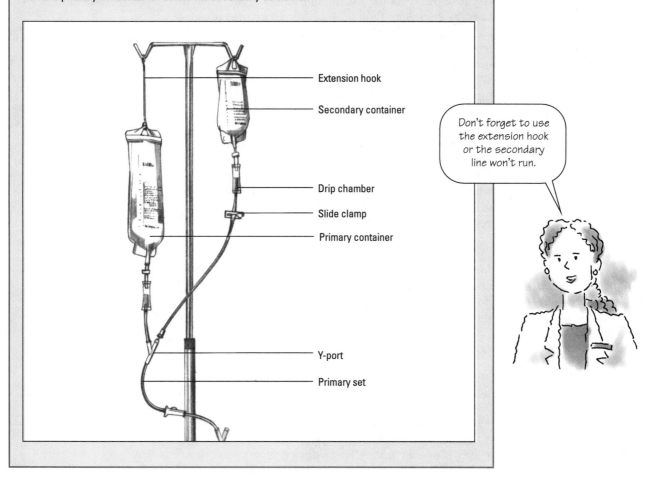

Extension hook

Secondary container

Drip chamber

Slide clamp

Primary container

Y-port

Primary set

Don't forget to use the extension hook or the secondary line won't run.

• Secure the needle or needleless device to the secondary tubing. Then, using an alcohol swab, clean the injection port on the primary tubing.
• Remove the cover from the secondary tubing; making sure the needle or needleless device is secure. If using a needle, secure it with tape to prevent it from dislodging. Insert the full length of the device into the center of the injection port.

• Lower the primary infusion with the supplied extension hook below the level of the secondary medication container, open the flow clamp of the secondary set, and allow the medication to infuse as prescribed.

Closing readjustment

Because the secondary container hangs higher than the primary container, fluid flowing from it creates pressure on the backcheck valve and completely shuts off fluid flow from the primary container. After the secondary infusion is completed, the primary fluid automatically flows again. When this happens, close the clamp on the secondary tubing and readjust the flow rate of the primary infusion.

Clamp and unclamp

If the primary tubing doesn't have a backcheck valve, you must clamp the primary line; you don't need to lower the primary container. Remember to open the primary clamp when the piggyback infusion is completed. Otherwise, the venous access device may clog and the patient may not receive the volume of I.V. fluid prescribed.

Fight phlebitis

Many drugs pose a high risk of phlebitis. So be sure to check the I.V. site carefully before administering each dose. If necessary, change the site before you administer the medication.

Heparin or saline lock

For intermittent I.V. drug infusion with a heparin lock (also called an intermittent infusion device), you need the following supplies:
• drug solution in its container
• administration set
• 20G 1″ needle or needleless device
• alcohol swab.
    You also need two 3-ml syringes filled with heparin or saline flush solution (depending on facility policy) each connected to a needleless device or 20G 1″ needle. (See *Using a heparin lock*, page 191, and *Hints for handling a heparin lock*, page 192.)

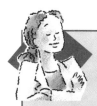

Peak technique

Using a heparin lock

After assembling your equipment, use the following step-by-step guidelines to safely administer a medication using a heparin lock.

Attach, secure, clean, stabilize

• Attach the minibag to the administration set and prime the tubing with the drug solution.

• Secure the 20G needle or needleless device to the I.V. tubing device and prime the needle or needleless device with the drug solution.

• Using an alcohol swab, clean the cap on the heparin lock.

• Stabilize the heparin lock with the thumb and index finger of your nondominant hand, as shown at right.

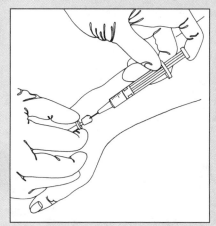

Insert, flush, secure, infuse

• Insert the needle or needleless device of one of the syringes containing flush solution into the center of the injection cap. Don't force it; if you feel resistance, insert the needle or device at a different angle. Pull back on the plunger slightly and watch for blood return. If blood appears, begin to slowly inject the flush solution. If you feel any resistance or the patient complains of pain or discomfort, stop immediately because the venous access device should be replaced.

• If you don't feel any resistance, watch for signs of infiltration as you slowly inject the flush solution. If you note signs of infiltration, remove the venous access device and insert a new device in a new location; if you don't note any signs, you're ready to give the medication.

• Insert the needle or needleless device attached to the administration set into the heparin lock.

• Regulate the drip rate, and infuse the medication, as ordered.

Discontinue and clean

• To discontinue the infusion, close the I.V. flow clamp and withdraw the needle or needleless device.
• Clean the injection cap and flush the heparin lock again.

Volume-control set

You can use a volume-control set as either:

 a primary line

 a secondary line.

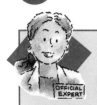

Advice from the experts

Hints for handling a heparin lock

Here are helpful hints for using a heparin lock.

Check carefully
Before accessing the lock, check the I.V. site carefully and change it if necessary.

Large enough and small enough
Access the intermittent cap with a needle or needleless device of the appropriate gauge and length. A 20G needle is large enough that it won't break and small enough that it won't cause leaks. A 1″ needle allows a secure connection without the risk of puncturing the catheter or tubing. However, when possible, use a needleless system.

Avoiding stress
When the injection cap serves as a heparin lock, stabilize the cap while accessing and removing the I.V. tubing and needle or needleless device to prevent stress at the insertion site. Stress increases the risks of phlebitis and catheter dislodgment.

Be present
You must be present when the infusion runs out so you can disconnect the tubing and flush

the device. Otherwise clots will form in the heparin lock.

Every 6 to 24 hours
Flush the device after each use and when it's not in use with the type and volume of solution recommended by facility policy. The flush solution may be saline or diluted heparin. Flushing may be required every 6 to 24 hours.

Time for new tubing
Follow your facility's policy for tubing changes. If you have to reconnect used tubing, make sure the tubing needle-adapter hasn't been contaminated. Always use a sterile needle or needleless device.

Medications
You can also give medications by direct injection through a heparin lock. In this case, flush the heparin lock, inject the medication as ordered, and flush the heparin lock again.

Memory jogger
To remember how to prime the volume-control set, fill the chamber with at least 20 ml of fluid; then use the mnemonic OSCAR:

Open the flow-regulating clamp.

Squeeze and hold the drip chamber.

Close the regulating clamp directly below the drip chamber.

And...

Release the drip chamber.

Get it together

When using a volume-control set as a primary line, gather the following supplies:
• I.V. solution
• medication in a syringe with a 20G 1″ needle or needleless device
• alcohol swabs
• a label.

When using a volume-control set as a secondary line, gather the following supplies:
• I.V. solution
• adhesive tape (for piggybacking)

• medication in a syringe with a 20G 1″ needle or needle-less device
• alcohol swabs
• a label.

Perform the procedure

To perform the procedure, follow these steps:
• Check the I.V. line for patency and the I.V. site for signs of infiltration or phlebitis.
• If you're using the volume-control set as a primary line, prime the tubing with the I.V. solution. Then insert the adapter of the set into the venipuncture device or heparin lock.
• If you're using the volume-control set as a secondary line, attach the 20G 1″ needle or needleless device to the adapter on the set and prime the tubing and needle with the I.V. solution. Then wipe the injection site on the primary tubing with an alcohol swab, and insert the needle or needleless device into the injection port. If using a needle, tape the connection. Needleless devices have a locking mechanism.
• To add medication to the chamber, wipe the injection port on the volume-control set with an alcohol swab and inject the medication. (See *Adding to a volume-control set*, and *Tips for adding medications*, page 194.)
• Place a label on the chamber indicating the drug, dose, time, and date. Don't write directly on the chamber with ink (the plastic can absorb the ink). Also, don't place the label over the numbers of the chamber. Then open the upper clamp; fill the fluid chamber with the prescribed amount of solution to dilute the medication. Close the clamp. Gently rotate the chamber to mix the medication and the solution.
• If you're using the volume-control set as a secondary line, either stop the primary infusion or set a low drip rate so the line will be open when the secondary infusion is completed. Then open the lower clamp of the volume-control set, and adjust the drip rate as ordered.
• After the infusion is completed and if the patient can tolerate the extra fluid, open the upper clamp and let 10 ml of I.V. solution flow into the chamber and through the tubing to flush it and complete delivery of the medication to the patient.
• If you're using the volume-control set as a secondary line, close the lower clamp and reset the flow rate on the

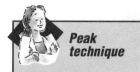

Peak technique

Adding to a volume-control set

After wiping the injection port with an alcohol swab, inject the medication, using a syringe, as shown below.

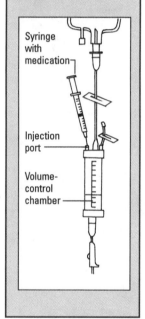

Syringe with medication

Injection port

Volume-control chamber

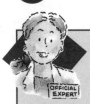

Advice from the experts

Tips for adding medications

When adding medications to a volume-control set, check for an immediately visible incompatibility. Especially when using multiple lines, make sure all drugs are compatible. Also, follow these tips.

Tangle-proofing

To prevent confusion when using multiple secondary lines, don't let them become tangled. Tag the lines below the drip chamber and at the connection site to the primary line. This clearly identifies the source and tubing connection for each drug.

Pump it up

When possible, use a pump or controller to achieve more accurate dosage control. Put a time strip on the secondary container to help monitor the administration rate.

Secure, patent, and firmly stable

Maintain a secure, patent venous access device. To avoid interrupting drug therapy when you change the I.V. site, establish the new site before disconnecting the old one. Also, firmly stabilize the connection to the primary tubing with tape or a locking device to prevent a broken needle or dislodgment.

Secondary and primary

If attaching the secondary line to the primary line with a needle in an injection port, use a 20G 1″ needle. A larger-gauge needle may cause leaks. A longer needle may pierce the tubing. A needleless system eliminates these concerns.

primary line. If you're using the set as a primary line, close the lower clamp, refill the chamber to the prescribed amount of primary solution, and restart the infusion.

Try this instead

Instead of using the volume-control set as a primary line, you can mix the medication in the primary solution, then use the volume-control chamber to closely regulate the amount of fluid and the drug dosage the patient receives.

Maintaining the membrane

If you're using a volume-control set with a membrane for intermittent drug administration, fill the chamber with fluid before adding the medication. This prevents the membrane from becoming sticky and difficult to operate. Be sure to read the manufacturer's instructions for priming volume-control sets.

Keeping air out of an empty chamber

The infusion stops when the fluid chamber is empty. If the set doesn't have a membrane or shut-off valve, refill the fluid chamber quickly to prevent air from filling the set.

Continuous infusion

A continuous infusion of medication allows you to carefully regulate drug delivery over a prolonged period. A continuous infusion may be given through a peripheral or central venous line. Sometimes, before you start a continuous infusion, a loading dose is given to achieve peak serum levels quickly.

A continuous infusion enhances the effectiveness of some drugs, such as lidocaine and heparin. Delivery of these drugs is commonly regulated with an I.V. pump or controller.

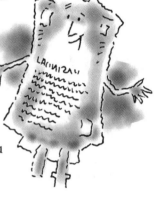

Go with the flow! Continuous infusion enhances the effectiveness of such drugs as lidocaine and heparin.

Primary line

To give a continuous infusion through a primary line, you need to assemble:
• the prescribed medication in I.V. solution
• an administration set
• gloves.

You may also need an infusion pump or controller. If so, make sure you have the correct administration set for the pump or controller.

Get ready

Preparations for giving a continuous infusion through a primary line include the following:
• First, make sure the I.V. solution container is labeled with the name and dosage of the medication.
• Attach the administration set to the solution container and prime the tubing with the I.V. solution.
• Attach the administration set to the pump or controller, if appropriate.
• If necessary, perform or assist with the venipuncture.

Continuous infusions are often regulated with an I.V. pump or controller.

Thanks for the help, guys.

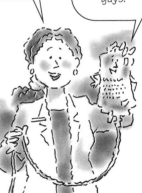

Perform the procedure

To begin the infusion, follow these steps:
• Put on gloves.

• Remove the protective cap at the end of the administration set.
• Attach the set to the venipuncture device.
• Begin the infusion and regulate the flow to the ordered rate. Remember to frequently monitor the patient and the flow rate.
• When the infusion is completed, hang another solution container or change solutions, as ordered.

Eyes on intake, output, and electrolytes

Maintain accurate intake and output records, and be alert for excessive fluid retention and fluid overload. When a patient receives small amounts hourly, his total daily volume can be excessive without any obvious signs.

Remember, too, that giving a large volume of fluid can seriously change a patient's electrolyte levels. Make sure you check the patient's laboratory results to make sure his electrolyte levels stay within normal limits.

Stop and go

Check the flow rate at regular intervals to ensure that the medication is delivered as ordered. Also, check I.V. sites frequently for signs of complications. If you note tenderness, redness, swelling, or leakage of infusate, discontinue the infusion and treat the site according to facility policy. Restart the infusion in another vein.

Secondary line

To give a continuous infusion through a secondary line, make sure you have the following supplies:
• the prescribed medication in I.V. solution
• administration set
• 20G 1″ needle or needleless device
• alcohol swabs
• 1″ adhesive tape.

You may also need an infusion pump or controller. If so, make sure you have the correct administration set for the pump or controller. (See *Infusing medication through a secondary line*.)

Documentation

After you administer a drug I.V., always document the procedure. Note the following:

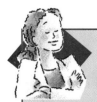

Peak technique

Infusing medication through a secondary line

After assembling the necessary equipment, follow the step-by-step technique below to safely administer medication through a secondary line.

Attach, prime, label, clean
• Attach the administration set to the solution container and prime the tubing with the I.V. solution. If appropriate, attach the administration set to the pump or controller.

• Secure the 20G 1″ needle or needleless device to the administration set, and prime the needle with the I.V. solution.

• Place labels with the name of the drug under the drip chamber and at the end of the tubing.

• Clean the injection port on the primary tubing with an alcohol swab.

Insert, adjust, monitor, remove
• Insert the full length of the needle or needleless adapter into the center of the injection port. Secure the needle with tape to prevent mistakenly dislodging the needle.

• Regulate the drip rate of the secondary solution and adjust the rate of the primary solution.

• Frequently monitor the patient and the infusion rate.

• When the secondary infusion is completed, remove the needle from the injection port. Adjust the flow rate of the primary solution.

• date and time of each infusion
• drug and dosage
• access site
• duration of administration
• patient's response
• your name.

Patient-controlled analgesia

PCA therapy allows your patient to control I.V. delivery of an analgesic (usually morphine) and maintain therapeutic serum levels of the drug. The computer-controlled PCA machine holds a syringe of medication that is attached directly to the patient's I.V. line. The patient can then push a button to receive a dose of analgesic through the I.V.

Lock-out time

A timing unit prevents the patient from accidentally overdosing by imposing a lock-out time between doses — usually 6 to 10 minutes. During this interval, the patient won't receive any analgesic despite pushing the button.

Who uses PCA therapy?

PCA therapy is indicated for patients who require parenteral analgesia. It's commonly used by patients after surgery and by patients with chronic diseases, particularly those with terminal cancer or sickle cell anemia.

Eligibility

To receive PCA therapy, a patient must:
• be mentally alert
• be able to understand and comply with instructions and procedures
• have no history of an allergy to the analgesic.

Not for everyone

Patients not eligible for therapy include those with:
• a limited respiratory reserve
• a history of drug abuse or chronic sedative or tranquilizer use
• a psychiatric disorder.

PCA "pluses"

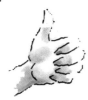

Patients receiving PCA therapy use less narcotics for pain relief than other patients. Also on the upside, PCA therapy provides the following advantages:
• It eliminates the need for I.M. analgesics.
• It provides individualized pain relief; each patient receives the appropriate dosage for his size and pain tolerance.
• It gives the patient a sense of control over pain.
• It allows the patient to sleep at night while minimizing daytime drowsiness.

PCA "minuses"

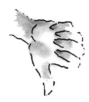

The main adverse effect of narcotic analgesics is respiratory depression. Therefore, you must routinely monitor your patient's respiratory rate. In addition to the effects on the respiratory system, narcotic analgesics can also lower blood pressure. Also, if the narcotic analgesic makes your patient nauseated, he may need an antiemetic drug.

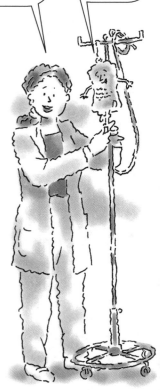

Patients who receive PCA therapy use less narcotics for pain relief...

...and feel a greater sense of control over their pain.

When your patient is receiving PCA therapy, make sure you check for infiltration into S.C. tissue and catheter occlusion, which may cause the drug to back up in the primary I.V. tubing.

The full story

The doctor's order for PCA may include:
• a loading dose, which is given by bolus and is programmed by the infusion device
• a lock-out interval, during which the PCA device can't be activated (such as every 6 to 10 minutes)
• the maintenance dose, if a continuous infusion of narcotic analgesia is ordered
• the amount the patient will receive when the device is activated (such as 10 mg meperidine [Demerol] or 1 mg morphine)
• the maximum amount the patient can receive within a specified time. This is usually the amount the patient can receive on demand or the maintenance dose over 60 minutes.

Evaluating a PCA

In evaluating a PCA pump, first consider its cost and the cost of its operation. Ask the following questions:
• Does it include expensive refill cassettes or less expensive syringes?
• Consider the pump's complexity. How easy is it to operate, both for you and the patient?
• Operating the pump should be a straightforward procedure but not so simple that anyone can manipulate the program. What kind of lock-out mechanism is employed by the device?
• Evaluate the equipment size and portability. An ambulatory patient should have a small, portable PCA pump. Can the pump be used on an I.V pole and be carried or worn as well?

Available features

PCA pumps are available with a variety of features:
• Some pumps provide both continuous infusion and bolus doses. Others provide only bolus doses.
• PCA pumps that provide both continuous infusion and bolus doses may offer a wide range of volume settings.

In evaluating a PCA pump, consider cost, complexity, ease of operation, size, and portability.

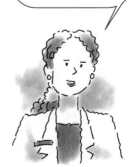

• The pump may have a panel that displays the amount delivered or, if necessary, an alarm message.

• You can program certain pumps to record the concentration in either milligrams (mg) or milliliters (ml), allowing greater flexibility in choosing rates.

• With some pumps, you can vary the length of the lockout interval from 5 to 90 minutes.

• Some pumps can be programmed to store and retrieve information such as the total dose allowed in a specified length of time.

• Most pumps can provide the total volume infused to include the narcotic analgesia in intake and output measurements.

Managing PCA therapy

With PCA, the patient self-administers drug delivery by pressing a button on a hand-held controller that is connected to the pump. Before the device can be used, it must be programmed to deliver specified doses at specified time intervals.

Continuous infusion plus bolus doses

If the patient is using a pump that provides continuous infusion and bolus doses, make sure that he understands that he is receiving medication continuously, but that he can give himself intermittent bolus doses for incidental pain (from coughing, for example) using the patient control button.

Remember this rule

If you program the pump to deliver a continuous infusion plus bolus doses, remember this rule: The cumulative doses per hour administered by PCA shouldn't exceed the total hourly dose ordered by the doctor. For example, if the patient needs a total of 6 mg of morphine over 1 hour, the doctor may begin therapy with a continuous infusion of 3 mg/hour, allowing a bolus dose of 0.5 mg every 10 minutes.

Continuing with continuous infusion

A PCA pump that provides continuous infusion in addition to bolus doses will provide analgesia regardless of whether the patient uses the control button This type of PCA is useful for helping patients cope with steady pain

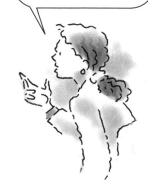

If a PCA pump delivers a continuous infusion plus bolus doses, remember this rule.

that gradually increases or decreases, incidental pain, or pain that is worse at different times. If the patient's pain is intermittent, he may not need continuous infusion.

Check the record first

Before allowing the patient to self-administer narcotic analgesics with a PCA, review his medication regimen. Concurrent use of two central nervous system (CNS) depressants may cause drowsiness, oversedation, disorientation, and anxiety.

Inform and reassure

Inform the patient how often he can self-administer the pain medication. Reassure him that the lock-out interval will prevent him from administering medication too frequently.

Determining doses

You and the doctor may determine the initial trial bolus dose and time interval between boluses, according to the patient's condition and activity level. The doctor orders ranges of dosing. Then you can enter these prescribed ranges into the PCA pump's program.

Push the button

Once safe limits are set, the patient can push the button to receive a dose when he experiences pain. Explain to him how the PCA device works.

Making adjustments

You and the doctor may decide to change either the dose or the lock-out interval after close monitoring and thorough assessment of the patient.

Determining the lock-out interval

The following are general guidelines for determining an appropriate lock-out interval. These guidelines apply for both pumps that provide bolus doses only and pumps that provide bolus doses plus continuous infusions.
• For I.V. boluses, set the lock-out interval as prescribed by the doctor. Typically, pain relief after an I.V. narcotic bolus takes 6 to 10 minutes.
• For S.C. boluses, set the lock-out interval for 30 minutes or more. Typically, pain relief after an S.C. bolus takes 30 to 60 minutes.

• For spinal boluses, set the lock-out interval for 60 minutes or more. Typically, pain relief after a spinal bolus takes 30 to 60 minutes.

Until pain subsides

If the patient hasn't been receiving narcotics, first program the pump to deliver the drug until his pain is relieved (the loading dose). Then set the pump's hourly infusion rate to equal the total number of milligrams per hour ordered by the doctor. Check the patient's response every 15 to 30 minutes for 1 to 2 hours.

Monitor amount, rate, and relief...

During therapy, monitor and record the following:
• amount of analgesic infused
• patient's respiratory rate
• patient's assessment of pain relief.

    If the patient doesn't feel that pain has been sufficiently relieved, notify the doctor, who may increase the dosage.

...and vital signs

Remember to monitor vital signs, especially when first initializing therapy. Encourage the patient to practice coughing and deep breathing. This promotes ventilation and prevents pooling of secretions, which could lead to respiratory difficulty.

PCA complications

The primary complication of PCA administration is respiratory depression. If the patient's respiratory rate declines to 10 or fewer breaths per minute, call his name, touch him, and have him breathe deeply. If he's confused or restless or he can't be roused, stop the infusion, notify the doctor, and prepare to give oxygen. Administer a narcotic antagonist, such as naloxone, if prescribed.

Uh-oh! Anaphylaxis, nausea, tolerance

Infiltration into S.C. tissue and catheter occlusion may also occur in PCA therapy. There are other possible complications. These include:
• anaphylaxis
• nausea
• vomiting
• constipation

- postural hypotension
- drug tolerance.

A note about nausea

If prescribed, give the patient who experiences nausea an antiemetic such as chlorpromazine. If the patient has persistent nausea and vomiting during therapy, the doctor may change the medication.

Patient teaching

Make sure the patient and caregiver fully understand the following:
- how the pump works
- when to contact the doctor
- signs and symptoms of adverse reactions
- signs and symptoms of drug tolerance.
    Tell the patient that he'll be able to control his pain and that the pump is safe and effective. Also remind him that a narcotic analgesic relieves pain best when it's taken before the pain becomes intense.

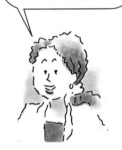

A narcotic analgesic works best when it's taken before the pain becomes intense.

Good advice

Because a narcotic analgesic may cause postural hypotension, tell the patient to get up slowly from his bed or a chair. Instruct him to eat a high-fiber diet, drink plenty of fluids, and take a stool softener if one has been prescribed. Caution him against drinking alcohol because this may enhance CNS depression.

Don't keep it a secret

The patient should notify the doctor if he fails to achieve adequate pain relief.
    The patient's caregiver should report signs of an overdose:
- slow or irregular breathing
- pinpoint pupils
- loss of consciousness.
    Teach the caregiver how to maintain respiration until help arrives should the need arise.

Did it work?

Evaluate the effectiveness of the drug at regular intervals. Ask these questions:
- Is the patient getting relief?

• Does the dosage need to be increased because of persistent or worsening pain?
• Is the patient developing a tolerance to the drug?
• Is the patient's condition stable?

Patients with special needs

When giving I.V. medications to a pediatric or elderly patient, be aware of special considerations.

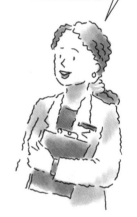

A child's venipuncture device may stay in place longer than an adult's...

Pediatric patients

Neonates and infants have precise fluid requirements. Keep in mind the following considerations when you give I.V. medications to children:
• Small children can't tolerate the large amount of fluid recommended for diluting many drugs.
• Because the drug dosage is based on the child's weight, each patient has a different normal dosing.
• Because of the small drug volume and slow delivery, you must make sure that no drug remains in the I.V. tubing before you change it.

Intermittent infusion

The most common method of giving I.V. drugs to pediatric patients is by intermittent infusion, using a volume-control set.

Out-of-reach, tamper-proof, and anti-free-flow

When setting up the equipment for a pediatric patient, take steps to ensure safety:
• Keep flow-control clamps out of the child's reach.
• Use tamper-proof pumps so the child can't change the rate inadvertently.
• Use an infusion pump with an anti-free-flow device that prevents inadvertent bolus infusions if the pump door is accidentally opened.

Especially careful

In many cases, a child's venipuncture device must stay in place longer than an adult's. Be especially careful to protect the I.V. site from accidental dislodgment or contami-

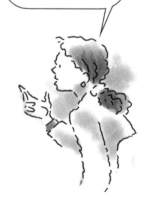

...so be especially careful to protect the I.V. site from dislodgment or contamination.

nation. Also, use aseptic technique whenever you're administering I.V. medications.

Retrograde administration

Retrograde administration offers one method for dealing with infants' precise fluid requirements. This method uses a coiled, low-volume tubing and a displacement syringe to prevent fluid overload.

Advantages

Retrograde administration allows you to administer an I.V. antibiotic over a 30-minute period without increasing the volume of fluid delivered to the patient. This method requires only one tubing to administer all I.V. fluids and medications. Also, you don't have to change the primary flow rate to administer I.V. drugs.

Disadvantages

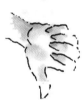

On the downside of retrograde administration, drug delivery is unpredictable, particularly with flow rates of less than 5 ml/hour. Also, the low-volume tubing must be able to hold the entire diluted drug volume. If any is displaced into the syringe, it must be discarded.

The drug must be diluted in a volume equal to half that used at the milliliter-per-hour rate of the primary infusion; this allows for a 30-minute drug infusion. Therefore, if the primary rate is changed, the diluted drug volume must be changed, too.

Syringe pump

A syringe pump is especially useful for giving intermittent I.V. medications to pediatric patients. It provides the greatest control for small-volume infusions.

Make sure the pump you use is tamper-proof, has a built-in guard against uncontrolled flow rates, and has an alarm sensitive to low-pressure occlusion. It should operate accurately with syringe sizes from 1 to 60 ml using low-volume tubing.

Intraosseous infusion

When venous access can't be established in an emergency, intraosseous infusion may be administered. This type of infusion is the infusion of I.V. medication into a bone.

Intraosseous infusion is usually performed by emergency personnel. It's a simple, quick, and relatively safe method for short-term emergency administration of lifesaving I.V. fluids and medications.

Drugs used in intraosseous infusion may be given by continuous or intermittent infusion or by direct injection. Intraosseous infusion is as quick and effective as the I.V. route. However, intraosseous infusion should be used only until venous access can be established.

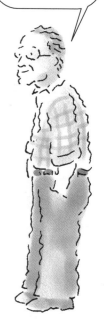

> Intraosseous infusion offers a way to administer lifesaving I.V. fluids and medications...

> ...but use it only until venous access can be established.

Elderly patients

When administering an I.V. analgesic to an elderly patient, watch closely for signs of respiratory depression or CNS depression, including confusion. Also, when giving a drug that can cause renal toxicity, monitor the patient closely for this complication. Remember, the aging process alone means many elderly patients have decreased functioning in several of their biological systems.

Fragile veins and fluid overload

Because many elderly patients have fragile veins, they're prone to infiltration and phlebitis. Carefully assess the I.V. site for signs and symptoms of these complications. If necessary, restart the infusion before you give a medication I.V.

Many I.V. drugs are particularly irritating to fragile veins, so you may have to dilute a drug in a larger volume than you normally would. Remember, though, elderly patients are prone to fluid overload. Keep accurate intake and output records, and include all fluids given for I.V. drug administration.

> I'm prone to irritation, phlebitis, and fluid overload.

Managing complications

To protect any patient receiving I.V. medication therapy, watch for signs and symptoms of these serious complications:
• hypersensitivity
• extravasation
• infiltration
• phlebitis
• infection. (See *Managing complications of I.V. drug therapy.*)

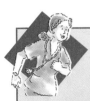

Running smoothly

Managing complications of I.V. drug therapy

Use the following chart to correct possible complications of I.V. drug administration.

Complications	Signs and symptoms	Nursing interventions
Circulatory overload	• Neck vein distention or engorgement • Respiratory distress • Increased blood pressure • Crackles • Positive fluid balance	• Stop infusion, and place patient in the semi-Fowler's position, as tolerated. • Reduce patient's anxiety. • Administer oxygen as ordered. • Notify doctor. • Administer diuretics as ordered.
Hypersensitivity	• Itching, urticarial rash • Tearing eyes, runny nose • Bronchospasm • Wheezing • Anaphylactic reaction	• Stop infusion. • Maintain patent airway. • Administer antihistaminic steroid, anti-inflammatory, and antipyretic medications as ordered. • Give 0.2 to 0.5 ml of 1:1000 aqueous epinephrine S.C.; repeat at 3-minute intervals and as needed. • Monitor vital signs.
Infiltration (peripheral I.V.)	• Swelling • Discomfort • Burning • Tightness • Cool skin • Blanching • Slow flow rate	• Stop infusion and remove the device. • Apply ice or warm pack. • Elevate limb. • Check pulse and capillary refill. • Restart I.V. and infusion. • Document patient's condition and interventions. • Check site frequently.
Phlebitis (peripheral I.V.)	• Redness or tenderness at tip of device • Puffy area over the vein • Elevated temperature	• Stop infusion and remove the device. • Apply warm pack. • Document patient's condition and interventions. • Insert a new I.V. catheter using a larger vein or small device and restart the infusion.
Systemic infection	• Fever • Malaise	• Stop infusion. • Notify doctor. • Remove device. • Culture site and device. • Administer medications as prescribed. • Monitor vital signs.

(continued)

Managing complications of I.V. drug therapy *(continued)*

Complications	Signs and symptoms	Nursing interventions
Venous spasm	• Pain along vein • Sluggish flow rate when clamp is completely open • Blanched skin over vein	• Apply warm soaks over vein and surrounding tissue. • Slow flow rate.
Speed shock	• Headache • Syncope • Flushed face • Tightness in chest • Irregular pulse • Shock • Cardiac arrest	• Stop infusion. • Call doctor. • Give dextrose 5% in water at a keep-vein-open rate.

Hypersensitivity

Before you administer a drug, take steps to find out if your patient may be prone to hypersensitivity:
• Ask the patient if he has any allergies, including ones to food or pollen.
• Ask if he has a family history of allergies. Patients with a personal or family history of allergies are more likely to develop a drug hypersensitivity.
• If your patient is an infant under 3 months old, be sure to ask about the mother's allergy history because maternal antibodies may still be present.

Follow through

After giving an I.V. medication, follow through with these precautions:
• Stay with the patient for 5 to 10 minutes to detect early signs and symptoms of hypersensitivity: sudden fever, joint swelling, rash, hives, bronchospasm, and wheezing.
• If the patient is receiving a drug for the first time, check him every 5 to 10 minutes or according to your facility's policy. Otherwise, check every 30 minutes for a few hours.

Now what?

At the first sign of hypersensitivity, discontinue the infusion and notify the doctor immediately. Remember, imme-

> At the first sign of hypersensitivity, STOP the infusion.

diate severe reactions are life-threatening. If necessary, assist with emergency treatment or resuscitation.

Infiltration

This complication often stems from improper placement or dislodgment of the catheter. In elderly patients, infiltration may occur because the veins are thin and fragile.

Raising the risk

The risk of infiltration increases when the venous access device remains in the vein for more than 2 days or when the tip is positioned near a flexion area. In these cases, patient movement may cause the device to telescope within the vein or slip out or through the lumen of the vessel.

Routine but comforting

If only a small amount of an isotonic solution or nonirritating drug infiltrates, the patient usually experiences only mild discomfort. Routine comfort measures in this case include:
• warm soaks
• elevating the extremity.

Damage delays healing...and worse

Extravasation of vesicant drugs, such as various antineoplastic drugs and sympathomimetics, can produce severe local tissue damage, which may:
• cause discomfort
• delay healing
• produce infection and disfigurement
• lead to loss of function and possibly amputation.

Now what?

If you suspect extravasation, stop the I.V. infusion at once and elevate the patient's arm. Notify the doctor immediately and follow treatment for extravasation according to the drug manufacturer's recommendations. Subsequent treatment varies, depending on the drug and your facility's policy. (See *Treating extravasation* and *Preventing extravasation,* page 210.)

Don't be fooled: Myths about extravasation

Frequently, nurses test for blood return to determine if extravasation is occurring. However, the absence of blood

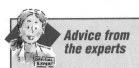
Advice from the experts

Treating extravasation

When extravasation occurs, emergency treatment is required. Follow your facility's protocol. Essential steps are described below.

Stop, estimate, instill
• Stop the I.V. flow and remove the I.V. line, unless you need the catheter in place to infiltrate the antidote.
• Estimate the amount of extravasated solution and notify the doctor.
• Instill the appropriate antidote according to facility protocol.

Elevate, record, apply
• Elevate the extremity.
• Record the extravasation site, the patient's symptoms, the estimated amount of infiltrated solution, and the treatment. Also record the time you notified the doctor and his name. Continue documenting the appearance of the site and associated symptoms.
• Following manufacturer's recommendations, apply either ice packs or warm compresses to the affected area.

Advice from the experts

Preventing extravasation

Extravasation — the infiltration of a potentially necrotizing drug into the surrounding tissue — can occur when a vein is punctured or when there is leakage around an I.V. site. If vesicant (blistering) drugs or fluids extravasate, severe local tissue damage may result.

To prevent extravasation when you're giving vesicants, adhere strictly to proper administration techniques and follow these guidelines described below.

Site selection, venipuncture, and infusion

• Don't use an existing I.V. line unless its patency is assured. Perform a new venipuncture to ensure correct needle placement and vein patency.

• Select the site carefully. Use a distal vein that allows successive venipunctures. To avoid tendon and nerve damage from possible extravasation, avoid using the back of the hand. Also, avoid the wrist and fingers (they're hard to immobilize) and areas previously damaged or that have poor circulation.

• Probing for a vein may cause trauma. Stop and begin again at another site.

• Start the infusion with dextrose 5% in water (D_5W) or normal saline solution.

Check it out

Check for infiltration before giving the medication. Apply a tourniquet above the needle to occlude the vein, then see if the flow continues. If the flow stops, the solution isn't infiltrating. Al-

ternatively, simply lower the I.V. container and watch for blood backflow. The latter method is less reliable because the needle may have punctured the opposite vein wall though still resting partially in the vein. Flush the needle to ensure patency. If swelling occurs at the I.V. site, the solution is infiltrating.

During and after administration

• Give the drugs by slow I.V. push through a free-flowing I.V. line or by small-volume infusion (50 to 100 ml).

• Give vesicants last when multiple drugs are ordered. If possible, avoid using an infusion pump to administer vesicants. A pump will continue the infusion if infiltration occurs.

• During administration, observe the infusion site for erythema or infiltration. Tell your patient to report any burning, stinging, pain, or sensation of sudden "heat" at the site.

• Use a transparent semipermeable dressing to allow frequent inspection of the I.V. site.

• After drug administration, instill several milliliters of D_5W or normal saline solution to flush the drug from the vein and to preclude drug leakage when the catheter is removed.

return doesn't always indicate extravasation. Blood return may not be possible if:
• you're using a small needle in a small vein or in one with low venous pressure
• the tip of the venous access device is lodged against the vein wall.
    Here is the truth about other common misconceptions:
• Extravasation doesn't always cause a hard lump. When the needle tip is completely out of the vein wall, a lump may form. However, if fluid leaks out of the vein slowly (as it may when the catheter tip partially punc-

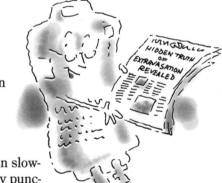

tures the vein wall), extravasation may produce only a flat, diffuse swelling.

• The patient may not always experience coldness or discomfort with extravasation. He may feel cold if extravasation occurs during rapid administration of a medication, but rarely will a patient feel cold from extravasation during a slow infusion.

Phlebitis

Postinfusion phlebitis is a common complication of I.V. therapy. It's often associated with drugs or solutions that:
• are acidic
• are alkaline
• have high osmolarity.
   Other contributing factors include:
• vein trauma during insertion
• using a vein that is too small
• using a vascular access device that is too large
• prolonged use of the same I.V. site.

When does it happen?

Phlebitis can follow any infusion — or even an injection of a single drug — but it's more common after continuous infusions. Typically, phlebitis develops 2 to 3 days after the vein is exposed to the drug or solution. Phlebitis develops more rapidly in distal veins than in the larger veins close to the heart.

Drugs given by direct injection generally don't cause phlebitis when administered at the correct dilution and rate. However, phenytoin and diazepam, which are frequently given by direct injection, can produce phlebitis after one or more injections at the same I.V. site.

Likely culprits

When piggybacked, certain irritating I.V. drugs are likely to cause phlebitis. These include:
• erythromycin
• tetracycline
• nafcillin sodium
• vancomycin
• amphotericin B.
   Large doses of potassium chloride (40 mEq/L or more), amino acids, dextrose solutions (10% or more), and multivitamins can also cause phlebitis.

Reducing the risk

If ordered, and if the patient's condition can tolerate it, add 250 to 1,000 ml of diluent to irritating drugs to help reduce the risk of irritation. You still should change the I.V. site every 48 hours or more frequently if necessary. If peripheral access is limited, suggest the placement of a central line to reduce the number of needle sticks, especially for long-term therapy.

Phlebitis can also result from motion and pressure of the venous access device. Also, particles in drugs and I.V. solutions can produce phlebitis, but you can reduce this risk by using filter needles and in-line filters.

> Why gamble? Adding diluent to irritating drugs helps reduce the risk of irritation.

Reducing the risk even further...

To help prevent phlebitis, the pharmacist can alter drug osmolarity and pH without affecting the primary medication. Additional measures you can take include the following:
• Use proper venipuncture technique.
• Dilute drugs correctly.
• Monitor administration rates.
• Observe the I.V. site frequently.
• Change the infusion site regularly.

Inspecting and detecting

To detect phlebitis, inspect the I.V. site several times daily. Use a transparent semipermeable dressing so you can see the skin distal to the tip of the access device as well as the insertion site. (See *Detecting and classifying phlebitis.*)

> Give phlebitis the one-two punch. Move the venipuncture site. Apply warm soaks.

Fighting phlebitis

If you suspect phlebitis, follow these steps to care for your patient:
• At the first sign of redness or tenderness, move the venipuncture device to another site, preferably on the opposite arm.
• To ease your patient's discomfort, apply warm packs or soak the arm in warm water, and elevate the extremity.

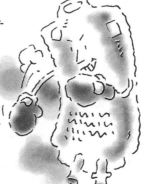

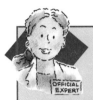

Advice from the experts

Detecting and classifying phlebitis

If you detect postinfusion phlebitis early, it can be treated effectively. If undetected, however, phlebitis can cause local infection, severe discomfort and, possibly, sepsis.

A brief explanation

Here's a brief explanation of how the signs and symptoms of phlebitis develop. As platelets aggregate at the damage site, a clot begins to form and histamine, bradykinin, and serotonin are released. Increased blood flow to the injury site and clot formation at the vein wall cause redness, tenderness, and slight swelling.

If you don't remove the venous access device at this stage, the vein wall becomes hard and tender and may develop a red streak 2″ to 6″ (5 to 15 cm) long. Left untreated, phlebitis may produce exudate at the I.V. site, accompanied by elevated white blood cell count and fever. It can also produce pain at the I.V. site, but a lack of pain doesn't eliminate the possibility of phlebitis.

How to classify it

According to the 1998 Intravenous Nurses Society Revised Standards of Practice, the degrees of phlebitis are classified as follows:

0 = no clinical symptoms

1+ = erythema with or without pain, edema may or may not be present, no streak formation, no palpable cord

2+ = erythema with or without pain, edema may or may not be present, streak formation, no palpable cord

3+ = erythema with or without pain, edema may or may not be present, streak formation, palpable cord.

Infection

A patient receiving I.V. medication therapy may develop a local infection at the I.V. site. Monitor your patient for signs and symptoms of infection, such as:
- extreme redness
- discharge at the site.

Protect yourself

Keep in mind that you're at risk for exposure to serious infection. If your patient has the hepatitis B virus, human immunodeficiency virus, or another blood-borne pathogen, it can be transmitted to caregivers through:
- poor technique
- failure to use standard precautions.

To protect yourself, follow the precautions for handling blood and body fluids recommended by the CDC.

Protect yourself some more

Remember to treat all patients as potentially infected and take appropriate precautions. Also, if you administer I.V.

drugs and solutions, you should receive the hepatitis B vaccine (if you don't already have hepatitis B antibodies).

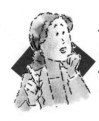

Quick quiz

1. I.V. medication may be indicated when:
    A. the patient needs a slower, more controlled therapeutic effect.
    B. the medication can't be absorbed by the GI tract.
    C. the medication given orally is stable in gastric juices.

Answer: B. I.V. medication has a rapid effect and may be indicated if the medication can't be absorbed by the GI tract, is unstable in gastric juices, or causes pain or tissue damage when given I.M. or S.C.

2. The route of medication preferred in emergencies is:
    A. I.V.
    B. S.C.
    C. I.M.

Answer: A. The I.V. route allows therapeutic levels to be achieved rapidly.

3. Loading dose, lock-out interval, and maintenance doses are basic to:
    A. I.V. therapy
    B. PCA therapy
    C. morphine continuous I.V. drips.

Answer: B. These concepts are basic to therapy with PCA.

Scoring

☆☆☆   If you answered three questions correctly, wow! Whether you used a direct, intermittent, or continuous approach, you caught the essence of this chapter.

☆☆   If you answered two correctly, you're right in line—no significant absorption problems.

☆   If you answered fewer than two questions correctly, don't panic. Three more quick quizzes to go.

Transfusions

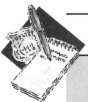

Just the facts

This chapter will help you sharpen your transfusion skills. In this chapter you'll learn:

♦ blood composition and physiology

♦ administering whole blood, blood components, plasma, and plasma fractions

♦ special considerations for pediatric and elderly patients

♦ common complications of transfusion.

Understanding transfusion therapy

The circulatory system is the body's main mover of blood and its components. The bloodstream carries oxygen, nutrients, hormones, and other vital substances to all other tissues and organs of the body. When illness or injury decreases the volume, oxygen-carrying capacity, or vital components of blood, transfusion therapy may be the only solution.

When illness or injury decreases the volume, oxygen-carrying capacity, or vital components of blood...

... transfusion therapy may be the only solution.

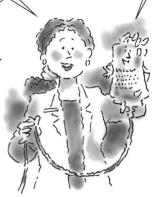

Purpose of transfusion therapy

Transfusion therapy is the introduction of whole blood or blood components directly into the bloodstream. It's used mainly to:
• restore and maintain blood volume
• improve the oxygen-carrying capacity of blood

• replace deficient blood components and improve coagulation.

Pump up the volume

The average adult body contains about 5 L of blood. However, hemorrhage, trauma, or burns can send blood volume plunging. Restoring and maintaining the volume of blood in the body is important because blood is a major player in maintaining fluid balance. When blood transfusion is contraindicated in a patient, fluid infusions can restore circulatory volume. Unlike blood, however, fluid infusions can't improve oxygen-carrying capacity or replace deficient components.

Pump up the volume. Pump up the volume. Yeah!

Carry on

Breathe in and air surges into the lungs. Blood then harvests oxygen from the air mixture and carries it throughout the body. The oxygen-carrying capacity of blood may be depleted from respiratory disorders, sepsis, carbon monoxide poisoning, acute anemia due to blood loss, or sickle cell disease. I.V. transfusion of the correct blood components can restore blood's role in oxygen delivery.

Get it together

Blood's coagulation capacity can be depleted by hemorrhage, liver failure, bone marrow suppression, platelet depletion (thrombocytopenia), medication- and disease-induced coagulopathies, or vitamin K deficiency. I.V. transfusion is used to replace the blood's missing coagulation components.

Transfusing blood products

There are two ways to administer blood and blood products:
• through a peripheral I.V. line
• through a central venous (CV) line.

A peripheral matter

Blood products can be transfused through a peripheral I.V. line, but it's not the best idea if large volumes must be transfused quickly. The small diameter of the vein and peripheral resistance (resistance to blood flow in the vein) can slow the transfusion.

The central point

Large volumes of blood products can be delivered quickly through a CV line because of the large size of the blood vessels and their decreased resistance to infusion.

The right to transfuse

Most states allow RNs (but not LPNs) to administer blood and blood components. In some states, LPNs may regulate transfusion flow rates, observe patients for reactions, discontinue transfusions, and document procedures.

The good and the bad

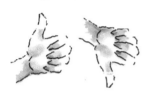

Because of careful screening and testing, the supply of blood is safer today than it has ever been. Even so, a patient who receives a transfusion is still at risk for life-threatening complications, such as a hemolytic reaction (which destroys red blood cells), and exposure to infectious diseases, such as human immunodeficiency virus (HIV) and hepatitis. Therefore, the doctor, the nurse, and the patient (when able) must weigh the benefits of a transfusion against the risks. (See *Protect yourself*.)

Blood physiology

Blood contains two basic components:

 cellular elements

 plasma.

Cells and plasma

The cellular (or formed) elements make up about 45% of blood volume. They include:
• erythrocytes, or red blood cells (RBCs)
• leukocytes, or white blood cells (WBCs)
• thrombocytes (platelets).

Plasma part by part

Plasma, the liquid component of blood, makes up about 55% of blood volume. Plasma consists of:

- water (serum)
- protein (albumin, globulin, and fibrinogen).
     Other elements in plasma include:
- lipids
- electrolytes
- vitamins
- carbohydrates
- nonprotein nitrogen compounds
- bilirubin
- gases.

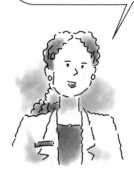

Plasma, the liquid component of blood, consists of blood's noncellular components.

Blood products

Generally, only a patient who has lost a massive amount of blood in a short time requires a whole blood transfusion. Most patients can be treated with individual blood products — the separate components that make up whole blood.

Component parts

Current technology allows freshly donated whole blood to be separated into its component parts:
- RBCs
- plasma
- platelets
- leukocytes
- plasma proteins, such as immune globulin, albumin, and clotting factors.

The availability of blood components usually makes it unnecessary to transfuse whole blood.

Partial components but full solutions

Individual blood components can be used to correct specific blood deficiencies. The availability of blood components usually makes it unnecessary to transfuse whole blood.

Compatibility

Recipient blood is choosy about donor blood. Any incompatibility can cause serious adverse reactions. The most severe is a hemolytic reaction, which destroys RBCs and may become life-threatening. Before a transfusion, testing helps to detect incompatibilities between recipient and donor blood.

Are you my type?

Typing and crossmatching establish the compatibility of donor and recipient blood. This precaution minimizes the risk of a hemolytic reaction. The most important tests include the following:
- ABO blood typing
- Rh typing
- crossmatching
- direct antiglobulin test
- antibody screening test
- screening for such diseases as hepatitis B and C, HIV, human T-cell leukemia virus type I (HTLV-1) and type II (HTLV-2 or hairy cell leukemia), syphilis and, for certain patients, cytomegalovirus (CMV).

> Each blood group in the ABO system is named for antigens that are carried on a person's RBCs.

ABO blood type

There are four blood types in the ABO system:
- A
- B
- AB
- O.

Antigens

An antigen is a substance that can stimulate the formation of an antibody. RBCs carry antigens, which can initiate an immune response. Each blood group in the ABO system is named for antigens — A, B, both of these, or neither — that are carried on a person's RBCs. An antigen may induce formation of a corresponding antibody if given to a person who doesn't normally carry the antigen.

Antibodies

An antibody is an immunoglobulin molecule synthesized in response to a specific antigen. The ABO system includes two naturally occurring antibodies: anti-A and anti-B. One, both, or neither of these antibodies may be found in the plasma. The interaction of corresponding antigens and antibodies of the ABO system can cause agglutination (clumping together). (See *Blood type compatibility*, page 220.)

O, you're everybody's type

Because group O blood lacks both A and B antigens, it can be transfused in limited amounts in an emergency to

Now I get it!

Blood type compatibility

Precise typing and crossmatching of donor and recipient blood helps avoid transfusing incompatible blood, which can be fatal. The chart below shows ABO compatibility for both recipient and donor.

Blood group	Antibodies present in plasma	Compatible red blood cells	Compatible plasma
Recipient			
O	Anti-A and anti-B	O	O, A, B, AB
A	Anti-B	A, O	A, AB
B	Anti-A	B, O	B, AB
AB	Neither anti-A nor anti-B	AB, A, B, O	AB
Donor			
O	Anti-A and anti-B	O, A, B, AB	O
A	Anti-B	A, AB	A, O
B	Anti-A	B, AB	B, O
AB	Neither anti-A nor anti-B	AB	AB, A, B, O

any patient — regardless of the recipient's blood type — with little risk of adverse reaction. That's why people with group O blood are called universal donors.

Any donor will do

A person with AB blood type has neither anti-A nor anti-B antibodies. This person may receive A, B, AB, or O blood, making him a universal recipient.

Additional antigens

The major antigens, such as those in the ABO system, are inherited. Blood transfusions can introduce other antigens and antibodies into the body. Most are harmless, but any could cause a transfusion reaction.

Not a good match

A hemolytic reaction occurs when donor and recipient blood types are mismatched. This could happen, for example, if blood containing anti-A antibodies is transfused to a recipient who has blood with A antigens.

As little as 10 ml

A hemolytic reaction can be life-threatening. With as little as 10 ml infused, symptoms can occur quickly — including headache, chest pain, chills, back pain, and fever. Because this reaction is so fast, always adhere strictly to your facility's policy and procedures for assessing vital signs during transfusions.

A bad match

When mismatching occurs, antigens and antibodies of the ABO system do battle. Antibodies attach to the surfaces of the recipient's RBCs, causing the cells to clump together (agglutinate).

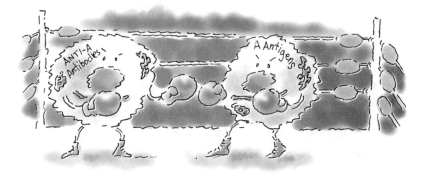

Eventually, the clumped cells can plug small blood vessels. This antibody-antigen reaction activates the body's complement system, a group of enzymatic proteins that cause RBC destruction (hemolysis). RBC hemolysis releases free hemoglobin (an RBC component) into the bloodstream, which can damage renal tubules and lead to kidney failure.

Rh blood group

Another major blood antigen system, the Rhesus (Rh) system, has two groups:
• Rh-positive
• Rh-negative.

D is the difference

The Rh system consists of different inherited antigens — D, C, E, c, or e. These antigens are highly immunogenic — they have a high capacity for initiating the body's immune response.

D or D factor is the most important Rh antigen. The presence or absence of D is one of the factors that determines whether a person has Rh-positive or Rh-negative blood.

Rh-positive blood contains a variant of the D antigen or D factor; Rh-negative blood doesn't have this antigen. A person with Rh-negative blood who receives Rh-positive blood will gradually develop anti-Rh antibodies. The first exposure won't cause a reaction because anti-Rh antibodies are slow to form. Subsequent exposures, however, may pose a risk of hemolysis and agglutination.

A person with Rh-positive blood doesn't carry anti-Rh antibodies because they would destroy his own RBCs.

Nearly 95% of Blacks, Native Americans, and Asians have Rh-positive blood; about 85% of Whites have Rh-positive blood. The rest of the population has Rh-negative blood.

Two ways

There are two ways Rh-positive blood can get into Rh-negative blood:
• by transfusion
• during a pregnancy in which the fetus has Rh-positive blood.

Problem in pregnancy

Rh factor incompatibility can cause a problem in pregnancy if a mother has Rh-negative blood and her fetus inherits Rh-positive blood from the father. During her first pregnancy, the woman becomes sensitized to Rh-positive fetal blood factors, but her antibodies usually aren't sufficient to harm the fetus.

In a subsequent pregnancy with an Rh-positive fetus, increasing amounts of the mother's anti-Rh antibodies attack the fetus, destroying RBCs. As the fetus's body produces new RBCs, cell destruction escalates, releasing bilirubin (a red cell component). The fetal liver's inability to properly process and excrete bilirubin can cause jaundice (soon after birth), other liver problems and, possibly, brain damage. Severely affected infants may develop life-threatening hemolytic disease.

Preventing formation of anti-Rh antibodies

Giving Rh immune globulin (RhoGAM) by I.M. injection prevents the formation of anti-Rh antibodies, thereby pre-

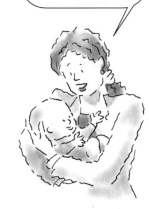

Rh incompatibility rarely affects a first child, but it could affect a second child if not treated.

venting development of hemolytic disease in newborns. This drug is also given to people who are Rh-positive and receive Rh-negative blood products.

> The histocompatibility system controls compatibility between transplant or transfusion recipients and donors...

HLA blood group

Human leukocyte antigens (HLAs) are essential to immunity. HLA is part of the histocompatibility system. This system controls compatibility between transplant or transfusion recipients and donors.

The HLA system:
- is responsible for graft success or rejection
- may be involved with host defense against cancer
- may be involved when WBCs or platelets fail to multiply after being transfused (if this happens, the HLA system could trigger a fatal immune reaction in the patient).

> ...the closer the HLA match...

Make me a match

Generally, the closer the HLA match between donor and recipient, the less likely the tissue or organ will be rejected.

HLA testing benefits patients receiving massive, multiple, or frequent transfusions. HLA evaluation is also conducted for patients who:
- will receive platelet and WBC transfusions
- will undergo organ or tissue transplant
- have severe or refractory febrile transfusion reactions.

> ...the less likely the tissue or organ will be rejected.

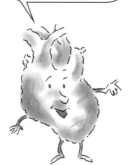

Administering transfusions

There are two kinds of transfused blood: autologous (from the recipient himself) and homologous (from a donor). Autologous blood reduces the risks normally associated with transfusions, but may not be available. Homologous blood undergoes rigorous screening and testing to ensure its quality. Part of this screening involves the donors themselves (see *Who can and can't give blood*, page 224.)

Your primary responsibility

Whatever the source of the blood or blood products, your primary responsibility is to prevent a potentially fatal hemolytic reaction by making sure the patient receives the correct product. Whether you transfuse whole blood, cellular components, or plasma, you will follow the same basic procedure. Always begin by checking, verifying, and inspecting. (See *Check, verify, and inspect.*)

Whole blood and cellular products

Before a transfusion, you need to send for the blood or cellular components ordered. Then gather and set up the appropriate equipment.

Cellular products

The patient's condition dictates which type of cellular product is needed in transfusion therapy. (See *Guide to cellular products*, pages 226 to 228.)

Commonly transfused cellular products include:
- whole blood
- packed RBCs
- leukocyte-poor RBCs
- WBCs
- platelets.

Whole or packed

To replenish decreased blood volume or to boost the blood's oxygen-carrying capacity, the doctor orders a transfusion of either whole blood or packed RBCs.

If your patient is receiving whole blood or packed RBCs (blood from which 80% of the plasma has been removed), don't send for the blood until just before you gather the equipment; RBCs deteriorate after 4 hours at room temperature.

Whole blood transfusions are used to increase blood volume. They're usually needed because of massive hemorrhage (loss of more than 25% of total blood) resulting from trauma or vascular or cardiac surgery.

Packed RBCs are transfused to maintain or restore oxygen-carrying capability. They can also replace RBCs lost because of a GI bleed, dysmenorrhea, surgery, trauma, or chemotherapy.

Who can and can't give blood

Donors must be screened to reduce the risks associated with transfusions.

Eligible
- Those ages 17 years or older
- Those who weigh at least 110 lb (50 kg)
- Those who are free from skin disease
- Those who haven't donated in the last 56 days
- Those whose hemoglobin level is at least 12.5 g/dl (women) or 13.5 g/dl (men)

Ineligible
- Those who have human immunodeficiency virus or acquired immunodeficiency syndrome
- Men who have had sex with another man since 1977
- Those who have ever taken illegal drugs I.V.
- Those who have had sex with a prostitute in the last 12 months
- Those who have had sex with anyone in the above categories
- Those who have had hepatitis
- Those with certain types of cancer (other than minor skin cancer)
- Those with hemophilia
- Those who have received clotting factor concentrations.

Centrifugal force, filters, washing

Leukocyte-poor RBCs are transfused when a patient has had a febrile, nonhemolytic transfusion reaction, caused by WBC antigens reacting with the patient's WBC antibodies or platelets. Several methods are used to remove leukocytes from blood:
- centrifugal force along with filtration and the addition of sedimentary agents, such as dextran and hydroxyethyl starch
- leukocyte removal filters
- washing the cells in a special solution (the most expensive and the least effective method; it also removes about 99% of the plasma).

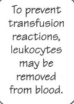

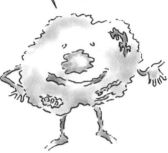

> To prevent transfusion reactions, leukocytes may be removed from blood.

Granulocytes to go

Transfusion of granulocytes (leukocytes containing granules) may be ordered to fight antibiotic-resistant septicemia and other life-threatening infections or when granulocyte supply is severely low (granulocytopenia). This therapy is repeated for 4 to 5 days or longer, as ordered, unless the bone marrow recovers or severe reactions occur.

(Text continues on page 228.)

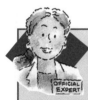

Advice from the experts

Check, verify, and inspect

Before administering any blood or blood product, take the following steps.

Check
Check to make sure an informed consent form was signed. Then double-check the patient's name, medical record number, ABO and Rh status (and other compatibility factors), and blood bank identification number against the label on the blood bag. Also check the expiration date on the bag.

Verify
Ask another nurse or doctor to verify all information, according to facility policy. (Some facilities routinely require double identification.) Make sure both you and the nurse or doctor who checked the blood or blood product have signed the blood confirmation slip. If even a slight discrepancy exists, don't administer the blood or blood product. Instead, immediately notify the blood bank.

Inspect
Inspect the blood or blood product to detect any abnormalities. Then confirm the patient's identity by checking the name, room number, and bed number on his wristband.

Guide to cellular products

Blood component	Indications	Nursing considerations
Whole blood Complete (pure) blood Volume: 500 ml	• To restore blood volume in hemor-rhaging, trauma, or burn patients	• Cross-typing is ABO identical. • Group A receives A; group B receives B; group AB receives AB; group O receives O. Rh type must match. • Use straight-line or Y-type I.V. set; can infuse rapidly in emergencies, but adjust the rate to the patient's condition and the transfusion order, and don't infuse over more than 4 hours. • Whole blood is seldom administered because its components can be extracted and administered separately. • Is used frequently in emergency treatment.
Packed red blood cells (RBCs) Same RBC mass as whole blood with 80% of the plasma removed Volume: 250 ml	• To restore or maintain oxygen-carrying capacity • To correct anemia and surgical blood loss • To increase RBC mass	• Cross-typing: Group A receives A or O; group B receives B or O; group AB receives AB, A, B, O; group O receives O. Rh type must match. • Use straight-line or Y-type I.V. set; can infuse rapidly in emergencies. Adjust the rate to the patient's condition and the transfusion order, and don't infuse over more than 4 hours. • RBCs have the same oxygen-carrying capacity as whole blood without the hazard of volume overload. • Using packed RBCs avoids potassium and ammonia buildup that sometimes occurs in the plasma of stored blood. • Packed RBCs shouldn't be used for anemic conditions correctable by nutrition or drug therapy.

Guide to cellular products *(continued)*

Blood component	Indications	Nursing considerations
Leukocyte-poor RBCs Same as packed RBCs except leuko-cytes (70%) are removed Volume: 200 ml	• To restore or maintain oxygen-carry-ing capacity • To correct anemia and surgical blood loss • To increase RBC mass • To prevent febrile reactions from leukocyte antibodies • To treat immunosuppressed patients	• Cross-typing: Group A receives A or O; group B receives B or O; group AB receives AB, A, B, O; group O receives O. Rh type must match. • Use straight-line or Y-type I.V. set. May require a Pall filter (40-micron fil-ter) for hard-spun, leukocyte-poor RBCs. Infuse over 1½ to 4 hours. • Cells expire 24 hours after washing. • RBCs have the same oxygen-carrying capacity as whole blood without the hazard of volume overload. • Leukocyte-poor RBCs shouldn't be used for anemic conditions correctable by nutrition or drug therapy.
White blood cells (leukocytes) Whole blood with all the RBCs and 80% of the plasma removed Volume: 150 ml	• To treat a patient with life-threatening granulocytopenia (granulocyte count usually less than 500/µl) who's not re-sponding to antibiotics (especially if he has positive blood cultures or persistent fever greater than 101° F [38.3° C])	• Cross-typing: Group A receives A or O; group B receives B or O; group AB re-ceives AB, A, B, O; group O receives O. Rh type must match. Preferably human leukocyte antigen (HLA)–compatible but not necessary unless patient is HLA-sensitized from previous transfusions. • Use straight-line set with standard in-line blood filter. Dosage is 1 unit daily for 4 to 6 days or until infection clears. • White blood cell infusion induces fever and chills. To prevent this reac-tion, premedicate the patient with anti-histamines, acetaminophen, steroids, or meperidine hydrochloride. Administer an antipyretic if fever occurs but don't discontinue transfusion. Flow rate may be reduced for patient comfort. • Because reactions are common, ad-minister slowly over 2 to 4 hours. Check vital signs and assess the patient every 15 minutes throughout the transfusion. • Give transfusion in conjunction with antibiotics to treat infection.

(continued)

Guide to cellular products *(continued)*

Blood component	Indications	Nursing considerations
Platelets Platelet sediment from RBCs or plasma Volume: 35 to 50 ml/unit; 1 unit of platelets = 7×10^7 platelets	• To treat thrombocytopenia caused by decreased platelet production, increased platelet destruction, or massive transfusion of stored blood • To treat acute leukemia and marrow aplasia • To restore platelet count in a preoperative patient with a count of 100,000/µl or less	• Cross-typing: ABO compatibility isn't necessary but is preferable with repeated platelet transfusions. Rh type match is preferred. • Use a component drip administration set; infuse 100 ml over 15 minutes. Administer at 150 to 200 ml/hour, or as rapidly as patient can tolerate; don't exceed 4 hours. • Platelet transfusions usually aren't indicated for conditions of accelerated platelet destruction, such as idiopathic thrombocytopenic purpura or drug-induced thrombocytopenia. • Patients with a history of platelet reaction require premedication with antipyretics and antihistamines. • Avoid administering platelets when the patient has a fever. • A blood platelet count may be ordered 1 hour after platelet transfusion to determine platelet transfusion increments.

Because some RBCs normally remain in WBC concentrates, granulocytes are tested for compatibility (ABO, Rh, and HLA).

Platelets plus

Platelets can be transfused to:
• control or prevent bleeding or correct an extremely low platelet count (20,000/µl or less) in a patient who doesn't have disease that destroys platelets
• increase the number of platelets in a patient who's receiving a platelet-destroying therapy, such as chemotherapy, or who has a hematologic disease, such as aplastic anemia or leukemia.

Selecting equipment

Before beginning a transfusion, gather the following equipment:
• gloves, gown, and mask to wear when handling blood products
• in-line or add-on filters as specified by the doctor's order or as appropriate for the product being infused
• I.V. pole
• transfusion component, exactly as ordered
• venipuncture equipment, if necessary.

Normal saline only

No I.V. solution other than normal saline (0.9% sodium chloride) should be given with blood. If a primary line has been used to deliver any solution other than normal saline, a blood administration set shouldn't be affixed or "piggy-backed" to it without first flushing the line.

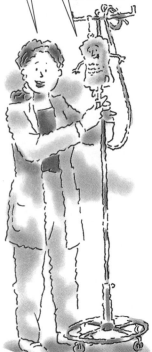

Only normal saline, an isotonic solution, should be given with blood.

Some other isotonic solutions may cause cells to clump.

Filters and their features

Always use blood filters on blood products to avoid infusing fibrin clots or cellular debris that forms in the blood bag. There are many types of filters, each with unique features and indications. A standard blood administration set comes with a 170-micron filter, which traps particles that are 170 microns or larger. This filter doesn't remove smaller particles, called microaggregates, which form after only a few days of blood storage.

Microaggregates form from degenerating platelets and fibrin strands, and may contribute to formation of microemboli (small clots that obstruct circulation) in the lungs. To remove microaggregates, the doctor may order a 20- to 40-micron filter, called a microaggregate filter. This filter removes smaller particles, but is costly and may slow the infusion rate — a particular problem when seeking to deliver a massive, rapid transfusion.

Filter tips

Filters may be used to screen out leukocytes during the transfusion of RBCs or platelets. Here are some tips:
• Use new tubing and a new filter for each unit of blood you transfuse.
• Never use a microaggregate filter to transfuse WBC concentrates or platelets; the filter will trap them. Instead, use a leukocyte reduction filter.

Heat it up

A blood warmer may be ordered in the following situations:
• to prevent hypothermia; for example, from large volumes of blood administered quickly
• to prevent arrhythmias from hypothermia (86° F [30° C])
• when antibodies called cold agglutinins are present because they react at temperatures below 68° F (20° C) and can cause agglutination of the blood.

Pump it up

In some facilities, an infusion pump is used to regulate the administration of blood and blood products. Always check the manufacturer's instructions to find out whether a particular pump can be used to administer blood or blood products.

Starting the transfusion

So far, you've identified the patient, inspected and verified the blood product, obtained baseline vital signs, and assembled the necessary equipment and supplies. Now you're ready to begin the transfusion. (See *Transfusing blood.*)

After you begin the transfusion, assess the patient and monitor vital signs according to the patient's transfusion history and your facility's policy — usually every 15 minutes for the 1st hour.

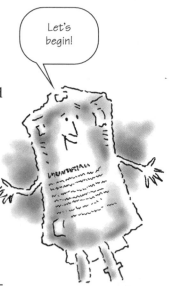

Let's begin!

Yikes! Fever, chills, headache

Watch for these signs of a transfusion reaction:
• fever
• chills
• rigors
• headache
• nausea.

If you detect any of these signs, quickly stop the transfusion and reestablish the normal saline infusion. *Note:* If you're using a Y-set, don't restart the infusion by opening the clamp; you'll just deliver more of the blood that's causing the problem. Instead, use a new bag and tubing to restart the infusion. (See *Monitoring a blood transfusion,* page 233.)

Peak technique

Transfusing blood

To begin transfusing blood, follow the steps described below.

Let's begin

• Explain the procedure to the patient.

• Wash your hands and put on the gloves, gown, goggles, and mask.

• If you're using a straight-line set, insert the set's tubing spike into the bag of saline solution.

• Hang the bag on the I.V. pole, and prime the filter and tubing with saline solution to reduce the risk of microclots forming in the tubing. Leave the bag of saline solution attached to the tubing until you're ready to start the transfusion.

Check, recheck, and verify

• Check, recheck, and verify the expiration date of the blood or cellular component. Also, double-check that you're giving the right blood or cellular component to the right patient, as shown below.

• Observe the blood or cellular component for abnormal color, clumping of red blood cells (RBCs), gas bubbles, and extraneous material that might indicate bacterial contamination. If you see any of these, return the bag to the blood bank.

Ready to start

• When you're ready to start the transfusion, prepare the equipment. When using a straight-line set, disconnect the blood administration set from the saline solution and clamp the open port of the saline solution. Then open the port on the blood bag and insert the spike on the blood administration set into the port.

• Next, remove the clamp from the saline solution and insert the spike on the regular administration set into the bag of saline solution and prime the line, as shown below.

Check and double-check

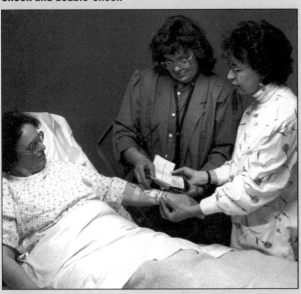

Priming the solution

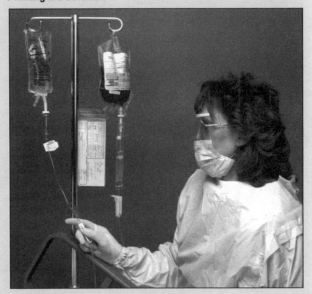

(continued)

Transfusing blood *(continued)*

• When using a Y-type set, close all the clamps on the set. Then insert the spike of the line you're using for the saline solution into the bag of saline solution. Next, open the port on the blood bag and insert the spike of the line you're using to administer the blood or cellular component into the port. Hang the bag of saline solution and blood or cellular component on the I.V. pole.

• Open the clamp on the line of saline solution, and squeeze the drip chamber until it's half full of saline solution. Then remove the adapter cover at the tip of the blood administration set, open the main flow clamp, and prime the tubing with saline solution. Close the clamp and recap the adapter.

The transfusion itself

To transfuse the blood or cellular component, follow these steps:

• Take the patient's vital signs to serve as baseline values. Recheck vital signs after 15 minutes (or according to hospital policy).

• If the patient doesn't have an I.V. device in place, perform a venipuncture, using a 20G or larger catheter.

• Attach the prepared blood administration set to the venous access device (VAD) and flush it with saline solution.

• When using a Y-type set, open both the clamp on the saline solution line and the main flow clamp.

• When administering whole blood or white blood cells, gently invert the bag several times during the procedure to mix the cells. (During the transfusion, gently agitate the bag to prevent the viscous cells from settling.)

• After you've flushed the VAD, begin to transfuse the blood.

• Adjust the flow clamp closest to the patient to deliver a slow rate (usually about 20 gtt/minute) for the first 10 to 30 minutes, as shown below. The type of blood product given and the patient's clinical condition determine the rate of transfusion. A unit of RBCs may be given over a period of 1 to 4 hours; platelets and coagulation factors may be given more quickly than RBCs and granulocytes.

• Usually, a transfusion doesn't take longer than 4 hours because the risk of contamination and sepsis increases after that. Discard or return to the blood bank any blood or blood products not given within this time, as hospital policy directs.

Hanging the bag

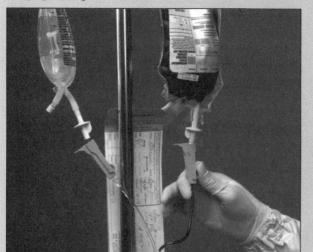

Adjusting the clamp

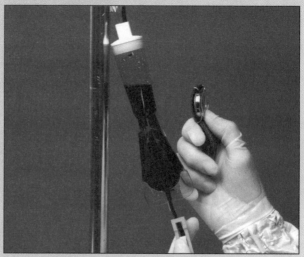

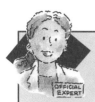

Advice from the experts

Monitoring a blood transfusion

To help avoid transfusion reactions and safeguard your patient, follow these guidelines:

• Record vital signs before the transfusion, 15 minutes later, after the transfusion, and more frequently if warranted by the patient's condition and transfusion history or the hospital's policy. Most acute hemolytic reactions occur during the first 30 minutes of the transfusion, so watch your patient extra carefully during the first 30 minutes.

• Always have sterile normal saline solution (NSS), an isotonic solution, set up as a primary line along with the transfusion.

• Act promptly if your patient develops wheezing and bronchospasm. These signs may indicate an allergic reaction or anaphylaxis. If, after a few milliliters of blood are transfused, the patient becomes dyspneic and shows generalized flushing and chest pain (with or without vomiting and diarrhea), he could be having an anaphylactic reaction. Stop the blood transfusion immediately, start the NSS, check and document vital signs, and call the doctor.

• If the patient develops a transfusion reaction, return the remaining blood together with a post-transfusion blood sample and any other required specimens to the blood bank.

Next, check and record the patient's vital signs. Notify the doctor immediately and don't dispose of the blood. If no signs of a reaction appear within 15 minutes, adjust the flow clamp to achieve the ordered infusion rate. Monitor the patient throughout the entire transfusion, according to your facility's policy and procedures. (See *Transfusion don'ts*, page 234.)

Under pressure

A pressure cuff on the blood container can increase the flow rate. If you use one, be sure it's equipped with a pressure gauge and exerts uniform compression against all parts of the container. Check the manufacturer's guidelines before using these devices for administration of blood or blood components. (See *The pressure is on*, pages 235 and 236.)

A positive pressure set also helps infuse the blood more rapidly. It looks like straight-line blood tubing but it has a bulb between the filter and the patient. This bulb fills with blood and can be squeezed to "pump" blood into the patient.

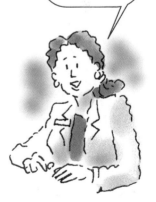

Monitor the patient throughout the entire transfusion.

Advice from the experts

Transfusion don'ts

A blood transfusion requires extreme care. Here are some tips on what not to do when administering a transfusion.

• Don't add any medications to the blood bag.

• Never give blood products without checking the order against the blood bag label — the only way to tell if the request form has been stamped with the wrong name. Most life-threatening reactions occur when this step is omitted.

• Don't transfuse the blood product if you discover any discrepancy in the blood number, blood slip, or patient identification number.

• Don't piggyback blood into the port of an existing infusion set. Most solutions, including dextrose in water, are incompatible with blood, so administer blood only with normal saline solution (NSS).

• Don't hesitate to stop the transfusion if your patient shows any changes in vital signs, is dyspneic or restless, or develops chills, hematuria, or pain in the flank, chest, or back. Your patient could go into shock, so don't remove the I.V. device that's in place. Keep it open with a slow infusion of NSS; call the doctor and the laboratory.

Terminating the transfusion

After a transfusion is complete, follow these steps:
• Flush the blood tubing with an adequate amount of normal saline, according to the patient's condition.
• On a Y-type set, close the clamp on the blood line and open the clamp on the saline line.
• Discard the tubing, filter, and blood bag per your facility's policy.
• Reassess the patient's condition and vital signs.
　　Make sure you record the following:
• date and time of the transfusion
• identification number on the blood bag
• type and amount of blood transfused
• volume of normal saline solution infused
• status of the venous access device
• patient's vital signs and clinical symptoms of a reaction (or the absence of any signs)
• how the patient tolerated the procedure.

Peak technique

The pressure is on

Rapid blood replacement requires transfusing blood under pressure. First, select the proper equipment—a pressure cuff or a positive-pressure set. A pressure cuff is placed over the blood bag like a sleeve and inflated, as shown. The pressure gauge, attached to the cuff, is calibrated in millimeters of mercury (mm Hg). A positive-pressure set is a gravity administration set containing a built-in pressure chamber that increases the flow rate when the chamber is compressed, as shown on the next page.

Prepare, prime, correct

To use either of these devices, prepare the patient and set up the equipment as you would with a straight-line blood administration set. Prime the filter and tubing with saline solution to remove all air from the administration set. Connect the tubing to the needle or catheter hub.

   Note: By increasing the pressure, you also increase the speed at which complications, such as infiltration, can occur. Therefore, watch the patient closely.

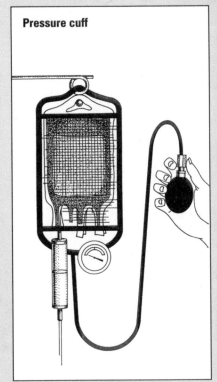

Pressure cuff

Using a pressure cuff

To use a pressure cuff:

• Insert your hand into the top of the pressure cuff sleeve and pull the blood bag up through the center opening. Then hang the blood bag loop on the hook provided with the sleeve.

• Hang the pressure cuff and blood bag on the I.V. pole. Open the flow clamp on the tubing.

• To set the flow rate, turn the screw clamp on the pressure cuff counterclockwise. Compress the pressure bulb of the cuff to inflate the bag until you achieve the desired flow rate. Then turn the screw clamp clockwise to maintain this constant flow rate.

• As the blood bag empties, the pressure decreases, so check the flow rate regularly and adjust the pressure in the pressure cuff as necessary to maintain a consistent rate. Don't allow the cuff needle to exceed 300 mm Hg; excessively high pressure can cause hemolysis and damage the component container or rupture the blood bag.

(continued)

The pressure is on (continued)

Positive-pressure set

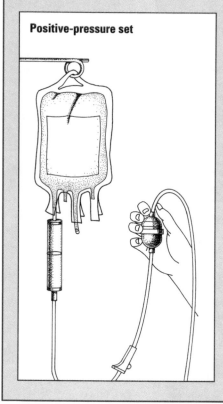

Using a positive-pressure set
To use a positive-pressure set:

• Open the upper and lower flow clamps on the administration set.

• Manually compress and release the pump chamber to force blood down the tubing and to the patient. Allow the pump chamber to refill completely before compressing it again.

• Continue to compress and release the chamber until the blood bag empties or until rapid administration is no longer necessary.

Plasma and plasma fractions

Plasma and plasma fractions are the anticoagulated clear portion of blood that's been run through a centrifuge. They make up about 55% of the blood, and are used in transfusion therapy to:
• correct blood deficiencies such as low platelet count
• control bleeding tendencies that result from clotting factor deficiencies
• increase the patient's circulating blood volume.

Plasma products

Before a transfusion, obtain the plasma or plasma fractions ordered. Commonly transfused plasma products include:
• fresh frozen plasma

- albumin
- cryoprecipitate
- prothrombin complex.

The patient's condition dictates which plasma product is needed. (See *Guide to plasma products,* pages 238 and 239.)

Plasma proxy

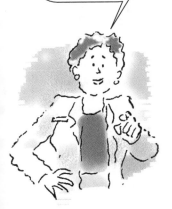

In an emergency, using plasma substitutes may allow time to get the patient's blood typed and crossmatched.

Plasma substitutes may be used to maintain blood volume in an emergency, such as acute hemorrhage and shock. Plasma substitutes lack oxygen-carrying and coagulation properties but using them allows time to get the patient's blood typed and crossmatched.

Depending on the circumstances, you may give:
- a synthetic volume expander such as dextran in saline solution
- a natural volume expander such as plasma protein fraction and albumin.

Selecting equipment

Gather the following infusion equipment:
- in-line or add-on filters or a filter system designated for the ordered component (usually a 170-micron filter) (*Note:* Never use a microaggregate filter to infuse platelets or plasma; it could remove essential components from the transfusion.)
- normal saline solution
- I.V. pole
- clean gloves
- ordered plasma or plasma fractions
- venipuncture equipment, if necessary.

Starting the transfusion

Before you begin a transfusion, review the procedure. (See *Transfusing plasma or plasma fractions,* page 240.)

When you're ready to begin the transfusion, follow these steps:
- Be sure the patient has a functional venous access device (20G or greater), or insert one as needed.
- Put on gloves and other protective equipment that your facility requires.
- Verify that you have the correct blood product and that it matches the number designated for the patient.

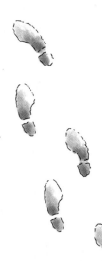

Guide to plasma products

Blood component	Indications	Nursing considerations
Fresh frozen plasma (FFP) Uncoagulated plasma separated from red blood cells (RBCs). FFP is rich in co-agulation factors V, VIII, IX. Volume: 200 to 250 ml	• To expand plasma volume • To treat postsurgical hemorrhage or shock • To correct an undetermined coagulation factor deficiency • To replace a specific factor when that factor alone isn't available • To correct factor deficiencies resulting from hepatic disease	• Cross-typing: ABO compatibility isn't necessary but is preferable with repeated platelet transfusions. Rh type match is preferred. • Use a straight-line set and administer as rapidly as tolerated. • Large-volume transfusions of FFP may require correction for hypocalcemia. Citric acid in FFP binds calcium.
Albumin 5% (buffered saline) **Albumin 25% (salt-poor)** Human albumin is a small plasma protein separated from plasma. Volume: 5% = 12.5 g/250 ml; 25% = 12.5 g/50 ml	• To replace volume in treatment of shock from burns, trauma, surgery, or infections • To replace volume and prevent marked hemoconcentration • To treat hypoproteinemia (with or without edema)	• Cross-typing isn't necessary. • Use a straight-line set; rate and volume depend on the patient's condition and response. • Reactions to albumin (fever, chills, nausea) are rare. • Albumin shouldn't be mixed with protein hydrolysates and alcohol solutions. • Albumin is often given as a volume expander until crossmatching for whole blood is complete. • Albumin is contraindicated as expander in severe anemia; administer cautiously in cardiac and pulmonary disease because of risk of heart failure from circulatory overload.
Factor VIII (cryoprecipitate) Cold insoluble portion of plasma recovered from FFP Volume: approximately 30 ml (freeze dried); dose calculated by body weight	• To treat a patient with hemophilia A • To control bleeding associated with factor VIII deficiency • To replace fibrinogen or factor VIII	• Cross-typing: ABO compatibility isn't necessary but is preferable. • Use the manufacturer-supplied administration set; administer with a filter. Standard dose recommended for treatment of acute bleeding episodes in hemophilia is 15 to 20 units/kg. • Half-life of factor VIII (8 to 10 hours) necessitates repeat transfusions at these intervals to maintain normal levels. • Administer I.V. as rapidly as tolerated, but don't exceed 6 ml/minute; monitor pulse rate while infusing.

Guide to plasma products *(continued)*

Blood component	Indications	Nursing considerations
Factors II, VII, IX, X complex (prothrombin complex) Lyophilized commercially prepared solution drawn from pooled plasma	• To treat a congenital factor V deficiency and other bleeding disorders resulting from an acquired deficiency of factors II, VII, IX, and X	• Cross-typing: No ABO or Rh matching is necessary. • Use a straight-line set; dosage is based on desired level and patient's body weight. • Risk of hepatitis is very high. • Coagulation assays are performed before administration and at suitable intervals during treatment. • Administration is contraindicated when the patient has hepatic disease resulting in fibrinolysis. • Administration is contraindicated when the patient has intravascular coagulation and isn't undergoing heparin therapy.

• Check the expiration date of the plasma or plasma fraction.
• Double-check that you're giving the right plasma or plasma fraction.
• Inspect the plasma or plasma fraction for cloudiness and turbidity, which could indicate possible contamination.
• Spike the bag with component-specific tubing (if the blood bank provided it) or with the blood tubing specified by your facility's policy and procedures.
• Prime the tubing.
• Explain the procedure to the patient.
• Obtain baseline vital signs and continue to check vital signs frequently, according to your facility's policy.
• Attach the plasma, fresh frozen plasma, albumin, factor VIII concentrate, prothrombin complex, platelets, or cryoprecipitate to the patient's flushed venous access device.
• Begin the transfusion and adjust the flow rate as ordered.
• Take the patient's vital signs and assess him frequently for signs of a transfusion reaction, such as fever, chills, or nausea. If a reaction occurs, quickly stop the infusion and start a normal saline infusion at a keep-vein-open rate. Check and record the patient's vital signs. Notify the doctor.

• After the infusion, flush the line with saline solution according to your facility's policy. Then disconnect the I.V. line. If therapy will continue, hang the original I.V. solution and adjust the flow rate as ordered.

• Record the type and amount of plasma or plasma fraction administered, duration of transfusion, baseline vital signs, any adverse reactions, and how the patient tolerated the procedure.

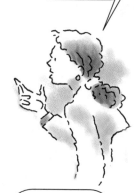

Autotransfusion is reinfusion of the patient's own blood.

Specialized transfusion methods

Specialized methods for administering blood include:
• autotransfusion
• hemapheresis.

Autotransfusion involves collecting, filtering, and reinfusing the patient's own blood. Hemapheresis involves collecting and removing specific blood components, then returning the remaining components to the donor.

Many patients prefer autotransfusion because it eliminates the risk of infectious disease. They can begin giving blood 4 to 6 weeks before surgery; the units are collected, labeled, and stored until needed.

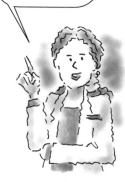

Hemapheresis involves collecting and removing specific blood components, then returning remaining components to the donor.

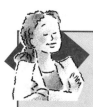

Peak technique

Transfusing plasma or plasma fractions

To transfuse plasma or plasma fractions, follow these steps:

• Obtain baseline vital signs.

• Flush the patient's venous access device with normal saline solution.

• Attach the plasma, fresh frozen plasma, albumin, factor VIII concentrate, prothrombin complex, platelets, or cryoprecipitate to the patient's venous access device.

• Begin the transfusion and adjust the flow rate as ordered.

• Take the patient's vital signs and assess him frequently for signs of a transfusion reaction, such as fever, chills, or nausea.

• After the infusion, flush the line with 20 to 30 ml of saline solution. Then disconnect the I.V. line. If therapy is to continue, resume the prescribed infusate and adjust the flow rate, as ordered.

• Record the type and amount of plasma or plasma fraction administered, duration of transfusion, baseline vital signs, and any adverse reactions.

Blood can also be collected during surgery. It's treated with an anticoagulant and collected in a sterile container that is fitted with a filter. The blood is reinfused as whole blood or processed before infusion. Salvaged blood can't be stored because the filtering and processing can't remove bacteria completely.

Both hemapheresis and autotransfusion must be performed by skilled personnel. Only nurses who are familiar with the procedures should monitor and evaluate a patient's condition throughout the transfusion.

Patients with special needs

Pediatric and elderly patients require special care during transfusion therapy. For instance, transfusing blood into a newborn requires specialized skills because the newborn's physiologic requirements differ vastly from those of an older infant, child, or adult.

Pediatric patients

Transfusions in children differ significantly from transfusions in adults.

Equipment

Blood units for pediatric patients are prepared in half-unit packs, and a 24G or 22G thin-walled catheter is used to administer the blood.

Rate

The rate of the infusion also differs. Usually, a child receives 5% to 10% of the total transfusion in the first 15 minutes of therapy. To maintain the correct flow rate, be sure to use an electronic infusion device.

Amount

A child's normal circulating blood volume determines the amount of blood transfused. The average blood volume for children and infants older than 1 month is 75 ml/kg. The proportion of blood volume to body weight decreases with age.

Good communication

Whenever you transfuse blood in an infant or child, explain the procedure, its purpose, and the possible compli-

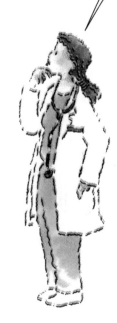

Pediatric and elderly patients require special care during transfusion therapy.

cations to the parents or legal guardian. If appropriate, also include the child in the explanation. Ask the parents for the child's transfusion history and obtain their consent.

A watchful eye

Closely monitor the child, particularly during the first 15 minutes to detect early signs of a reaction. Use a blood warmer, when indicated, to prevent hypothermia and cardiac arrhythmias, especially if you're administering blood through a central line.

Grown-up indications

In massive hemorrhage and shock, the indications for blood component transfusion in children remain similar to those for adults, although accurate assessment is difficult. Draw blood from a central vein to get a more accurate hemoglobin and hematocrit measurement, or use blood pressure readings to assess blood volume.

Elderly patients

An elderly patient with preexisting heart disease may be unable to tolerate rapid transfusion of an entire unit of blood without exhibiting shortness of breath or other signs of heart failure. The patient may be better able to tolerate half-unit blood transfusions.

Delayed reaction

Age-related slowing of the immune system puts an older adult at risk for delayed transfusion reactions. Because greater quantities of blood products transfuse before signs or symptoms appear, the patient may experience a more severe reaction. Also, an elderly patient tends to be less resistant to infection.

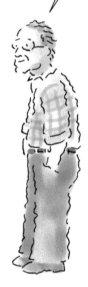

At my age, rapid transfusion of an entire unit of blood may be too much.

Complications

Always take steps to prevent transfusion complications and know how to manage them when they arise. (See *Correcting transfusion problems.*)

Transfusion reactions

Usually attributed to major antigen-antibody reactions, transfusion reactions may occur up to 96 hours after the transfusion begins. Transfusion reactions occur more commonly with the administration of platelets, WBCs, and cryoprecipitate than with whole blood, RBCs, or plasma.

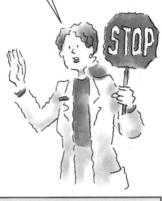

When you detect signs or symptoms of an acute transfusion reaction, stop the infusion immediately.

Stop immediately!

Whenever you detect signs or symptoms of an acute transfusion reaction, immediately stop the transfusion. Then follow these steps:
• Change the I.V. tubing to prevent infusing any more blood. Save the blood tubing and bag for analysis.
• Administer normal saline solution to keep the vein patent (open).

Running smoothly

Correcting transfusion problems

A patient who receives excellent care can still encounter problems during a transfusion. Here's how to proceed when common transfusion problems occur.

It stopped!
If the transfusion stops:
• Check that the I.V. container is at least 3′ (1 m) above the level of the I.V. site.
• Make sure the flow clamp is open.
• Make sure the blood completely covers the filter. If it doesn't, squeeze the drip chamber until it does.
• Gently rock the bag back and forth, agitating any blood cells that may have settled on the bottom.
• Untape the dressing over the I.V. site to check the placement of the cannula in the vein. Reposition the device, if necessary.
• If using a straight-line blood administration set, flush the line with saline solution and restart the transfusion. If using a Y-type blood administration set, close the flow clamp to the patient and lower the blood bag. Next, open the saline clamp and allow some saline solution to flow into the blood bag. Rehang the blood bag, open the flow clamp to the patient, and reset the flow rate.

Hematoma
If a hematoma develops at the I.V. site:
• Immediately stop the infusion.
• Remove the needle or catheter and cap the tubing with a new needle and guard.
• Notify the doctor and expect to place ice on the site for 24 hours; after that, apply warm compresses.
• Promote reabsorption of the hematoma by having the patient gently exercise the affected limb.
• Document your observations and actions.

An empty bag
If the blood bag empties before the next one arrives:
• Hang a container of saline solution and administer it slowly.
• If using a Y-type set, close the blood line clamp, open the saline clamp, and let the saline solution run slowly until the new blood arrives. Make sure you decrease the flow rate or clamp the line before attaching the new unit of blood.

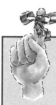

Memory jogger

To remember what to do in the event of a transfusion reaction, think of the acronym SPIN:

Stop the infusion

Pulse and other vital signs (check 'em)

Infuse normal saline solution

Notify the doctor

• Take and record the patient's vital signs.
• Notify the doctor.
• Obtain a urine specimen and blood sample and send them to the laboratory.
• Prepare for further treatment.
• Complete a transfusion reaction report and an incident report, according to your facility's policies and procedures.

The doctor or blood bank may eliminate some of these steps if a patient has a history of frequent mild reactions.

The rundown on reactions

Hemolytic, febrile, and allergic reactions can follow any transfusion. (See *Managing transfusion reactions.*) Certain complications typically result from multiple or massive transfusions. These include:
• hypothermia
• bleeding tendencies
• hemosiderosis (accumulation of an iron-containing protein).

Transfusion of blood products that have been processed and preserved increases the patient's risk of complications, especially if the patient receives frequent transfusions of large amounts.

Hemolytic reactions

An acute hemolytic reaction is life-threatening. It occurs as a result of incompatible blood. It also can occur as a result of improper storage of blood. It almost always results from a clerical error, such as mislabeling or failing to properly identify the patient. It may progress to shock and renal failure.

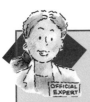

Advice from the experts

Managing transfusion reactions

If your patient experiences a transfusion reaction, stop the infusion and consult the chart below for further steps and tips for preventing future reactions.

Reaction	Nursing interventions	Prevention
Reactions from any transfusion		
Hemolytic	• Monitor blood pressure. • Treat shock as indicated by patient's condition, using I.V. fluids, oxygen, epinephrine, a diuretic, and a vasopressor. • Obtain posttransfusion reaction blood and urine samples for evaluation. • Observe for signs of hemorrhage resulting from disseminated intravascular coagulation.	• Before transfusion, check donor and recipient blood types to ensure blood compatibility; also identify patient with another nurse or doctor present. • Transfuse blood slowly for first 15 to 20 minutes; closely observe patient for the first 30 minutes of the transfusion.
Febrile	• Relieve symptoms with an antipyretic, antihistamine, or meperidine (Demerol).	• Premedicate with an antipyretic, an antihistamine and, possibly, a steroid. • Use leukocyte-poor or washed red blood cells (RBCs).
Allergic	• Administer antihistamines. • Monitor for anaphylactic reaction and administer epinephrine and steroids, if indicated.	• Premedicate with antihistamine if patient has a history of allergic reactions. • Observe patient closely for the first 30 minutes of the transfusion.
Plasma protein incompatibility	• Treat for shock by administering oxygen, fluids, epinephrine and, possibly, a steroid, as ordered.	• Transfuse only IgA-deficient blood or well-washed RBCs.
Bacterial contamination	• Treat with a broad-spectrum antibiotic and a steroid.	• Observe blood before transfusion for gas, clots, and dark purple color. • Use air-free, touch-free methods to draw and deliver blood. • Maintain strict storage control. • Change the blood tubing and filter every 4 hours. • Infuse each unit of blood over 2 to 4 hours; terminate the infusion if the time period exceeds 4 hours. • Maintain sterile technique when administering blood products.

(continued)

Managing transfusion reactions (continued)

Reaction	Nursing interventions	Prevention
Reactions from multiple transfusion		
Hemosiderosis	• Perform a phlebotomy to remove excess iron.	• Administer blood only when absolutely necessary.
Bleeding tendencies	• Administer platelets. • Monitor platelet count.	• Use only fresh blood (less than 7 days old) when possible.
Elevated blood ammonia level	• Monitor ammonia level. • Decrease the amount of protein in the diet. • If indicated, give neomycin sulfate or lactulose.	• Use only RBCs, fresh frozen plasma, or fresh blood, especially if patient has hepatic disease.
Increased oxygen affinity for hemoglobin	• Monitor arterial blood gas levels and give respiratory support as needed.	• Use only RBCs or fresh blood if possible.
Hypothermia	• Stop transfusion. • Warm patient with blankets. • Obtain an electrocardiogram (ECG).	• Warm blood to 95° to 98° F (35° to 37° C), especially before massive transfusions.
Hypocalcemia	• Monitor potassium and calcium levels. • Use blood less than 2 days old if administering multiple units. • Slow or stop transfusion, depending on reaction. Expect a worse reaction in hypothermic patients or patients with elevated potassium levels. • Slowly administer calcium gluconate I.V.	• Infuse blood slowly.
Potassium intoxication	• Obtain an ECG. • Administer sodium polystyrene sulfonate (Kayexalate) orally or by enema.	• Use fresh blood when administering massive transfusions.

Febrile reactions

Nonhemolytic febrile reactions are characterized by a temperature increase of 1.8° F. Such reactions are related to a transfusion and not caused by disease. They usually result from the patient's anti-HLA antibodies reacting against antigens on the donor's WBCs or platelets. Febrile reactions may occur in approximately 1% of transfusions. They can occur immediately or within 2 hours after completion of a transfusion.

Signs and symptoms of febrile reactions include the following:
- fever
- chills
- headache
- nausea and vomiting
- hypotension
- chest pain
- dyspnea
- nonproductive cough
- malaise.

Allergic reactions

An allergic reaction is the second most common transfusion reaction. It occurs because of an allergen in the transfused blood.

Oh my! Itching, hives, fever, chills...

Signs of an allergic reaction may include:
- itching
- hives
- fever
- chills
- face swelling
- wheezing
- throat swelling.

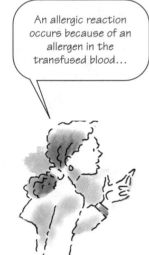

An allergic reaction occurs because of an allergen in the transfused blood...

An allergic reaction may progress to an anaphylactic reaction. This reaction can occur immediately or within 1 hour after infusion. Severe anaphylactic reactions produce bronchospasm, dyspnea, pulmonary edema, and hypotension. Treatment includes immediate administration of epinephrine, corticosteroids, and antihistamines.

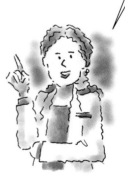

.... and may progress to an anaphylactic reaction.

Plasma protein incompatibility

A plasma protein incompatibility usually results from blood that contains IgA proteins being infused into a IgA-deficient recipient who has developed anti-IgA antibodies. The reaction can be life-threatening and usually resembles anaphylaxis. Signs and symptoms include:
- flushing and urticaria

- abdominal pain
- chills
- fever
- dyspnea and wheezing
- hypotension
- shock
- cardiac arrest.

Bacterial contamination

Blood and blood products may be contaminated during the collection process. As storage times and temperature increase, growth of microorganisms also increases. The resulting transfusion reaction is most often related to the endotoxins produced by gram-negative bacteria.

Yikes! Chills, cramping, kidney failure...

Signs and symptoms of bacterial contamination include:
- chills
- fever
- vomiting
- abdominal cramping
- diarrhea
- shock
- kidney failure.

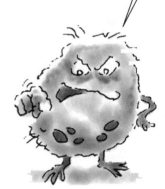

As storage time and temperature increase, growth of microorganisms also increases.

Reactions from multiple transfusions

Reactions from multiple transfusions include:
- hemosiderosis
- bleeding tendencies
- elevated blood ammonia levels
- increased oxygen affinity for hemoglobin
- hypothermia
- hypocalcemia
- potassium intoxication.

Hemosiderosis

Accumulation of an iron-containing pigment (hemosiderin) may be associated with RBC destruction in patients who receive many transfusions. In hemosiderosis, the patient's iron plasma level is greater than 200 mg/dl.

Bleeding tendencies

A low platelet count — which can develop in stored blood — can cause bleeding tendencies. Signs and symptoms may include abnormal bleeding, oozing from a cut or break in the skin surface, and abnormal clotting values.

Elevated blood ammonia level

Blood ammonia levels can increase in patients receiving transfusions of stored blood. Signs and symptoms of high blood ammonia levels include forgetfulness and confusion. The patient may also have a sweet mouth odor. High ammonia levels can cause behaviors that range from stuporlike to combative.

High ammonia levels can cause behaviors that range from stuporlike to combative.

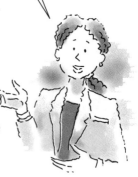

Increased oxygen affinity for hemoglobin

A blood transfusion can cause a decreased level of 2,3-diphosphoglycerate (2,3-DPG). Found on RBCs but scarce in stored blood, 2,3-DPG affects the oxyhemoglobin dissociation curve. This curve represents hemoglobin saturation and desaturation in graph form. Levels of 2,3-DPG (as well as other factors) cause the curve to shift either to the right (causing a decrease in oxygen affinity) or to the left (causing an increase in oxygen affinity).

A shift to the left

When 2,3-DPG levels are low, they produce a shift to the left. This causes an increase in the oxygen's hemoglobin affinity, so the oxygen stays in the patient's bloodstream and isn't released into other tissues. Signs of this reaction include a depressed respiratory rate, especially in patients with chronic lung disease.

Transfusing large amounts of cold blood can cause hypothermia, which can lead to cardiac arrest.

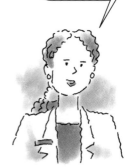

Hypothermia

A rapid infusion of large amounts of cold blood can cause hypothermia. The patient may experience shaking chills, hypotension, and cardiac arrhythmias, which may become life-threatening. Cardiac arrest can occur if core temperature falls below 86° F (30° C).

Hypocalcemia

If blood is infused too rapidly, citrate toxicity can occur. (Citrate is used to preserve blood.) Because citrate binds with calcium, calcium deficiency results. It can also follow normal citrate metabolism that is hindered by a liver disorder.

Oh, my! Tingling, cramps, hypertension...

Signs and symptoms of calcium deficiency include:
- tingling in the fingers
- muscle cramps
- nausea
- vomiting
- hypotension
- cardiac arrhythmias
- seizures.

Potassium intoxication

Some cells in stored RBCs may leak potassium into the plasma. Intoxication usually doesn't occur with transfusions of 1 to 2 qt of blood; larger volumes, however, may cause potassium toxicity.

Yikes! Colic, weakness, tall T waves...

Signs and symptoms of potassium toxicity may include:
- irritability
- intestinal colic
- diarrhea
- muscle weakness
- oliguria
- renal failure
- ECG changes with tall, peaked T waves
- bradycardia that may proceed to cardiac arrest.

Transmission of disease

Unlike a transfusion reaction, an infectious disease transmitted during a transfusion may go undetected until days, weeks, or months later, when signs and symptoms appear. Remember, all blood products are potential carriers of infectious disease, including:
- hepatitis
- HIV
- CMV.

Steps to prevent disease transmission include laboratory testing of blood products and careful screening of potential donors. Neither of these precautions is foolproof.

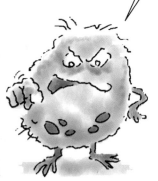

Remember, all blood products are potential carriers of infectious disease.

Laboratory testing

Hepatitis C (non-A, non-B) accounts for most posttransfusion hepatitis cases. The test that detects hepatitis C can produce false-negative results and may allow some contamination to go undetected.

HIV screening determines the presence of antibodies and antigens to HIV. The Food and Drug Administration requires that the antigen test be used in conjunction with the antibody test to reduce the risk of exposure from blood transfusions. False-negative results can occur, particularly during the incubation period of about 6 to 12 weeks after exposure. The Centers for Disease Control and Prevention estimates that undetected infection occurs in 1 out of every 450,000 to 660,000 donations per year.

Many facilities screen blood for CMV. Blood with CMV is especially dangerous for an immunosuppressed, seronegative patient.

Facilities also test blood for the presence of syphilis, although the routine practice of refrigerating blood kills the syphilis organism. This has virtually eliminated the risk of transfusion-related syphilis.

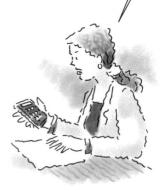

The chances of getting HIV infection from a blood transfusion are about 0.000002%—or one in a half-million.

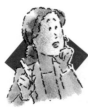

Quick quiz

1. The blood group type designated to be the universal donor is:
  A. A.
  B. B.
  C. O.
Answer: C. Group O blood type lacks both A and B antigens; for this reason, people with group O blood are called universal donors.

2. The size of the micron filters that come with standard blood transfusion sets is:
  A. 60 microns.
  B. 170 microns.
  C. 100 microns.
Answer: B. The standard blood administration set comes with a 170-micron filter.

3. The type of transfusion that involves collecting, filtering, and re-infusing the patient's own blood is called:

    A. autotransfusion.

    B. hemapheresis.

    C. plasmapheresis.

Answer: A. Autotransfusion involves collecting, filtering, and re-infusing the patient's own blood.

4. Fresh frozen plasma must be transfused within:

    A. 4 hours.

    B. 6 hours.

    C. 8 hours.

Answer: A. Plasma must be transfused within 4 hours because it doesn't contain preservatives.

5. If you detect any signs of a transfusion reaction, the first thing you should do is:

    A. slow down the infusion rate.

    B. stop the infusion.

    C. notify the doctor.

Answer: B. If you detect signs of a transfusion reaction, stop the transfusion and quickly take and record the patient's vital signs. Then start infusing saline solution at a slow rate and notify the doctor.

6. You should start a blood transfusion at a slow rate in order to:

    A. maintain blood volume.

    B. observe for the effect of any transfusion reaction.

    C. prevent clot formation at the tip of the venipuncture device.

Answer: B. Always start the transfusion at a slow rate to observe for the effects of any transfusion reaction.

Scoring

☆☆☆   If you answered five or six questions correctly, congrats! The information recipient (you) and the information donor (this chapter) are clearly compatible.

☆☆   If you answered three or four questions correctly, good going! The micron filter of your mind has allowed the key particles of information to successfully transfuse.

☆   If you answered fewer than three questions correctly, don't fret. Perhaps the flow rate on your information infusion device was set too low.

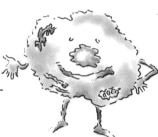

I'm having a reaction against all these puns.

Chemotherapy infusions

Just the facts

In this chapter, you'll learn:

♦ how chemotherapy works against cancer

♦ the types of chemotherapeutic agents

♦ how to administer chemotherapy

♦ the adverse effects of chemotherapy

♦ how to avoid dangerous exposure to chemotherapeutic drugs.

Understanding I.V. chemotherapy

Chemotherapy, along with surgery and radiation, is a mainstay of cancer treatment. Its most common route is I.V., using peripheral or central veins, though it's also administered by oral, subcutaneous (S.C.), intrathecal, I.M., intra-arterial, and intracavitary routes.

Chemotherapeutic drugs may be administered in the doctor's office, a clinic, the patient's home, or a hospital. Wherever treatments take place, the same basic principles of I.V. therapy apply. Because of rapid changes in health care delivery, emphasis on patient teaching is increasing.

I'm capable of delivering a precise dose, but everything has its price.

Precise but with a price

Suppressing rapidly dividing cancer cells with chemotherapy requires effective delivery of a precise dosage of toxic drugs. The I.V. route achieves this, but not without a potentially high price.

Benefits

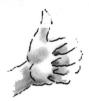

The advantages of I.V. chemotherapy are the same as those for any I.V. fluid or drug. These include complete absorption, systemic distribution, and accurate dosing.

Dosing is accurate because it doesn't depend on the variable rates of absorption associated with oral, rectal, S.C., or I.M. routes. Infusion causes less discomfort than either an I.M. or S.C. injection. Indeed, many chemotherapeutic drugs are so toxic that direct contact with the tissues could cause necrosis.

Risks

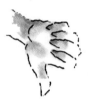

What are the prices that I.V. chemotherapy can exact? Although chemotherapy is intended to control or eliminate cancer cells, it can also damage healthy cells. Bleeding and infection may result from thrombocytopenia and a decrease in white blood cells. Chemotherapy may also lead to phlebitis and sclerosing of the veins. Because delivery is immediate, any adverse reaction, including hypersensitivity, is more pronounced.

How chemotherapy works

Healthy and cancerous cells pass through similar life cycles and are similarly vulnerable to chemotherapeutic drugs. Some of these drugs are cycle-specific; they're designed to disrupt a specific biochemical process, making them effective only during specific phases of the cell cycle. Other drugs are cycle-nonspecific; their prolonged action is independent of the cell cycle, allowing them to act on both reproducing and resting cells.

Cycle-specific drugs are effective only during a specific phase of the cell cycle...

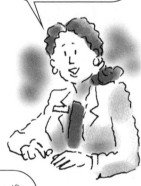

A full-scale attack

Because tumor cells are active in various phases of the cell cycle, chemotherapy typically employs more than one drug. This way, each drug can target a different site or take action during a different phase of the cell cycle.

... cycle-nonspecific drugs act independently of the cell cycle.

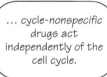

Targeting cells

During a single administration of a cycle-nonspecific chemotherapeutic drug, a fixed percentage of both normal and malignant cells die, while a percentage of normal and malignant cells survive.

When cycle-specific chemotherapy is administered, cells in the resting phase survive and eventually reproduce. (See *The cell cycle and chemotherapeutic drugs.*)

The challenge is to provide a drug dose large enough to kill the greatest number of cancer cells but small enough to avoid irreversibly damaging normal tissue or causing toxicity. In many cases, this challenge is met by prescribing smaller doses of different chemotherapeutic

The cell cycle and chemotherapeutic drugs

All cells cycle through five phases. Chemotherapeutic drugs that are active on cells during one or more of these phases are called cycle-specific. The illustration below tells what happens at each phase of the cell cycle and gives examples of cycle-specific drugs that are active during each phase.

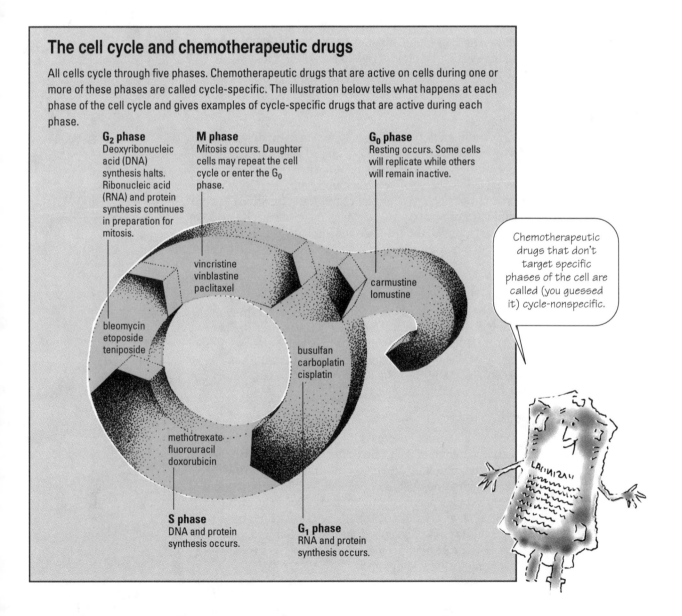

G_2 phase
Deoxyribonucleic acid (DNA) synthesis halts. Ribonucleic acid (RNA) and protein synthesis continues in preparation for mitosis.

M phase
Mitosis occurs. Daughter cells may repeat the cell cycle or enter the G_0 phase.

G_0 phase
Resting occurs. Some cells will replicate while others will remain inactive.

vincristine
vinblastine
paclitaxel

carmustine
lomustine

bleomycin
etoposide
teniposide

busulfan
carboplatin
cisplatin

methotrexate
fluorouracil
doxorubicin

S phase
DNA and protein synthesis occurs.

G_1 phase
RNA and protein synthesis occurs.

Chemotherapeutic drugs that don't target specific phases of the cell are called (you guessed it) cycle-nonspecific.

drugs. Given in combination, the drugs potentiate each other, and the tumor responds as it would to a larger dose of a single drug. Combination chemotherapy is also less likely to cause toxicity. In addition, because different drugs work at different stages of the cell cycle or employ different mechanisms to kill cancer cells, using several drugs decreases the likelihood that the tumor will develop resistance to the chemotherapy.

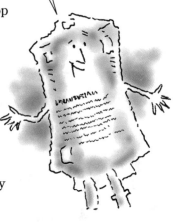

My challenge is to provide a drug dose large enough to kill the greatest number of cancer cells...

Hit me with your best shot

Drug selection depends on the patient's age, overall condition, and allergies or sensitivities as well as the stage of the cancer. Doctors strive to select the most effective drugs for the first round of chemotherapy because that is when cancer cells respond best.

Carefully planned cycles

Eradicating a tumor calls for repeated drug doses, usually over several days. This is considered a single course of chemotherapy and is repeated on a cyclic basis, often every 3 to 4 weeks. Treatment cycles are carefully planned so normal cells can regenerate. Specifically, the timing of repeat treatment cycles depends on the cycle of the target cells, the return of normal blood count, and the point at which the drug reaches its lowest serum level.

At least three

Most patients require at least three treatment cycles before they show any beneficial response. Even then, evaluating chemotherapy's effectiveness can be difficult because undetectable cancer cells may still be present. Because of this difficulty, doctors administer another treatment cycle after the cancer seems to have been eradicated.

...but small enough to avoid irreversibly damaging normal tissue or causing toxicity.

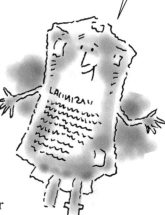

Which tumors respond to what

How well a tumor responds to chemotherapy depends on the percentage of cells killed, the rate of regrowth, and the development of resistant cells. Rapidly growing cancers, such as acute leukemias and lymphomas, respond best to cycle-specific chemotherapy. Slower growing cancers, such as GI and pulmonary tumors, which have fewer cells undergoing division at any given moment, respond better to cycle-nonspecific drugs but are less responsive to chemotherapy in general.

Tumor response also depends on the size of the tumor. Generally, small tumors respond to drugs that affect deoxyribonucleic acid synthesis, especially cycle-specific drugs. This is because small tumors have a higher percentage of actively dividing cells than large tumors. Large tumors respond better to cycle-nonspecific drugs. Once the large tumor shrinks, the doctor may switch to a cycle-specific drug.

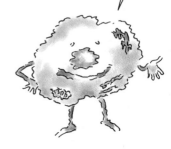

Rapidly growing cancers respond best to cycle-specific chemotherapy.

Chemotherapeutic drugs

Chemotherapeutic drugs are categorized according to their pharmacologic action and the way in which they interfere with cell production. In addition to the way they interfere with cell production, chemotherapeutic drugs are also categorized by their pharmacologic action.

Cycle-specific drugs are divided into antimetabolites and vinca alkaloids. Cycle-nonspecific drugs are divided into alkylating agents, nitrosoureas, antineoplastics, and antibiotics as well as a miscellaneous category.

Other drugs used to inhibit tumor cell growth include steroids, hormones, and antihormones. These drugs work in the intracellular environment. Steroids, which normally act as anti-inflammatory agents, make malignant cells vulnerable to damage from cycle-specific drugs. Hormones alter the cell's environment by affecting its membrane's permeability. Antihormones affect hormone-dependent tumors by inhibiting the production of those hormones or neutralizing their effect. (See *Common chemotherapeutic drugs*, page 258.)

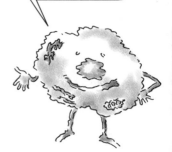

Slower growing cancers respond better to cycle-nonspecific chemotherapy.

Cure and more

Doctors order chemotherapeutic drugs not just to cure a cancer, but also to prevent metastasis or relieve symptoms. Drugs may be given alone or in combinations called protocols. (See *Sample chemotherapy protocols*, pages 259 and 260.)

The search for new cancer treatments is ongoing. Each year, the National Cancer Institute screens about 15,000 potential new compounds for chemotherapeutic action. Specific areas of research include biological therapy, immunotherapy, and cellular therapy.

(Text continues on page 260.)

Common chemotherapeutic drugs

Compare the characteristics and toxic effects of these commonly used chemotherapeutic drugs.

Category	Characteristics	Toxic effects
Cycle-specific		
Antimetabolites • cytarabine • fluorouracil • mercaptopurine • methotrexate • thioguanine	• Interfere with nucleic acid synthesis • Attack during S phase of cell cycle	• Effects on bone marrow, central nervous system (CNS), and GI, renal, and hematopoietic systems • Myelosuppression
Plant alkaloids • vinblastine • vincristine • vindesine	• Prevent mitotic spindle formation • Cycle-specific to M phase	• CNS effects, effects on GI and peripheral nervous systems • Myelosuppression • Tissue damage
Enzymes • asparaginase	• Blocks asparagine in protein synthesis • Useful only in leukemias	• Serious hypersensitivity reactions
Cycle-nonspecific		
Alkylating agents • altretamine • busulfan • chlorambucil • cisplatin • cyclophosphamide • dacarbazine • melphalan	• Disrupt deoxyribonucleic acid (DNA) replication	• Infertility • Secondary carcinoma • Tissue necrosis
Antibiotics • bleomycin • dactinomycin • daunorubicin • doxorubicin • mitomycin • plicamycin	• Bind with DNA to inhibit synthesis of DNA and RNA	• Effects on GI, renal, and hepatic systems • Effects on bone marrow • Tissue damage (except bleomycin)
Hormones and steroid drugs		
Hormones and hormone inhibitors • Adrenal suppressants • Androgens • Antiandrogens • Antiestrogens (tamoxifen) • Corticosteroids • Estrogens • Progestins	• Interfere with binding of normal hormones to receptor proteins, manipulate hormone levels, and alter hormone environment • Mechanism of action not always clear • Therapy usually palliative and not cytotoxic or curative	• No known toxic effect

Sample chemotherapy protocols

Chemotherapeutic drugs are often given in combinations called protocols. Here are the protocols typically given for some common cancers.

Specific cancers	Protocols	Drugs
Bladder cancer	CISCA	• cisplatin • cyclophosphamide • Adriamycin (doxorubicin)
Breast cancer	AC	• Adriamycin (doxorubicin) • cyclophosphamide
	CFM	• cyclophosphamide • fluorouracil • mitoxantrone
Colon cancer	F-CL	• fluorouracil • calcium leucovorin
Gastric cancer	EAP	• etoposide • Adriamycin (doxorubicin) • Platinol (cisplatin)
Acute lymphocytic leukemia, induction	DVP-ASP	• daunorubicin • vincristine • prednisone • asparaginase
Acute lymphocytic leukemia, maintenance	MM	• mercaptopurine • methotrexate
Acute myelocytic leukemia, induction	CD	• cytarabine • daunorubicin
Acute myelocytic leukemia, consolidation	MC	• mitoxantrone • cytarabine
Chronic lymphocytic leukemia, blast crisis	CVP (COP)	• cyclophosphamide • vincristine (Oncovin) • prednisone
Lung cancer, small-cell	CAE	• cyclophosphamide • Adriamycin (doxorubicin) • etoposide
Lung cancer, non-small-cell	CAP	• cyclophosphamide • Adriamycin (doxorubicin) • Platinol (cisplatin)

Both generic and trade names may be used in protocol abbreviations.

When trade names are used, you'll find the generic name in parentheses.

(continued)

Sample chemotherapy protocols *(continued)*

Specific cancers	Protocols	Drugs
Lymphoma (Hodgkin's disease)	ABVD	• Adriamycin (doxorubicin) • bleomycin • vinblastine • dacarbazine
Lymphoma, malignant	BACOP	• bleomycin • Adriamycin (doxorubicin) • cyclophosphamide • Oncovin (vincristine) • prednisone
Pediatric acute myelocytic leukemia, induction	DA	• daunorubicin • ARA-C (cytarabine)
Sarcomas, bony and soft tissue	ICEM	• ifosfamide • carboplatin • etoposide • mesna
Wilms' tumor	VA	• vincristine • actinomycin-D (dactino-mycin)

Biological therapy

Biological therapy consists mostly of administration of drugs known as biological response modifiers (BRMs), which alter the body's response to cancer. In addition to beneficial effects, some BRMs cause direct cytotoxicity.

Immunotherapy

In cancer immunotherapy, drugs are used to enhance the body's ability to destroy cancer cells. Cancer immunotherapy seeks to evoke effective immune response to human tumors by altering the way cells grow, mature, and respond to cancer cells. Immunotherapy may include administration of monoclonal antibodies, immunomodulatory cytokines, and tumor vaccines.

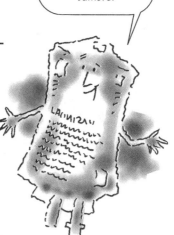

Some drugs try to pump up the immune system's response to tumors.

Monoclonal antibodies

Monoclonal antibodies provide an important diagnostic tool. Serum assays with monoclonal antibodies are commonly used to monitor solid tumors. For example, a monoclonal antibody called CA-125 is used to monitor ovarian cancer. A monoclonal antibody called prostate-specific antigen is used to monitor prostate cancer.

The use of monoclonal antibodies in treating cancer remains investigational. Research into the use of monoclonal antibodies includes trials of antibodies conjugated to drugs, radioisotopes, and toxins.

Immunomodulatory cytokines

Immunomodulatory cytokines are intracellular messenger proteins (proteins that deliver messages within cells). They include interferon, interleukins, tumor necrosis factor, and colony-stimulating factors.

Interferon

Interferon is subdivided into categories. Type I interferon includes alpha and beta interferons. Type II includes gamma interferon. Interferon inhibits viral replication, has immunoregulatory effects, and may also directly inhibit tumor proliferation.

Interferon alpha is approved for treating chronic myeloid leukemia, hairy cell leukemia, and AIDS-related Kaposi's sarcoma. It's also used with low-grade malignant lymphoma, multiple myeloma, and renal cell carcinoma.

Interferon gamma is produced by lymphocytes and is used to treat chronic granulomatous disease. Its use as an antitumor agent remains investigational.

Interleukins

Interleukins are cytokines whose primary function is to deliver messages to leukocytes. Interleukin 2 (IL-2) is an approved anticancer agent. IL-2 stimulates the proliferation and cytolytic activity of T cells and natural killer cells. High doses of IL-2 have been effective in a few patients with metastatic renal cell carcinoma and melanoma. The other interleukins remain investigational for cancer therapy.

Tumor necrosis factor

Tumor necrosis factor (TNF) plays a role in the inflammatory response to tumors and cancer cells. In animal studies, TNF has sometimes produced impressive antitumor responses. Unfortunately, this drug's high toxicity and occasional low antitumor response has limited its clinical development.

Colony-stimulating factors

Colony-stimulating factors (CSFs) are cytokines that regulate hematopoietic growth and differentiation. CSFs have been helpful in the clinical care of patients receiving myelosuppressive chemotherapy. Examples of CSFs include:
• erythropoietin, which induces erythroid maturation (maturation of red blood cells) and increases the release of reticulocytes from the bone marrow
• granulocyte CSF
• granulocyte-macrophage CSF
• interleukin-3, which increases the number of erythroid, myeloid, and megakaryocytic precursors
• thrombopoietin, which supports megakaryocyte maturation and platelet production.

Cellular therapy

In cellular therapy, immune effector cells are transferred to a tumor-bearing host. Different lymphokines — such as lymphokine-activated killer cells — are used in this procedure. Lymphokines fight cancer by:
• stimulating the production of T cells
• activating the lytic (cell-destroying) mechanisms of macrophages
• promoting the migration of lymphoid cells from the bloodstream
• stimulating the release of other cytokines, such as TNF and interferon gamma.

Drug preparation

Many health care institutions use existing guidelines as a basis for their policies and procedures regarding chemotherapeutic drugs. Among the major sources for these guidelines are the following agencies and associations:

• The American Society of Hospital Pharmacists has published guidelines for the preparation of chemotherapeutic drugs since 1990.

• The Occupational Safety and Health Administration (OSHA) published its revised standards for controlling exposure to chemotherapeutic drugs in 1995.

• The Oncologic Nursing Society produced standards for nursing education, practice, and administration of chemotherapy in 1996.

• The Intravenous Nurses Society issued revised standards of practice for the safe delivery of antineoplastic drugs in infusion therapy in 1998.

Certification required

At the local level, most health care facilities require nurses and pharmacists involved in the preparation and delivery of chemotherapeutic drugs to complete a certification program covering the competent and safe delivery of antineoplastic drugs and care of the patient with cancer.

Protective measures

Preparation of chemotherapeutic drugs requires adherence to guidelines regarding work area and equipment, clothing, and specific safety measures. Preparation may be performed by an oncology-certified nurse, a pharmacist, or (in states that allow it) a pharmacy technician.

Area and equipment

Prepare chemotherapeutic drugs in a quiet, well-ventilated work space, away from heating or cooling vents, refrigerators, and people. A restricted area away from people is best. Do all admixing or compounding within a class II biological safety cabinet (BSC) or laminar airflow hood that is vented to the outside with the blower on at all times. If a class II BSC isn't available, OSHA recommends that you wear a special respirator.

Punctureproof, shatterproof, and leakproof

Have close access to a sink, alcohol sponges, and sterile gauze pads, as well as the OSHA-required hazardous waste containers, sharps containers, and chemotherapy spill kit. Hazardous waste containers should be made of punctureproof, shatterproof, leakproof plastic. Use them to dispose of all contaminated I.V. containers, tubing, filters, needles, and syringes. (For a list of other supplies needed to prepare chemotherapeutic drugs, see *Equipment for preparing chemotherapeutic drugs*.)

An absorbent, plastic-backed liner should cover the work surface. This liner must be changed immediately if there is a spill. Depending on your facility's policy, the liner should also be changed after each use of the work surface, at the end of the shift, or at the end of the day.

Clothing

Essential clothing includes a gown, gloves, and goggles or a face shield.

Disposable, water-resistant, and lint-free

Gowns should be disposable, water-resistant, nonpermeable, and lint-free. They should have long sleeves, knitted cuffs, and a closed front.

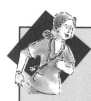

Running smoothly

Equipment for preparing chemotherapeutic drugs

Before preparing chemotherapeutic drugs, the following equipment should be in your work area:

- patient's medication order or record
- prescribed drugs
- appropriate diluent (if necessary)
- medication labels
- long-sleeved gown
- latex chemotherapy gloves
- face shield or goggles and face mask
- chemoabsorbent disposable pad and covers for the work surface
- 18G needles
- hydrophobic filter or dispensing pin
- syringes with luer-lock fittings and needles of various sizes
- I.V. tubing with luer-lock fittings
- 70% alcohol
- sterile gauze pads
- plastic bags with "hazardous drug" labels
- sharps disposal container
- hazardous waste container
- chemotherapy spill kit.

Essential accessories

Gloves designed for use with chemotherapeutic drugs are disposable, made of thick latex, and extend up the forearm to the elbow. They're also powder-free because powder can carry contamination from the chemicals into the surrounding air. Double gloving may be required when gloves aren't the best quality or when contact with the chemotherapeutic drug will be prolonged. Change gloves every hour (some sources suggest as frequently as every half-hour) and whenever a tear or puncture occurs. Wash your hands before putting on the gloves and after removing them.

> **Memory jogger**
>
> For correct clothing, remember the 3 G's: gown, gloves, goggles.

Extra care required

Take extra care to protect staff, patients, and the environment from unnecessary exposure to the chemotherapeutic drug. Don't leave the preparation area while wearing the personal protective gear you wore during drug preparation.

Not a good idea

Eating, drinking, smoking, or applying cosmetics in the preparation area violates OSHA recommendations.

Do it beforehand

Put on protective equipment before beginning work in the BSC. Before preparing the drugs, clean the internal surfaces of the cabinet with 70% alcohol and a disposable towel; do the same after you're finished and after any spill. Discard the towel into the leakproof chemical waste container. Change the absorbent pad on the work surface when you finish the preparation or whenever a spill occurs.

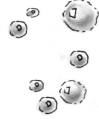

Wash thoroughly

If the drug comes in contact with your skin, wash the skin thoroughly with soap (not a germicidal agent) and water. If eye contact occurs, flood the eye with water or an isotonic eyewash for at least 5 minutes while holding the eyelid open.

Postexposure action

After any accidental exposure, obtain a medical evaluation as soon as possible. Document the exposure in your employee health record, describing the drug, concentration, and approximate amount to which you were exposed.

More advice

Some other safety precautions to keep in mind:
• Use aseptic technique when preparing all drugs.
• Vent vials with a hydrophobic filter, or use negative pressure techniques.
• Use a needle with a hydrophobic filter to remove solutions from vials.
• When you break ampules, wrap a sterile gauze pad or alcohol sponge around the neck of the ampule to decrease the chances of droplet contamination.
• Wear a face mask and goggles to protect yourself against splashes and aerosolized drugs.
• Don't clip needles, break syringes, or remove needles from syringes used in drug preparation. Place tubing, syringes, and all connected needles into the waste container for sharps disposal; don't remove or recap the needles.
• Use only syringes and I.V. sets that have luer-lock fittings. Label all chemotherapeutic drugs with a chemotherapy hazard label.

Transport tactics

Transport the medication in a sealable plastic bag, prominently labeled as a hazardous drug. Only employees who have been educated in the safe handling and disposal of chemotherapeutic drugs should come in contact with them.

The spiel on spills

Be sure your facility's protocol for spills is available in any area where chemotherapeutic drugs are handled, including patient care areas. Chemotherapy spill kits should be available as well. (See *Inside a chemotherapy spill kit*.)

If a spill occurs in or out of the preparation area, follow your facility's protocol, which is probably based on OSHA regulations. This protocol will likely instruct you to:
• Put on protective garments if you're not already wearing them.
• Isolate the area, and contain the spill with absorbent materials from the spill kit.
• Use the disposable dustpan and scraper to collect any broken glass; carefully place the dustpan, scraper, and

Inside a chemotherapy spill kit

A chemotherapy spill kit should contain:

• long-sleeved gown that's water-resistant and nonpermeable, with cuffs and back closure
• shoe covers
• two pairs of powder-free surgical gloves (for double gloving)
• respirator mask
• chemical splash goggles
• disposable dustpan and plastic scraper (for collecting broken glass)
• plastic-backed absorbent towels, or spill-control pillows
• dessicant powder or granules (for absorbing wet contents)
• disposable sponges
• two large cytotoxic waste disposal bags.

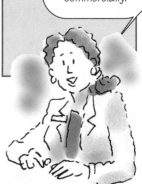

Low-cost spill kits are available commercially.

glass in a leakproof, punctureproof, plastic hazardous waste container.
• Place nonsharp materials in cytotoxic waste disposal bags.
• Prevent the aerosolization of the drug at all times.
• Clean the spill area three times with detergent solution followed by clear water.

Drug administration

Because dosage, route, and timing must be exact to avoid possibly fatal complications, only oncology-certified nurses should be involved in administering chemotherapeutic drugs or teaching patients or caregivers to give them. If you have the skill and educational background, follow these four steps:

 Perform a preadministration check.

 Obtain I.V. access.

 Give drugs.

 Conclude the treatment.

Performing a preadministration check

Before administering any chemotherapeutic drugs, get another registered nurse who's involved in the patient's therapy to help you double-check the order for the complete chemotherapy protocol.

Is the identity identical?

Confirm that the order and the drug label have identical information: the patient's name, the drug name and dosage, and the route, rate, and frequency of administration. If dosage depends on the results of certain laboratory tests, review the appropriate laboratory reports.

Which drugs by which route

Make sure that you understand clearly which drugs are to be given and by which route. Check whether the drug is classified as a vesicant, nonvesicant, or irritant. (See *Risks of tissue damage*, page 268.)

Before you give that drug!

Risks of tissue damage

To administer chemotherapy safely, you need to know each drug's potential for damaging tissue. In this regard, chemotherapeutic drugs are classified as vesicant, nonvesicant, or irritant.

Vesicants

Vesicants cause a reaction so severe that blisters form and tissue is damaged or destroyed. These drugs are subdivided according to whether they cause short-term or long-term injury. Short-term injury will eventually heal; long-term injury requires surgical excision.

Chemotherapeutic vesicants that cause short-term injury include:

- cisplatin
- etoposide
- mechlorethamine
- plicamycin
- vinblastine
- vincristine
- vinorelbine.

Chemotherapeutic vesicants that cause long-term injury include:

- dactinomycin
- daunorubicin
- doxorubicin
- epirubicin
- idarubicin
- mitomycin
- mitoxantrone
- nitrogen mustards.

Nonvesicants

Nonvesicants don't cause undue irritation or damage. Chemotherapeutic nonvesicants include:

- asparaginase
- bleomycin
- carboplatin
- cyclophosphamide
- cytarabine
- floxuridine
- fluorouracil
- ifosfamide.

Irritants

Irritants can cause a local venous response, with or without a skin reaction. These symptoms usually don't last long; tissue damage is uncommon and necrosis doesn't occur. Chemotherapeutic irritants include:

- carmustine
- dacarbazine
- streptozocin.

First or last

Sometimes an irritant or vesicant may be given first because that is when the vein is healthiest; other times it's given last so the maximum number of drugs can be administered through one site.

Confirm and verify

Confirm any written orders for needed antiemetics, fluids, diuretics, or electrolyte supplements to be given before, during, or after chemotherapy administration.

Verify the patient's level of understanding of treatment and adverse effects. If required, make sure that either the patient or a responsible family member has signed an informed consent form. (See *Preventing errors.*)

Advice from the experts

Preventing errors

Follow these precautions to prevent errors in chemotherapy administration:

• Only qualified personnel should write orders or administer chemotherapy. With rare exceptions, the administration of chemotherapy is not an emergency procedure.

• All orders should be double-checked by the personnel preparing and administering the drugs.

• Just one or two nurses should care for the patient, so they can communicate and work together to chart which drugs have been given and repeatedly check the "five rights" of drug administration (right drug, right patient, right time, right dosage, right route).

• Any aspect of the order that is contrary to customary practice or to what has been done for the patient in the past should be questioned, especially when unusually high doses or unusual schedules are involved.

• The nurse should not permit any distractions while checking an order or administering treatment.

• Orders for chemotherapy should be written only by the attending doctor or oncology fellow who is responsible for the patient's care and most familiar with the drug regimen and dosing schedule — not by a resident or an intern.

• Verbal orders for chemotherapy should not be given or taken.

Obtaining I.V. access

Assemble the equipment you'll need to start the I.V. and to prepare to administer the drug. (See *Equipment for administering chemotherapeutic drugs.*) The infiltration kit and the chemotherapy spill kit need not be in the room with you, but they should be immediately available because time is critical in determining the severity of an infiltration or a spill.

Put on a long-sleeved gown, latex chemotherapy gloves, and a face shield or goggles. Carefully check the doctor's order once again, prepare the proper dose using aseptic technique, and review the drug's potential adverse effects.

The right vein

Examine the possibilities for venous access. Don't use an existing peripheral I.V. line. If a permanent access device isn't in place, follow these suggestions:

  select a site where veins aren't damaged or distal to previously used areas

  avoid extremities that have impaired circulation

designate the line "For chemotherapy only."

When giving vesicants, avoid sites where damage to underlying tendons or nerves can occur (for example,

Running smoothly

Equipment for administering chemotherapeutic drugs

To administer chemotherapeutic drugs, gather the following equipment:

- prescribed drugs
- I.V. access supplies, if necessary
- sterile normal saline solution
- I.V. syringes and tubing with luer-lock connectors
- leakproof chemical waste container labeled "Caution: Biohazardous Waste"

- long-sleeved gown
- latex chemotherapy gloves
- face shield or goggles
- chemotherapy spill kit
- infiltration kit.

veins in the antecubital fossa, near the wrist, or in the back of the hand). Also, take into consideration the potential for drug incompatibilities, the frequency of administration, and the vesicant potential of the drug. Select the venous access device with the largest possible gauge (to accommodate the therapy and reduce the risk of infiltration), insert it into the vein, and then infuse 5 to 10 ml of sterile normal saline solution (NSS) to confirm vein patency before beginning the infusion.

Site-seeing encouraged

Apply a transparent dressing so the site can be observed at all times for early signs of infiltration and vein irritation.

Giving drugs

Before attaching the medication container, prime the I.V. line with NSS or dextrose 5% in water (D_5W), depending on facility and pharmacy protocols and compatibility with the chemotherapeutic drug. This helps prevent the possibility of splashing the drug.

Infusion pump insight

Avoid using an infusion pump to administer vesicants because the pump will continue the infusion after infiltration occurs. Instead, use a rate-controlling gravity device or an electronic infusion device.

Vesicant variations

For intermittent administration of a vesicant drug, instill the drug either into the side port of an infusing I.V. line or by direct I.V. push. Draw back on the plunger every few minutes to verify blood return and vein integrity, again according to facility policy and procedure. (See *Preventing infiltration*.)

If a vesicant drug is to be infused for longer than 1 hour or the infusion is continuous, administer it through a central venous line or an implanted vascular access device (VAD). Be sure to inspect these sites for infiltration as closely as you would a peripheral site.

Nonvesicant variations

Administer nonvesicant drugs and irritants in one of three ways: by direct I.V. push, through the side port of an infusing I.V. line, or as a continuous infusion.

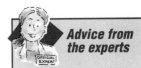

Advice from the experts

Preventing infiltration

Follow these guidelines when giving vesicants:

• Use only fresh sites.
• Use a distal vein that allows successive proximal venipunctures.
• Avoid using the hand, wrist, and antecubital space, damaged areas, or those with compromised circulation.
• Don't probe or "fish" for veins.
• Place a transparent dressing over the site.
• Start the push delivery or the infusion with normal saline solution (NSS) or dextrose 5% in water (D_5W).
• Avoid using an infusion pump.
• Test frequently for blood return; inspect the site for swelling and erythema.
• Tell patient to report burning, stinging, pain, pruritus, or temperature changes near the site.
• After drug administration, flush the line with 20 ml of NSS or D_5W.
• Administer vesicants in the order prescribed when infusing multiple drugs.

Investigating infiltration

Check for infiltration before and during the infusion by flushing the catheter with NSS to ensure patency. If swelling occurs at the I.V. site, the solution is infiltrating. Also, rely on the patient and his level of comfort; sudden discomfort during drug administration or flushing could indicate infiltration. Keep in mind the expression: "When in doubt, take it out!" (A less reliable way to check for infiltration is to lower the I.V. container and watch for blood return or backflow. The needle may have punctured the opposite vein wall yet still rest partially within the vein, producing backflow even in the presence of infiltration.)

Protection from sunlight

During infusion, some drugs need protection from direct sunlight to avoid breakdown. Cover the container and tubing with a brown bag or aluminum foil, taping it securely along the length of the tubing.

Monitor, instruct, observe

During the infusion, closely monitor the patient for signs of a hypersensitivity reaction or infiltration. Instruct the patient to report any burning, stinging, or pain at or near the site. Observe around the site for streaky redness along the vein and other skin changes.

In between administering drugs

Infuse 20 ml of sterile NSS or D_5W (depending on compatibility) between administration of different chemotherapeutic drugs and before discontinuing the I.V. line. This will flush the medication from the infusion delivery set, further preventing drug leakage and possible exposure when the catheter is removed.

Concluding treatment

After discontinuation of the I.V. line, take the following steps:

• Dispose of used needles, syringes, and all other waste material (including all protective coverings worn while administering the infusion) in the chemical waste container or in clearly labeled, leakproof, sealable plastic bags. All disposable equipment and unused medications are considered hazardous waste and should be disposed of according to your facility's policy.

• Wash your hands thoroughly with soap and warm water, even though you've worn gloves.
• Document each drug administered, including dose, route of administration, type and volume of solution, and adverse reactions.
• According to facility policy and procedures, wear protective clothing when handling all excreta from the patient for 48 hours after chemotherapy treatment. Dispose of all cleaning materials in the appropriate hazardous waste containers or hazardous linen collection bags. Observe standard precautions at all times.

Complications of chemotherapy

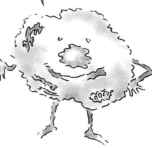

Properties that make chemotherapeutic drugs effective in killing cancer cells also make them toxic to normal cells.

The properties that make chemotherapeutic drugs effective in killing cancer cells also make them toxic to normal cells. No organ system is untouched by chemotherapy. Therefore, all administration protocols strive to time the treatments and adjust the doses in a way that maximizes the effects against cancer cells while allowing time for normal cells and tissues to recover between courses of treatment.

Immediate, short-term, and long-term

Complications resulting from chemotherapy can be categorized as immediate, short-term, and long-term, based on when exposure to the drug began.

Immediate adverse effects

Infiltration and hypersensitivity reactions are the most common reasons for immediate adverse effects of chemotherapy.

Infiltration

Infiltration occurs when a punctured vein or a leaky I.V. site allows passage of an I.V. fluid or drug solution into the tissues surrounding the vein. Infiltrated I.V. fluid such as NSS can be painless or, if more than a small amount of fluid escapes, can cause a sensation of tightness or pressure at the affected area. However, hypertonic fluids and many drugs can be irritating and even damaging to the veins and S.C. tissues surrounding them.

Drugs and I.V. fluids can be classified into three groups: vesicants, nonvesicants, and irritants. The last two don't pose much of a threat and can be handled easily. Vesicants are fraught with danger and require vigorous response.

Nonvesicants and irritants

A nonvesicant causes little or no discomfort when infusing and little or no damage if infiltration occurs. NSS is an example of a nonvesicant infusate.

An irritant causes a local venous response with or without an accompanying skin reaction. The patient may complain of burning, pain, aching along the vein, or itching. You may observe erythema surrounding the venipuncture site or along the vein path. Certain chemotherapeutic drugs are also associated with a response called a flare reaction, which involves urticaria and a stinging sensation. These symptoms usually resolve soon after the drug is discontinued. In some cases, an irritant may cause prolonged problems, such as persistent phlebitis, thrombosis development, and hyperpigmentation of the vein.

You can treat an irritated vein by applying ice, increasing the dilution of the infused medication, or decreasing the infusion rate of the drug. Premedication with an antihistamine or a corticosteroid may also help.

Vesicants

Infiltration with a vesicant (also called "extravasation") may cause blistering, tissue damage, even tissue necrosis. The irritation to the vein may be so severe that plasma escapes into the tissues, even though the infusion began with a fresh, intact vein. The degree of injury may vary, from short-term injury that will likely heal to long-term injury that doesn't heal and will require surgical debridement.

Initial signs of infiltration may resemble those of vein irritation: burning, pain, and erythema. Eventually, infiltration into the surrounding tissues will cause swelling and severe pain. (To distinguish between infiltration and other reactions, see *Assessing for infiltration, vein irritation, and flare reactions.*) You may still get a blood return if part or all of the catheter or needle tip remains inside the vein. Ulceration will not appear until 2 to 4 days after infiltration.

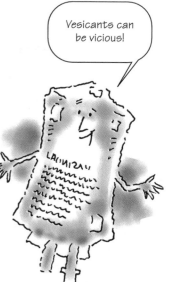

Vesicants can be vicious!

Yikes! An emergency!

If a vesicant has infiltrated, it's an emergency! Quickly take the following six steps — they're designed to limit the damage by cutting off the infusion, counteracting the effects of the drug, and containing the affected area:

☞ Stop the I.V. infusion and remove the I.V. device. The only exception is if you need the catheter to infuse an antidote into the affected area. Treatment for infiltration of specific drugs should be in accordance with manufacturer's guidelines.

Assessing for infiltration, vein irritation, and flare reactions

This chart tells you how to determine whether a patient who's receiving chemotherapy has experienced infiltration, vein irritation, or a flare reaction.

Assessment parameter	Infiltration	Vein irritation	Flare reaction
Blood return	Absent (in some cases, may be present)	Usually present	Usually present
Pain	Severe pain or burning lasting minutes to hours, eventually subsiding; usually occurs at the needle site while the drug is being given	Aching and tightness along the vein	Not present
Redness	Blotchy redness at needle site	Full length of vein may be reddened or darkened	Immediate blotches or streaks along the vein as drug is given; usually subsides within 30 minutes, with or without treatment
Swelling	At needle site, either immediately or hours later	Not likely	Not likely
Ulceration	Usually appears 48 to 96 hours after drug administration	Not likely	Not likely
Other	Change in quality of infusion; increased resistance; local tingling; sensory deficits (may appear as delayed manifestations)	None	Itching

Estimate the amount of infiltrated solution and notify the doctor.

Instill the appropriate antidote according to facility protocol. (See *Antidotes to vesicant infiltration*.) Usually, you'll give an antidote for vesicant infiltration either by instilling it through an existing I.V. device or by using a 1-ml syringe to inject small amounts S.C. in a circle around the infiltrated area.

Remove the venous access device.

Elevate the arm.

Apply ice packs to the affected area. The only exception is the vinca alkaloids, which require warm compresses.

Memory jogger

As soon as you spot an infiltration, think of the three C's:

Cut off (the infusion)

Counteract (effects of the drug)

Contain (the affected area).

Don't forget the paperwork!

Document the location of the infiltration site, the patient's symptoms, the estimated amount of infiltrated solution, and the treatment. Also record the time you notified the doctor and the doctor's name. Continue documenting the site's appearance and associated symptoms.

If ulceration occurs, apply antibiotic cream and change the dressing frequently. If severe necrosis occurs, the patient may need surgery and physical therapy.

Hypersensitivity reactions

Immediate hypersensitivity reactions range from urticaria at the site to anaphylaxis. A hypersensitivity reaction can occur at the initial dose of the drug or not until a later dose. (See *Hypersensitivity risk of chemotherapeutic drugs*, page 278.)

Hypersensitivity reactions generally happen within the first few minutes of infusion. Signs and symptoms are the same as those of any drug reaction. (See *Signs and symptoms of immediate hypersensitivity*, page 279.)

The specific treatment for a hypersensitivity reaction will depend on the severity of the reaction and the form it takes. Usually, you'll follow these six steps:

Stop the infusion immediately.

Stay with the patient.

Check the vital signs.

Call the doctor.

 Keep the I.V. line open with NSS.

Administer emergency drugs as ordered by the doctor.

Antidotes to vesicant extravasation

The chart below provides examples of antidotes you may administer in the event of infiltration by a vesicant.

Infiltrating agent	Antidote	Nursing considerations
• amsacrine • daunorubicin • doxorubicin • epirubicin • idarubicin	• dimethyl sulfoxide (DMSO)	• Apply a cold pack for at least 1 hour 4 times per day for 3 to 5 days. • DMSO 50% to 90% solution can be applied to the extravasation site every 6 hours for 14 days. Don't cover the application site; allow it to air dry. • Injection of sodium bicarbonate is contraindicated.
• mechlorethamine (nitrogen mustard)	• 10% sodium thiosulfate	• Mix 4 ml of 10% sodium thiosulfate with 6 ml of sterile water for injection. • Inject 4 ml of the solution into the existing I.V. line that extravasated. • After the injection through the I.V. line, remove the catheter. • Inject 2 to 3 ml of the solution subcutaneously (S.C.) clockwise into the infiltrated area using a 25G needle. Change the needle with each new injection. • Apply ice for 6 to 12 hours.
• etoposide • teniposide • navelbine • vinblastine • vincristine • vindesine	• hyaluronidase	• Inject 3 to 5 ml of hyaluronidase (150 units/ml) S.C. clockwise into the infiltrated area using a 25G needle; change the needle with each injection. • Apply heat for 1 hour and repeat 4 times per day for 3 to 5 days. • Application of cold is contraindicated. • Injection of hydrocortisone is contraindicated.

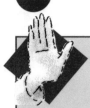

Before you give that drug!

Hypersensitivity risk of chemotherapeutic drugs

Note the risk levels associated with these chemotherapeutic drugs.

High risk	Moderate to low risk	Very low risk
• asparaginase	• Anthracyclines	• cytarabine
• paclitaxel	• bleomycin	• cyclophosphamide
	• carboplatin	• chlorambucil
	• cisplatin	• dacarbazine
	• cyclosporine	• fluorouracil
	• docetaxel	• ifosfamide
	• etoposide	• mitoxantrone
	• melphalan	
	• methotrexate	
	• procarbazine	
	• teniposide	

Memory jogger

When your patient has an immediate hypersensitivity reaction, guide your reactions with these three pairs of words:

• **st**op & **st**ay (stop the infusion and stay with the patient)

• **c**heck & **c**all (check vital signs and call the doctor)

• **o**pen & **o**rdered (keep the I.V. line open and administer ordered medications).

Epinephrine is the drug of choice for a severe hypersensitivity reaction. Others include antihistamines, corticosteroids, and bronchodilators. Once you've administered the drug, monitor vital signs every 2 minutes until the patient is stable, then every 5 minutes for the next 30 minutes, and then every 15 minutes for 1 to 2 hours — or follow facility policy and procedures for acute treatment of allergic reactions.

Throughout the episode, maintain the patient's airway, oxygenation, cardiac output, and tissue perfusion. Check that life support equipment is available in case the patient fails to respond. Document the reaction to the drug and the response to treatment.

Whether to continue

If the reaction was severe, the patient shouldn't receive the drug again. A milder reaction, such as a rash that responded to an antihistamine, may allow continuation of the drug once the patient's condition is stable. Future use will require premedication with an antihistamine and perhaps a corticosteroid. Be sure to check with the doctor for the pre-infusion treatments before subsequent therapy cycles.

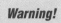

Warning!

Signs and symptoms of immediate hypersensitivity

An immediate hypersensitivity reaction to a chemotherapeutic drug will appear within 15 minutes after starting to administer the drug.

Organ system	Subjective complaints	Objective findings
Respiratory	• Dyspnea, inability to speak, tightness in chest	• Stridor, bronchospasm, decreased air movement
Skin	• Pruritus, urticaria	• Cyanosis, urticaria, angioedema
Cardiovascular	• Chest pain, increased heart rate	• Tachycardia, hypotension, arrhythmias
CNS	• Dizziness, agitation, anxiety	• Decreased sensorium, loss of consciousness
GI	• Abdominal pain, nausea	• Increased bowel sounds, diarrhea, vomiting.

Short-term adverse effects

Short-term adverse effects include — but aren't limited to — the adverse effects people commonly associate with chemotherapy, such as nausea and vomiting, hair loss, and diarrhea. Tissues that have a large proportion of frequently reproducing cells include bone marrow, hair follicles, and GI mucosa. Damage to these tissues produces myelosuppression, alopecia, stomatitis, and diarrhea.

Nausea and vomiting

Nausea and vomiting appear in three patterns: anticipatory, acute, and delayed. Each has its own cause. Because a single course of chemotherapy may span several weeks of daily treatments, expect to see a mix of these three patterns. Managing them is a difficult balancing act but is crucial because of the effects nausea and vomiting have on the patient's nutritional status, emotional well-being, and fluid and electrolyte balance.

Just thinking about it

The anticipatory pattern is a learned response from prior nausea and vomiting after a dose of chemotherapy. It's most likely to develop in people who experienced moderate to severe symptoms after the prior dose, have high anxiety levels, and are younger. Though anxiolytics and behavior modification techniques may help prevent this pattern, successful posttreatment control of nausea and vomiting is far more effective.

Within 24 hours

Acute nausea and vomiting occur within the first 24 hours of treatment. A major factor is the emetogenic (vomit-inducing) potential of the drug or drugs administered. For example, cisplatin has a high potential; more than 90% of patients receiving it will experience nausea and vomiting. Bleomycin, however, has a low potential; only 10% to 30% of patients are affected. Other factors contributing to occurrence and severity include the combination of drugs, doses and routes of administration, rates of administration, treatment schedules, and patient characteristics.

Pretreatment includes a serotonin antagonist and dexamethasone, administered I.V. or orally. Prochlorperazine may be effective with chemotherapeutic drugs that have low emetogenic potential. Again, nonpharmacologic techniques may also help, but they're no substitute for pharmacologic antiemetics.

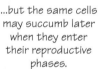

Healthy cells that reproduce frequently may survive the introduction of a chemotherapeutic drug during their resting phase...

Not out of the woods yet

Delayed nausea and vomiting is loosely designated as starting or continuing beyond 24 hours after chemotherapy has begun. Although its cause is less clearly understood than the anticipatory and acute patterns, the arsenal of drugs for treating it is larger. Besides serotonin antagonists and corticosteroids, various antihistamines and benzodiazepines as well as cannabinoids and metoclopramide are frequently effective.

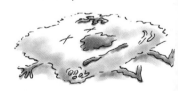

...but the same cells may succumb later when they enter their reproductive phases.

Myelosuppression

Myelosuppression is damage to the stem cells in the bone marrow. These cells are the precursors to cellular blood components — red and white blood cells and platelets — so their damage produces anemia, leukopenia, and thrombocytopenia. (See *Managing complications of chemotherapy*, page 282.)

Alopecia

Alopecia results from the destruction of rapidly dividing cells in the hair shaft or root. It may be minimal or severe. Regardless of degree, hair growth resumes in about 3 months — even, in many cases, if chemotherapy continues. Because so many patients find alopecia disturbing, reassurance about resumed hair growth is important.

Follicle fortification

Devices to prevent hair loss include scalp tourniquets and cooling caps. These devices attempt to limit superficial blood flow to the scalp during drug administration, thus partially protecting the hair follicles from the circulating drug. Such devices are apparently useful with certain drugs but are contraindicated with certain cancers. In addition, their use is controversial. Therefore, preparing the patient ahead of time and suggesting coping strategies if alopecia occurs are preferable.

Stomatitis

Stomatitis produces painful mouth ulcers 3 to 7 days after chemotherapy begins, with symptoms ranging from mild to severe. Because of the accompanying pain, stomatitis can lead to malnutrition and fluid and electrolyte imbalance if the patient is unable to chew and swallow adequate food and fluid. Treat stomatitis with scrupulous oral hygiene and topical anesthetic mixtures.

Diarrhea

Diarrhea — brought on because the rapidly dividing cells of the intestinal mucosa are killed — occurs in up to 75% of patients receiving chemotherapy. Complications of persistent diarrhea include weight loss, malnutrition, and dehydration. To minimize the effects of diarrhea, use dietary adjustments, antidiarrheal medications, and palliatives,

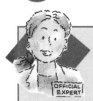

Advice from the experts

Managing complications of chemotherapy

This chart identifies some common adverse effects of chemotherapy and ways to minimize them.

Adverse effect	Signs and symptoms	Interventions
Anemia	Dizziness, fatigue, pallor, and shortness of breath after minimal exertion; low hemoglobin and hematocrit; may develop slowly over several courses of treatment	• Monitor hemoglobin, hematocrit, and red blood cell count; report dropping values; remember that dehydration from nausea, vomiting, and anorexia will cause hemoconcentration, yielding falsely high hematocrit readings. • Be prepared to administer a blood transfusion or erythropoietin. • Instruct the patient to take frequent rests, increase intake of iron-rich foods, and take a multivitamin with iron as prescribed.
Leukopenia	Susceptibility to infections; neutropenia (an absolute neutrophil count less than 1,500 cells/µl)	• Watch for the nadir, the point of lowest blood cell count (usually 7 to 14 days after last treatment). • Be prepared to administer colony-stimulating factors. • Institute neutropenic precautions in the hospitalized patient. • Include the following in patient and family teaching: good hygiene practices, signs and symptoms of infection, the importance of checking one's temperature regularly, how to prepare a low-microbe diet, and how to care for any vascular access devices. • Instruct the patient to avoid crowds, people with colds or respiratory infections, and fresh fruit, fresh flowers, and plants.
Thrombocytopenia	Bleeding gums, increased bruising, petechiae, hypermenorrhea, tarry stools, hematuria, coffee-ground emesis	• Monitor platelet count: under 50,000 cells/µl means a moderate risk of excessive bleeding; under 20,000 cells/µl means a major risk and the patient may need a platelet transfusion. • Avoid unnecessary I.M. injections or venipunctures; if either is necessary, apply pressure for at least 5 minutes; then apply a pressure dressing to the site. • Instruct patient to avoid cuts and bruises, shave with an electric razor, avoid blowing his nose, stay away from irritants that would trigger sneezing, and not use rectal thermometers. • Instruct patient to report sudden headaches (which could indicate potentially fatal intracranial bleeding).
Alopecia	Minimal: less than 25% Moderate: 25% to 50% Severe: more than 50% May occur suddenly 10 to 21 days after start of therapy; may include eyebrows, lashes, and body hair; regrowth will begin after 2 to 3 months	• Minimize shock and distress by warning patient of the possibility of hair loss, discussing why hair loss occurs, and describing how much hair loss to expect. • Suggest using hats, wigs, and artfully tied scarves. • For patients receiving drugs causing severe hair loss, suggest that shaving the head may be less stressful than watching the hair fall out. • Emphasize the need for appropriate head protection against sunburn and heat loss in the winter.

such as heat to the abdomen and barrier ointments to the rectal area.

Long-term adverse effects

Organ system dysfunction, especially in the hematopoietic and GI systems, is common after chemotherapy. These effects are usually temporary, but some systems suffer permanent damage that manifests itself long after chemotherapy. The renal, pulmonary, cardiac, reproductive, and neurologic systems all show a variety of temporary and permanent dysfunctions from exposure to chemotherapy.

A devastating effect

One devastating long-term effect of chemotherapy is secondary malignancy, frequently acute myeloid leukemia (AML), which follows treatment with an alkylating agent for multiple myeloma, Hodgkin's disease, and malignant lymphoma. The highest risk period for secondary AML is 2 to 10 years after chemotherapy. The prognosis is usually poor.

Teaching and documentation

Not only is cancer a frightening and frequently lethal disease, but also the only treatments for it — the only hopes for survival and cure — are ironically among the most noxious that humans have devised. Honor the courage of your patients by arming them with knowledge.

To give your patients some sense of control in the face of overwhelming odds, explain each procedure you do and teach them strategies for dealing with fear, pain, and the unwelcome adverse effects of chemotherapy. Keep in mind that a positive attitude and a strong emotional support system will enable your patients to better endure, if not actually overcome, the disease and its treatments.

In it for the long haul

Documentation is important for more than just legal reasons. Because the treatment for cancer can be prolonged, numerous health care providers and facilities may be involved over an extended period. Without clear and concise documentation of treatments given, actions taken, and pa-

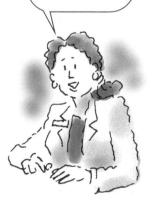

Honor the courage of your patients by arming them with knowledge.

tient responses, the chain of communication can become worthless. When that happens, the patient will most certainly experience additional suffering needlessly.

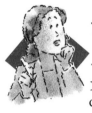

Quick quiz

1. The following are advantages of administering chemotherapy I.V., except:
   A. The drugs are completely absorbed and systemically distributed.
   B. The chances of acute nausea and vomiting are decreased.
   C. The dosage is highly accurate.
Answer: B. Administering chemotherapeutic drugs I.V. doesn't decrease the chance of nausea and vomiting.

2. A drug that is cycle-specific will attack normal and malignant cells during specific phases of cell development, except:
   A. the resting phase.
   B. metaphase.
   C. any of the cell's reproductive phases.
Answer: A. Cycle-specific drugs act primarily on proliferating cells; that is, when cells reproduce and divide (metaphase is one of the phases of cell reproduction). When cycle-specific chemotherapy is administered, cells in the resting phase survive.

3. OSHA requires that anyone administering chemotherapy must wear:
   A. special chemotherapy gloves.
   B. two pairs of latex surgical gloves.
   C. any type of latex gloves.
Answer: A. Chemotherapy gloves help prevent inadvertent exposure because they are thick and powderless and extend to the elbow.

Scoring

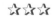 If you answered all three items correctly, congratulations! Now treat yourself to some extra time in your resting phase.

☆☆ If you answered less than three correctly, don't get discouraged. Sometimes it takes a few learning cycles before the information starts taking effect.

Parenteral nutrition

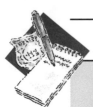

Just the facts

In this chapter, you'll learn:

♦ basic nutritional needs

♦ indications for parenteral nutrition

♦ nutritional solutions

♦ performing a nutritional assessment

♦ administering parenteral nutrition

♦ complications of parenteral nutrition.

Understanding parenteral nutrition

You may administer parenteral nutrition when illness or surgery prevents a patient from eating and metabolizing food. Common conditions that make parenteral nutrition necessary include:

- GI trauma
- pancreatitis
- ileus
- inflammatory bowel disease
- GI tract malignancy
- GI hemorrhage
- paralytic ileus
- GI obstruction
- short-bowel syndrome
- GI fistula
- severe malabsorption.

Critically ill patients may also receive parenteral nutrition if they're hemodynamically unstable or if GI tract blood flow is impaired.

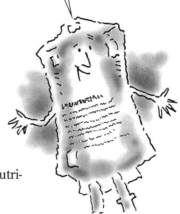

Consider using me to deliver parenteral nutrition if the patient is unable to eat or metabolize food.

Nutritional needs

Essential nutrients found in food provide energy, maintain body tissues, and aid body processes, such as growth, cell activity, enzyme production, and temperature regulation.

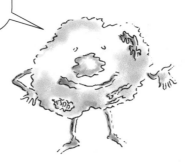

Nutrients in food are essential for me to remain active.

If forced to forgo food, you're going to need parenteral nutrition.

Food, metabolism, and energy

When carbohydrates, fats, and proteins are metabolized by the body, they produce energy, which is measured in calories (also called kilocalories). A normal healthy adult generally requires 2,000 to 3,000 calories a day. Specific requirements depend on an individual's size, sex, age, and level of physical activity.

Parenteral nutrients

A parenteral nutrition solution — also known as hyperalimentation, I.V. hyperalimentation, or I.V. feedings — may contain one or more of the following:
- dextrose
- proteins
- lipids
- electrolytes
- vitamins
- trace elements.

Depending on the type of therapy ordered, nutritional support solutions are administered through either a peripheral or central venous (CV) infusion device.

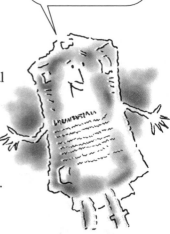

I offer calories and nutrients from dextrose, proteins, and electrolytes.

Central venous infusion

If a patient needs parenteral nutrition for more than 5 days, he usually requires total parenteral nutrition (TPN). TPN is delivered through a central line, usually placed in the subclavian vein, with the tip of the catheter in the superior vena cava.

Peripheral infusion

Peripheral parenteral nutrition (PPN) — also called partial parenteral nutrition — is the delivery of nutrients through a short catheter inserted into a peripheral vein. Generally, PPN provides fewer nonprotein calories than TPN because lower dextrose concentrations are used. A much larger volume of fluid must be infused for PPN to deliver the same number of calories as TPN. Therefore, most patients who require parenteral nutrition therapy receive TPN rather than PPN.

Benefits

Parenteral nutrition is an important support measure. Parenteral solutions can provide all needed nutrients when a patient is unable to take nutrients through the GI tract. This enables cells to function despite the patient's inability to take in or metabolize food.

Risks

Like all invasive procedures, parenteral nutrition incurs certain risks, including:
- catheter infection
- hyperglycemia (high blood glucose)
- hypokalemia (low blood potassium).
    Complications of parenteral nutrition can be minimized with careful monitoring of the catheter site, infusion rate, and laboratory test results.

A matter of access

Another disadvantage of parenteral nutrition is the need for vascular access. If peripheral access isn't possible because of poor vasculature, central access may be necessary, perhaps requiring surgical intervention.

It costs

Parenteral nutrition is expensive, about 10 times as expensive as enteral nutrition for the solutions alone. For this reason, it's used only when absolutely necessary.

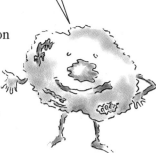

How did I survive when food intake stopped? Parenteral nutrition enabled me to keep functioning.

Nutritional deficiencies

The most common nutritional deficiencies involve protein and calories. Nutritional deficiencies may result from a nonfunctional GI tract, decreased food intake, increased metabolic need, or a combination of these factors.

Taking in less

Food intake may be decreased because of illness, decreased physical ability, or injury. Decreased food intake can occur with GI disorders such as paralytic ileus, surgery, or sepsis.

Up to twice the calories

Any increase in metabolic activity requires an increase in calorie intake. Fever commonly increases metabolic activity. The metabolic rate may also increase in victims of burns, trauma, disease, or stress; patients may require up to twice the calories of their basal metabolic rate (the minimum energy needed to maintain respiration, circulation, and other basic body functions).

Effects of protein-calorie deficiencies

When the body detects protein-calorie deficiency, it turns to its reserve sources of energy. Reserve energy is drawn from three sources, in order:

First, the body mobilizes and converts glycogen to glucose through a process called glycogenolysis.

Next, if necessary, the body draws energy from the fats stored in adipose tissue.

As a last resort, the body taps its store of essential visceral proteins (serum albumin and transferrin) and somatic body proteins (skeletal, smooth muscle, and tissue proteins). These proteins and their amino acids are converted to glucose for energy through a process called gluconeogenesis. When these essential body proteins break down, a negative nitrogen balance results (which means more protein is used by the body than is taken in). Starvation or disease-related stress contributes to this catabolic (destructive) state.

The body fights starvation by breaking down the proteins in bone, muscle, and other tissues. Parenteral nutrition can prevent this.

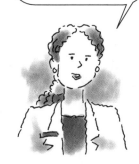

Protein-energy malnutrition

A deficiency of protein and energy (calories) results in protein-energy malnutrition (PEM), also called protein-calorie malnutrition. PEM refers to a spectrum of disorders that occur as a consequence of chronic inadequate protein or calorie intake or high metabolic protein and energy requirements.

Causes

Disorders that commonly lead to PEM include:
- cancer
- GI disorders
- chronic heart failure
- alcoholism
- conditions causing high metabolic needs, such as burns.

Consequences

The consequences of PEM may include the following:
- reduced enzyme and plasma protein production
- increased susceptibility to infection
- physical and mental growth deficiencies in children
- severe diarrhea and malabsorption
- numerous secondary nutritional deficiencies
- delayed wound healing
- mental fatigue.

Three forms

PEM takes three basic forms:

 iatrogenic PEM

 kwashiorkor

 marasmus.

Form #1

During hospitalization a patient's nutritional status often deteriorates because of inadequate protein or calorie intake, leading to iatrogenic PEM. Iatrogenic PEM affects more than 15% of patients in acute care centers. It's most common in patients hospitalized longer than 2 weeks.

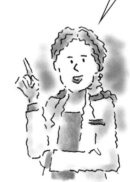

PEM occurs as a consequence of chronic inadequate protein or caloric intake or high metabolic protein and energy requirements.

Form #2

Kwashiorkor results from severe protein deficiencies without a calorie deficit. It occurs most often in children ages 1 to 3. In the United States, it's usually secondary to the following:
- malabsorption disorders
- cancer and cancer therapies
- kidney disease
- hypermetabolic illness
- iatrogenic causes.

Form #3

The third form of malnutrition, marasmus, is a prolonged and gradual wasting of muscle mass and subcutaneous fat. It's caused by inadequate intake of protein, calories, and other nutrients. Marasmus occurs most commonly in infants ages 6 to 18 months, after gastrectomy, and in patients with cancer of the mouth and esophagus.

Nutritional assessment

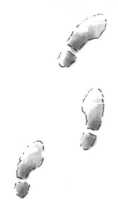

When illness or surgery compromises a patient's intake or alters his metabolic requirements, you'll need to assess the relationship between nutrients consumed and energy expended. A nutritional assessment provides insight into how well the patient's physiologic need for nutrients is being met. To assess nutritional status, follow these steps:
- Obtain a dietary history.
- Perform a physical assessment.
- Take anthropometric measurements.
- Review the results of pertinent diagnostic tests.
  Because poor nutritional status can affect most body systems, a thorough nutritional assessment helps you anticipate problems and intervene appropriately.

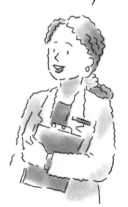

A nutritional assessment reveals the relationship between nutrients consumed and energy expended.

Dietary history

When obtaining a dietary history, check for signs of decreased food intake, increased metabolic requirements, or a combination of the two. Also check dietary recall, using either a 24-hour recall or diet diary. Note any factors that affect food intake and changes in appetite. Obtain a weight history, and observe for subtle signs of malnutrition. (See *Signs of poor nutrition*.)

Physical assessment

When performing a physical assessment, be sure to include the following:
- chief complaint
- present illness
- past medical history, including any previous major illnesses, injuries, hospitalizations, or surgeries
- allergies and history of intolerance to food and medications
- family history, including any familial, genetic, or environmental illnesses
- social history, including environmental, psychological, and sociologic factors that may influence nutritional status, such as alcoholism, living alone, or lack of transportation.

Anthropometry

Anthropometry compares the patient's measurements with established standards. It's an objective, noninvasive method for measuring overall body size, composition, and specific body parts. Commonly used anthropometric measurements include the following:
- height
- weight
- ideal body weight
- body frame size
- triceps skinfold thickness
- midarm circumference
- midarm muscle circumference.

Any finding of less than 90% of the standard measurement may indicate a need for nutritional support. (See *Taking anthropometric measurements*, pages 292 and 293.)

Diagnostic studies

Evidence of a nutritional problem often appears in the results of a diagnostic test. Tests are used to evaluate the following:
- visceral protein status

A nutritional problem often appears in the results of a diagnostic test.

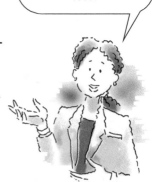

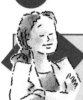

Peak technique

Taking anthropometric measurements

Follow the steps below to measure midarm circumference, triceps skinfold thickness, and midarm muscle circumference.

Midarm circumference
Locate the midpoint on the patient's upper arm using a nonstretching tape measure, and mark the midpoint with a marking pen.

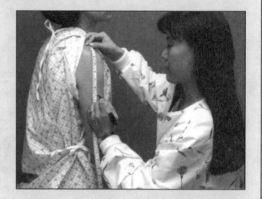

Triceps skinfold thickness
Determine the triceps skinfold thickness by grasping the patient's skin between thumb and forefinger approximately 1 cm above the midpoint. Place the calipers at the midpoint and squeeze the calipers for about 3 seconds. Record the measurement registered on the handle gauge to the nearest 0.5 mm. Take two more readings; then average all three to compensate for possible error.

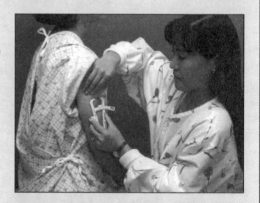

Midarm muscle circumference
At the midpoint, measure the midarm circumference. Calculate midarm muscle circumference by multiplying the triceps skinfold thickness (in centimeters) by 3.143 and subtracting the result from the midarm circumference.

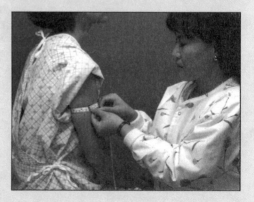

Taking anthropometric measurements (continued)

Interpreting your findings

Record all three measurements as percentages of the standard measurements using the following formula:

$$\frac{\text{Actual measurement}}{\text{Standard measurement}} \times 100$$

Compare the patient's percentage measurements with the standard. A measurement less than 90% of the standard indicates calorie deprivation; a measurement over 90% of the standard indicates adequate or more than adequate energy reserves.

Measurement	Standard	90%
Midarm circumference	Men: 29.3 cm Women: 26.5 cm	Men: 26.4 cm Women: 23.9 cm
Triceps skinfold thickness	Men: 12.5 mm Women: 16.5 mm	Men: 11.3 mm Women 14.9 mm
Midarm muscle circumference	Men: 25.3 cm Women 23.2 cm	Men: 22.8 cm Women: 20.9 cm

• lean body mass
• vitamin and mineral balance.

Diagnostic studies are also used to evaluate the effectiveness of nutritional support. (See *Detecting deficiencies,* pages 294 and 295.)

Indications for TPN

A patient may receive TPN for any of the following reasons:
• debilitating illness lasting longer than 2 weeks
• deficient or absent oral intake for longer than 7 days, as in cases of multiple trauma, severe burns, or anorexia nervosa
• loss of at least 10% of preillness weight
• serum albumin level below 3.5 g/dl
• poor tolerance of long-term enteral feedings
• chronic vomiting or diarrhea
• continued weight loss despite adequate oral intake
• GI disorders that prevent or severely reduce absorption, such as bowel obstruction, Crohn's disease, ulcerative colitis, short-bowel syndrome, cancer malabsorption syndrome, and bowel fistulas
• inflammatory GI disorders, such as wound infection, fistulas, or abscesses.

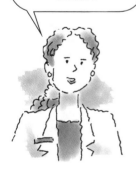

TPN is called for when lengthy or chronic illness leads to weight loss and decreased calorie and protein intake...

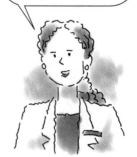

...PPN is used to help meet minimum calorie and protein requirements or to supplement oral or enteral feedings.

Detecting deficiencies

Laboratory studies help pinpoint nutritional deficiencies by aiding in the diagnosis of anemia, malnutrition, and other disorders. Check out this chart to learn about some commonly ordered diagnostic tests, their purposes, normal values, and implications. Albumin, prealbumin, transferrin, and triglyceride levels are the major indicators of nutritional deficiency.

Test and purpose	Normal values	Implications
Creatinine height index • Uses a 24-hour urine sample to determine adequacy of muscle mass	• Determined from a reference table of values based on a patient's height or weight	• Less than 80% of reference value: moderate depletion of muscle mass (protein reserves) • Less than 60% of reference value: severe depletion, with increased risk of compromised immune function
Hematocrit • Diagnoses anemia and dehydration	• Male: 42% to 50% • Female: 40% to 48% • Child: 29% to 41% • Neonate: 55% to 68%	• Increased values: severe dehydration, polycythemia • Decreased values: iron-deficiency anemia, excessive blood loss
Hemoglobin • Assesses blood's oxygen-carrying capacity to aid diagnosis of anemia, protein deficiency, and hydration status	• Older adult: 10 to 17 g/dl • Adult male: 13 to 18 g/dl • Adult female: 12 to 16 g/dl • Child: 9 to 15.5 g/dl • Neonate: 14 to 20 g/dl	• Increased values: dehydration, polycythemia • Decreased values: protein deficiency, iron-deficiency anemia, excessive blood loss, overhydration
Serum albumin • Helps assess visceral protein stores	• Adult: 3.5 to 5 g/dl • Child: same as adult • Neonate: 3.6 to 5.4 g/dl	• Decreased values: malnutrition; overhydration; liver or kidney disease; heart failure; excessive blood protein losses, such as from severe burns
Serum transferrin (similar to serum total iron binding capacity [TIBC]) • Helps assess visceral protein stores; has a shorter half-life than serum albumin and, thus, more accurately reflects current status	• Adult: 200 to 400 µg/dl • Child: 350 to 450 µg/dl • Neonate: 60 to 175 µg/dl	• Increased TIBC: iron deficiency, as in pregnancy or iron-deficiency anemia • Decreased TIBC: iron excess, as in chronic inflammatory states • Below 200 µg/dl: visceral protein depletion • Below 100 µg/dl: severe visceral protein depletion
Serum triglycerides • Screens for hyperlipidemia	• 40 to 200 mg/dl	• Increased values combined with increased cholesterol levels: increased risk of atherosclerotic disease • Decreased values: protein-energy malnutrition (PEM), steatorrhea

Detecting deficiencies *(continued)*

Test and purpose	Normal values	Implications
Skin sensitivity testing • Evaluates immune response compromised by PEM	• Immunocompetent patients exhibit a positive reaction within 24 hours, marked by a red area of 5 mm or greater at the test site	• Delayed, partial, or negative reaction (no response): may point to PEM
Total lymphocyte count • Diagnoses PEM	• 1,500 to 3,000/µl	• Increased values: infection or inflammation, leukemia, tissue necrosis • Decreased values: moderate to severe malnutrition if no other cause, such as influenza or measles, is identified
Total protein screen • Detects hyperproteinemia or hypoproteinemia	• 6 to 8 g/dl	• Increased values: dehydration • Decreased values: malnutrition, protein loss
Transthyretin (prealbumin) • Offers information regarding visceral protein stores; should be used in conjunction with the albumin level (Prealbumin has a shorter half-life [2 to 3 days] than albumin. This test is sensitive to nutritional repletion.)	• 16 to 40 mg/dl	• Increased values: renal insufficiency; patient on dialysis • Decreased values: PEM, acute catabolic states, postsurgery, hyperthyroidism
Urine ketone bodies (acetone) • Screens for ketonuria and detects carbohydrate deprivation	• Negative for ketones in urine	• Ketoacidosis: starvation

Indications for PPN

Patients who don't need to gain weight, yet need nutritional support, may receive PPN for as long as 2 to 3 weeks. It's used to help a patient meet minimum calorie and protein requirements. PPN therapy may also be used with oral or enteral feedings for a patient who needs to supplement low-calorie intake. PPN may also be given to a patient who's unable to absorb enteral therapy.

Putting PPN on hold

PPN shouldn't be used for patients with moderate to severe malnutrition or fat metabolism disorders, such as pathologic hyperlipidemia, lipid nephrosis, and acute pancreatitis caused by hyperlipidemia. In patients with severe liver damage, coagulation disorders, anemia, and pulmonary disease, and in those at increased risk for fat embolism, parenteral nutrition should be used cautiously.

Parenteral nutrition solutions

The solution you administer depends on the type of parenteral nutrition and the patient's status. (See *Parenteral solutions.*)

Dextrose plus...

Parenteral nutrition solutions may contain the following elements, each offering a particular benefit:
• *dextrose.* In parenteral nutrition solutions, most of the calories that can help maintain nitrogen balance come from dextrose. The number of nonprotein calories needed to maintain nitrogen balance depends on the severity of the patient's illness.

Dextrose is the basis for most solutions; it provides calories that maintain nitrogen balance.

Fats, in the form of lipid emulsions, provide other needed calories.

Amino acids, electrolytes, vitamins, and other nutrients are added to solutions to fulfill specific needs.

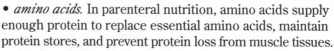

• *amino acids.* In parenteral nutrition, amino acids supply enough protein to replace essential amino acids, maintain protein stores, and prevent protein loss from muscle tissues.
• *fats.* Supplied as lipid emulsions, fats are a concentrated source of energy that prevent or correct fatty acid deficiencies. These are available in several concentrations and can provide 30% to 50% of a patient's daily calories.
• *electrolytes and minerals.* The amount of electrolytes and minerals added to the parenteral nutrition solution is based on an evaluation of the patient's serum chemistry profile and metabolic needs.

Parenteral solutions

Therapy and solution	Indications	Special considerations
Total parenteral nutrition (TPN) • Dextrose, 20% to 70% (1 L dextrose 25% = 850 nonprotein calories) • Crystalline amino acids, 2.5% to 15% • Electrolytes, vitamins, micronutrients, insulin, and heparin as ordered • Fat emulsion, 10% or 20% (can be given peripherally or centrally)	Long-term therapy (3 weeks or more) used to: • supply large quantities of nutrients and calories (2,000 to 2,500 calories/day or more) • provide needed calories, restore nitrogen balance, replace essential vitamins, electrolytes, minerals, and trace elements • promote tissue synthesis, wound healing, and normal metabolic function • allow bowel rest and healing, reduce activity in the pancreas and small intestine • improve tolerance to surgery if severely malnourished.	• Nutritionally complete • Requires minor surgical procedure for central venous (CV) catheter insertion (can be done by the doctor at patient's bedside) • Hypertonic solution may cause metabolic complications (glucose intolerance, electrolyte imbalances) *I.V. lipid emulsion* • May not be effective in severely stressed patients (such as those with sepsis or burns) • May interfere with immune mechanisms
Peripheral parenteral nutrition • Dextrose, 5% to 10% • Crystalline amino acids, 2.75% to 4.25% • Electrolytes, minerals, micronutrients, and vitamins as ordered • Fat emulsion, 10% or 20% • Heparin or hydrocortisone as ordered	Short-term therapy (3 weeks or less) used to: • maintain nutritional state in patients who can tolerate relatively high fluid volume, who usually resume bowel function and oral feedings in a few days, and who are not candidates for central venous catheters • provide approximately 1,300 to 1,800 calories/day.	• Nutritionally complete for short-term therapy • Should not be used in nutritionally depleted patients • Can't be used in volume-restricted patients because it requires high volumes of solution • Does not cause weight gain • Avoids insertion and maintenance of CV catheter, but patient must have good veins; I.V. site should be changed every 48 hours • Delivers less hypertonic solutions • May cause phlebitis • Less risk of metabolic complications *I.V. lipid emulsion* • As effective as dextrose for calorie source • Diminishes the risk of phlebitis if infused along with dextrose and amino acids • Irritates vein in long-term use

- *vitamins.* To ensure normal body functions and optimal nutrient use, the patient needs daily vitamins. A commercially available mixture of fat- and water-soluble vitamins, biotin, and folic acid may be added to the patient's parenteral nutrition solution.
- *micronutrients.* Also called trace elements, micronutrients promote normal metabolism. Most commercial solutions contain zinc, copper, chromium, selenium, and manganese.
- *water.* The amount of water added to a parenteral nutrition solution depends on the patient's fluid requirements and electrolyte balance.

Depending on the patient's condition, a doctor may also order additives for the parenteral nutrition solution, such as insulin or heparin. (See *Understanding common additives.*)

Now I get it!

Understanding common additives

Common parenteral nutrition solutions include dextrose 50% in water ($D_{50}W$), amino acids, and any of the additives listed here. These additives are used to treat a patient's specific metabolic deficiencies.

- Acetate prevents metabolic acidosis.
- Amino acids provide protein necessary for tissue repair.
- Calcium promotes development of bones and teeth and aids in blood clotting.
- Chloride regulates the acid-base equilibrium and maintains osmotic pressure.
- $D_{50}W$ provides calories for metabolism.
- Folic acid is needed for deoxyribonucleic acid formation and promotes growth and development.
- Magnesium aids carbohydrate and protein absorption.
- Micronutrients (such as zinc, manganese, and cobalt) help in wound healing and red blood cell synthesis.
- Phosphate minimizes the potential for developing peripheral paresthesia (numbness and tingling of the extremities).
- Potassium is needed for cellular activity and tissue synthesis.
- Sodium helps regulate water distribution and maintain normal fluid balance.
- Vitamin B complex aids the final absorption of carbohydrates and protein.
- Vitamin C helps in wound healing.
- Vitamin D is essential for bone metabolism and maintenance of serum calcium levels.
- Vitamin K helps prevent bleeding disorders.

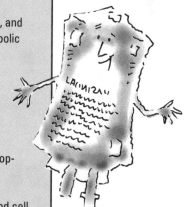

TPN solutions

Solutions for TPN are hypertonic, with an osmolarity of 1,800 to 2,600 mOsm/L. Electrolytes, minerals, vitamins, micronutrients, and water are added to the base solution to satisfy daily requirements. Lipids may be given as a separate solution or as an admixture with dextrose and amino acids.

The 3:1 solution

Daily allotments of TPN solution, including lipids and other parenteral solution components, are often given in a single 3-L bag, called a total nutrient admixture (TNA) or 3:1 solution. (See *Understanding total nutrient admixture,* page 300.)

Maintaining glucose balance without adding insulin

Glucose balance is extremely important in a patient receiving TPN. Adults use 0.8 to 1 g of glucose per kilogram of body weight per hour. That means a patient can tolerate a constant I.V. infusion of hyperosmolar (highly concentrated) glucose without adding insulin to the solution. As the concentrated glucose solution infuses, a pancreatic beta-cell response causes serum insulin levels to increase.

Start slow

To allow the pancreas to establish and maintain the necessary increased insulin production, start with a slow infusion rate and increase it gradually as ordered. Abruptly stopping the infusion may cause rebound hypoglycemia, which calls for an infusion of dextrose.

Off balance

Glucose balance may be further thrown off by the following:
• sepsis
• stress
• shock
• liver or kidney failure
• diabetes
• age
• pancreatic disease
• concurrent use of certain medications, including steroids.

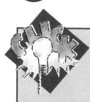

Now I get it!

Understanding total nutrient admixture

Total nutrient admixture (TNA) is a white solution that delivers 1 day's worth of nutrients in a single 3-L bag. Also called 3:1 solution, it combines lipids with other parenteral solution components. Here are some advantages and disadvantages of TNA.

Advantages
The benefits of TNA include:

• less need to handle the bag (less risk of contamination)

• requires less time

• less need for infusion sets and electronic infusion devices

• lower hospital costs

• increased patient mobility

• easier adjustment to home care.

Disadvantages
The disadvantages of TNA include:

• use of certain infusion devices precluded because of their inability to accurately deliver large volumes of solution

• 1.2-micron filter required (rather than a 0.22-micron filter) in order to allow lipid molecules through

• limited amount of calcium and phosphorus added because of the difficulty in detecting precipitate in the milky white solution

PPN solutions

PPN solutions usually consist of dextrose 5% in water (D_5W) to 10% dextrose and 2.75% to 4.25% crystalline amino acids. Alternatively, PPN solutions may be slightly hypertonic, such as dextrose 10% in water ($D_{10}W$), with an osmolarity no greater than 600 mOsm/L. Lipid emulsions, electrolytes, trace elements, and vitamins may be given as part of PPN to add calories and other needed nutrients.

Lipid emulsions

In an oral diet, lipids or fats are the major source of calories, usually providing about 40% of the total caloric intake. In parenteral nutrition solutions, lipids provide 9 kcal/g. I.V. lipid emulsions are oxidized for energy as needed. As a nearly isotonic emulsion, concentrations of 10% or 20% can be safely infused through peripheral or central veins. Lipid emulsions prevent and treat essential fatty acid deficiency and provide a major source of energy.

Administering parenteral nutrition

You may deliver parenteral nutrition one of two ways:

 continuously

 cyclically.

Over 24 hours

With continuous delivery, the patient receives the infusion over a 24-hour period. The infusion begins at a slow rate and increases to the optional rate as ordered. This type of delivery may prevent complications such as hyperglycemia due to a high dextrose load.

Cyclic delivery

A patient undergoing cyclic therapy receives the entire 24-hour volume of parenteral nutrition solution over a shorter period, perhaps 10, 12, 14, or 16 hours. Home care parenteral nutrition programs have boosted the use of cyclic therapy. This type of therapy may be used to wean the patient from TPN. (See *Switching from continuous to cyclic TPN,* page 302.)

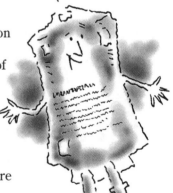

In continuous delivery, I have to work both day and night. In cyclic delivery, I get a few hours off.

Administering TPN

TPN solutions must be infused in a central vein, using one of the following:
• a peripherally inserted catheter, the tip of which lies in a central vein
• a CV catheter
• an implanted vascular access device.

The long haul

Long-term therapy requires use of one of the following:
• a Silastic CV catheter, such as a Hickman, Broviac, or Groshong catheter
• an implanted reservoir such as an Infus-A-Port
• an implanted vascular access device.

Concentration and dilution

Because TPN fluid has about six times the solute concentration of blood, peripheral I.V. administration can cause sclerosis and thrombosis. To ensure adequate dilution, the CV catheter is inserted into the superior vena cava, a wide-bore, high-flow vein. Usually, the catheter isn't advanced into the right atrium because of the risk of cardiac perforation and arrhythmias.

Preparing the patient

To increase compliance, make sure the patient understands the purpose of treatment, and enlist his help throughout the course of therapy.

TPN at home

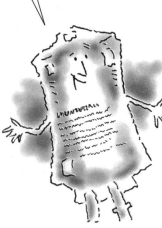

The TPN solution I'm filled with is highly concentrated. Infusion into a large vein ensures adequate dilution.

Understanding TPN and its goals helps a home care patient assume a greater role in administering, monitoring, and maintaining therapy. When instructing a home care patient, focus your teaching on the following:
• signs and symptoms of fluid, electrolyte, and glucose imbalances
• signs and symptoms of vitamin and trace element deficiencies and toxicities
• signs of catheter infection, such as fever, chills, discomfort on infusion, and redness or drainage at the catheter insertion site.

To help prevent glucose imbalance, teach the patient receiving his first I.V. bag of TPN how to regulate flow rate so he maintains the rate prescribed by the doctor. Explain that a gradual increase in flow rate allows the pancreas to establish and maintain the increased insulin production necessary to tolerate this treatment. Once the goal rate of the TPN infusion is met, there should be no reason to adjust the rate.

Finally, review the details of the administration schedule, the equipment the patient will use, and — to avoid in-

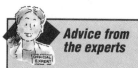

Advice from the experts

Switching from continuous to cyclic TPN

When switching from continuous to cyclic total parenteral nutrition (TPN), adjust the flow rate so the patient's blood glucose level can adapt to the decreased nutrient load. Do this by reducing the flow rate by one-half for 1 hour before stopping the infusion. Draw a blood glucose sample 1 hour after the infusion ends and observe the patient for signs of hypoglycemia, such as sweating, shakiness, and irritability.

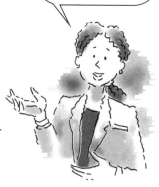

To maintain glucose balance, teach your home care patient to increase flow rate gradually.

compatibilities — the prescribed and over-the-counter medications he takes.

Compliance boosters

To safely maintain this therapy, the prescribed regimen must be adhered to by patients and caregivers. Your teaching efforts and return demonstrations by the patient help to boost compliance in all aspects of TPN therapy.

Preparing the equipment

Before TPN administration begins, the doctor inserts a venous access device. The access device may be a CV catheter or an implanted vascular access device. The location of the catheter tip is confirmed by X-ray.

Gather the TPN solution, a controller or pump, an administration set with a filter, alcohol swabs, gloves, and an I.V. pole. Be sure to wash your hands before preparing the TPN solution for administration, and prepare the administration set in a clean area.

Always use tubing with a filter when administering TPN. Filters are required by the Food and Drug Administration.

30-minute warm-up

The infusion of a chilled solution can cause discomfort, hypothermia, venous spasm, and venous constriction. Plan to remove the bag or bottle of TPN solution from the refrigerator about 30 minutes before hanging it to allow for warming.

Checking the order

Check the written order against the label on the bag. Make sure that the volumes, concentrations, and additives are included in the solution. Also check the infusion rate.

Inspecting infusate is imperative

Careful inspection of the infusate should be a habit. Check for clouding, floating debris, or change in color. Any of these phenomena could indicate contamination, problems with the integrity of the solution, or a pH change. If you see anything suspicious, notify the pharmacy. Inform the doctor that there may be a delay in hanging the solution; he may want to order $D_{10}W$ until a new container of TPN

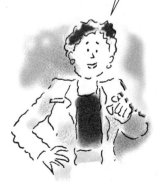

Check every solution for cloudiness, debris, or color changes.

solution is available. Also, be prepared to return the solution to the pharmacy.

Most TPN solutions contain lipid emulsions, which call for special precautions. (See *Administering lipid emulsions*.)

Beginning the infusion

Begin the infusion as ordered. Watch for swelling at the catheter insertion site. This may indicate extravasation of the TPN solution, which can cause necrosis (tissue damage). (See *Reducing the risk of infection*.)

Maintaining the infusion

If the patient tolerates the solution well the first day, the doctor usually increases intake to the goal rate by the second day. To maintain a TPN infusion, follow these key steps:
• Check the order provided by the doctor against the label on the TPN container.
• Label the container with the expiration date, time at which the solution was hung, glucose concentration, and total volume of solution. (If the bag or bottle is damaged and you don't have an immediate replacement, you can ap-

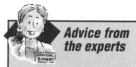

Advice from the experts

Reducing the risk of infection

Because a total parenteral nutrition (TPN) solution serves as a medium for bacterial growth and a central venous line provides systemic access, the patient receiving TPN risks infection and sepsis. To reduce the risk, always maintain strict aseptic technique when handling the equipment used to administer therapy.

Advice from the experts

Administering lipid emulsions

Most TPN solutions contain lipid emulsions. To safely administer them, follow these special precautions:

• Monitor the patient's vital signs and watch for signs and symptoms of an adverse reaction, such as fever, a pressure sensation over the eyes, nausea, vomiting, headache, chest and back pain, tachycardia, dyspnea, cyanosis, and flushing, sweating, or chills. If the patient has no adverse reactions to the test dose, begin the infusion at the prescribed rate.

• Before the infusion, always check the parenteral nutrition with lipids for separation or an oily appearance. If either condition exists, the lipid may have come out of emulsion and shouldn't be used.

• Because lipid emulsions are at high risk for bacterial growth, never rehang a partially empty bottle of emulsion.

proximate the glucose concentration until a new container is ready by adding 50% glucose to $D_{10}W$.)

• Maintain flow rates as prescribed, even if the flow falls behind schedule.

• Don't allow TPN solutions to hang for more than 24 hours.

• Change the tubing and filter every 24 hours, using strict aseptic technique. Make sure all tubing junctions are secure.

• Perform I.V. site care and dressing changes according to the facility's policy and protocol; usually every 48 hours, more often if the dressing becomes wet, soiled, or nonocclusive.

• Check the infusion pump's volume meter and time tape every 30 minutes (or more often, if necessary) to monitor for irregular flow rate. Gravity should never be used to administer TPN.

• Record vital signs when you initiate therapy and every 4 to 8 hours thereafter (or more often, if necessary). Be alert for increased body temperature — one of the earliest signs of catheter-related sepsis.

• Monitor your patient's glucose levels as ordered using glucose fingersticks or serum tests.

• Accurately record the patient's daily fluid intake and output, specifying the volume and type of each fluid. This record is a diagnostic tool that you can use to assure prompt, precise replacement of fluid and electrolyte deficits.

• Assess the patient's physical status daily. Weigh him at the same time each morning (after voiding), in similar clothing, using the same scale. Suspect fluid imbalance if the patient gains more than 1 lb (0.45 kg) per day. If ordered, obtain anthropometric measurements.

• Monitor the results of routine laboratory tests, such as serum electrolyte, blood urea nitrogen, and glucose levels, and report abnormal findings to the doctor so appropriate changes in the TPN solution can be made.

• Check serum triglyceride levels, which should be in the normal range during continuous TPN infusion. Typically, alanine aminotransferase, aspartate aminotransferase, alkaline phosphatase, cholesterol, triglyceride, plasma-free fatty acid, and coagulation tests are performed weekly.

• Monitor the patient for signs and symptoms of nutritional aberrations, such as fluid and electrolyte imbalances and glucose metabolism disturbances. Some patients may

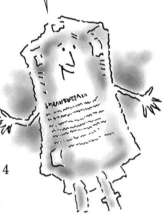

Need an emergency substitute for a damaged TPN bag? Try adding 50% glucose to $D_{10}W$.

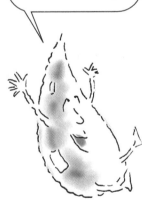

Gravity is great, but not for controlling TPN. Always use an infusion pump and check it every half hour — or more often, if necessary.

require supplementary insulin throughout TPN therapy; the pharmacy usually adds insulin directly to the TPN solution.

• Provide emotional support. Keep in mind that patients often associate eating with positive feelings and become disturbed when it's eliminated.

• Provide frequent mouth care for the patient.

• Document all assessment findings and nursing interventions.

A port of last resort

Avoid using a TPN infusion port for any other infusion. When using a single-lumen CV catheter, don't use the line to piggyback or infuse blood or blood products, give a bolus injection, administer simultaneous I.V. solutions, measure CV pressure, or draw blood for laboratory tests. In unavoidable circumstances, the TPN port may be used for electrolyte replacement or insulin drips because these infusions are often additives to the solution. Remember, never add medication to a TPN solution container. Also, avoid using add-on devices, which increase the risk of infection.

Administering PPN

Using an amino acid, dextrose, and lipid emulsion solution, PPN fulfills a patient's basic caloric needs without the risks involved in CV access. Because PPN solutions have lower tonicity than TPN solutions, a patient receiving PPN must be able to tolerate infusion of large volumes of fluid. Administer PPN through a peripheral vein.

Preparing the patient

Make sure the patient understands what to expect before, during, and after therapy.

The largest available vein

Select the patient's largest available vein as the insertion site. This enables the blood to adequately dilute the PPN solution, which can be irritating. When using a short-term catheter, rotate the site every 48 to 72 hours, or according to your facility's policy and procedures.

Preparing the equipment

To administer PPN, gather the following:
• ordered PPN solution (at room temperature)
• controller or pump
• administration set
• alcohol swabs
• I.V. pole
• venipuncture equipment if needed.

Checking the order

Check the written order against the written label on the Make sure that the solution is for peripheral infusion and that the volumes, concentrations, and additives are included in the solution. Also check the infusion rate.

A little lecture about lipids

In PPN therapy, lipid emulsions may or may not be part of the solution. If given separately, piggyback the lipid emulsion below the in-line filter close to the insertion site. This prevents the possibility of lipids clogging the filtration system. When giving lipids, use controllers that can accommodate lipid emulsions.

Beginning the infusion

Begin the PPN infusion as ordered. Watch for swelling at the peripheral insertion site. Swelling may indicate infiltration or extravasation of the PPN solution, which can cause tissue damage.

Maintaining the infusion

Caring for a patient receiving a PPN infusion involves the same steps required for any patient receiving a peripheral

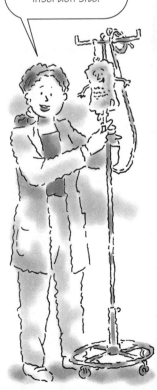

When giving lipid emulsions separately, piggyback the lipids below the in-line filter close to the insertion site.

I.V. infusion. You need to maintain the infusion rate and care for the tubing, dressings, infusion site, and I.V. devices. In addition, monitor the patient for these signs of sepsis:
- elevated temperature
- glucose in the urine (glycosuria)
- chills
- malaise
- increased white blood cells (leukocytosis)
- altered level of consciousness
- elevated glucose levels, measured by fingerstick or serum chemistry.

Insulin insight

Because the synthesis of lipase (a fat-splitting enzyme) increases insulin requirements, the insulin dosage of a diabetic patient may need to be increased, as ordered. Insulin is one of the additives that may be adjusted in the formulation of the PPN solution.

Hormone hint

For a patient with hypothyroidism, you may need to administer thyroid-stimulating hormone (TSH). TSH affects lipase activity and may prevent triglycerides from accumulating in the vascular system.

Bloated, metallic, greasy

Patients receiving lipid emulsions commonly report a feeling of fullness or bloating; occasionally, they experience an unpleasant metallic or greasy taste. Some patients develop allergic reactions to the fat emulsion.

Lipid letdowns

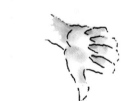

Early adverse reactions to lipid emulsion therapy occur in fewer than 1% of patients. Such reactions may include:
- fever
- difficulty breathing
- cyanosis
- nausea
- vomiting
- headache
- flushing
- sweating
- lethargy
- dizziness

- chest and back pain
- slight pressure over the eyes
- irritation at the infusion site.

Changes in laboratory test results may also reveal problems when a patient receives lipid emulsions. These problems include:

- hyperlipidemia
- hypercoagulability
- thrombocytopenia.

Considering clearance

The doctor monitors the patient's lipid emulsion clearance rate. Lipid emulsion may clear from the blood at an accelerated rate in a patient with severe burns, multiple trauma, or metabolic imbalance.

Precautions and complications

In this section, you'll find special considerations for administering parenteral nutrition to pediatric and elderly patients. You'll also find information about possible complications during therapy and pointers for discontinuing therapy safely.

Patients with special needs

Pediatric and elderly patients are particularly susceptible to fluid overload and heart failure. With these patients, be particularly careful to administer the correct volume of parenteral nutrition solution at the correct infusion rate.

Pediatric patients

Parenteral feeding therapy for children serves a dual purpose. It:

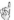 maintains a child's nutritional status

 fuels a child's growth.

An extra helping

Children have a greater need than adults for certain nutrients. This is an important consideration in accurately calculating solution components for pediatric patients. Overall, a child has greater need than an adult for the following nutrients:

- protein
- carbohydrates
- fat
- electrolytes
- micronutrients
- vitamins
- fluids.

As with adults, children receiving TPN should be evaluated carefully by the nurse, doctor, and nutritional support team. Keep in mind the following factors when planning to meet children's nutritional needs:

- age
- weight
- activity level
- size
- development
- caloric needs.

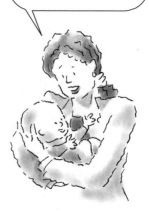

Because they're growing, children need more of some nutrients than adults.

Lipid liabilities in little ones

Administering PPN with lipid emulsions in a premature or low birth-weight infant may lead to lipid accumulation in the lungs. Thrombocytopenia (platelet deficiency) has also been reported in infants receiving 20% lipid emulsions.

Elderly patients

In an elderly patient, overinfusion can produce serious adverse effects, so always monitor flow rates carefully. The elderly are also at risk for fluid overload when TPN or PPN is given.

An elderly patient may have underlying clinical problems that affect the outcome of treatment. For example, he may be taking medications that can interact with the components in the parenteral nutrition solution. For this reason, ask the pharmacist about possible interactions with any drug the patient is taking.

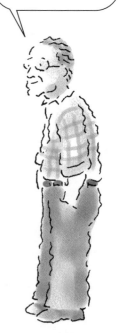

Elderly patients are subject to fluid overload and drug interactions. It's always something.

Complications

Patients receiving parenteral nutrition therapy face many of the same complications as patients undergoing any type of peripheral I.V. or CV therapy. (See *Handling TPN hazards,* pages 312 and 313.)

Complications of any parenteral nutrition therapy may result from problems that are:
• catheter-related
• metabolic
• mechanical.

Catheter-related problems

The most common catheter-related problems include:
• clotted catheter
• catheter dislodgment
• cracked or broken tubing
• pneumothorax and hydrothorax
• sepsis.

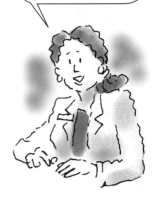

Common catheter-related complications include clotting, dislodgment, extravasation, and bleeding.

Clotted catheter

Suspect a clotted catheter if the infusion flow rate is interrupted. You may also notice that a greater pressure is needed to maintain the infusion at the desired infusion rate.

Catheter dislodgment

When the catheter comes out of the vein, catheter dislodgment may be obvious. You may note that the dressing is wet. The patient may report feeling cold or that his gown is wet. When the catheter is located peripherally, the area around the insertion site may be red or swollen due to subcutaneous extravasation of the PPN solution. With a centrally inserted catheter, there may be swelling around the insertion site, which may or may not be reddened. The most significant complications include bleeding from the insertion site or an air embolism.

Tubing trauma

If the catheter or vascular access device is damaged, infusate may leak from a cracked area or the insertion site. If the infusion tubing is damaged, the I.V. insertion site remains dry. Both situations require immediate attention because of the risk of bleeding, contamination, or air emboli.

Gasp! Air in the pleural cavity

Air in the pleural cavity (pneumothorax) usually results from trauma to the pleura during insertion of a CV access

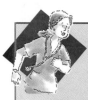

Running smoothly

Handling TPN hazards

Complications of total parenteral nutrition (TPN) therapy can result from catheter-related, metabolic, or mechanical problems. To help you treat these common complications, use this chart.

Complications	Interventions
Catheter-related complications	
Clotted catheter	• Reposition catheter. Attempt to aspirate clot. • If unsuccessful, instill urokinase to clear catheter lumen, as ordered.
Dislodged catheter	• Place a sterile gauze pad on the insertion site, and apply pressure.
Cracked or broken tubing	• Apply a padded hemostat above the break to prevent air from entering the line.
Pneumothorax and hydrothorax	• Assist with chest tube insertion. • Maintain chest tube suctioning, as ordered.
Sepsis	• Remove catheter and culture tip. • Give appropriate antibiotics.
Metabolic complications	
Hyperglycemia	• Start insulin therapy or adjust TPN flow rate as ordered.
Hypoglycemia	• Infuse dextrose as ordered.
Hyperosmolar hyperglycemic non-ketotic syndrome	• Stop dextrose. • Rehydrate with the ordered infusate.
Hypokalemia	• Increase potassium supplementation.
Hypomagnesemia	• Increase magnesium supplementation.
Hypophosphatemia	• Increase phosphate supplementation.
Hypocalcemia	• Increase calcium supplementation.
Metabolic acidosis	• Use acetate or lactate salts of sodium or hydrogen.
Liver dysfunction	• Use special hepatic formulations. • Decrease carbohydrates and add I.V. lipids.
Hyperkalemia	• Decrease potassium supplementation.

Handling TPN hazards (continued)

Complications	Interventions
Mechanical complications	
Air embolism	• Clamp catheter. • Place patient in Trendelenburg's position on the left side. • Give oxygen as ordered. • If cardiac arrest occurs, use cardiopulmonary resuscitation.
Venous thrombosis	• Remove catheter promptly. • Administer heparin, if ordered. • Venous flow studies may be done.
Too rapid an infusion	• Check the infusion rate. • Check the infusion pump if you're using one.
Extravasation	• Stop I.V. infusion. • Assess patient for cardiopulmonary abnormalities. Chest X-ray may be performed.
Phlebitis	• Apply gentle heat to the insertion site. • Elevate the insertion site, if possible.

device. The patient may have dyspnea and chest pain; he may also develop a cough. Auscultation reveals diminished breath sounds, and the patient may be sweating and appear cyanotic. Assessment may also reveal unilateral chest movement. Pneumothorax should be confirmed by X-ray for the best treatment results.

Sepsis alert

Sepsis, the most serious catheter-related complication, can be fatal. You can prevent it by providing meticulous, consistent catheter care.

If the patient is developing catheter-related sepsis, he may develop an unexplained fever, chills, and a red, indurated area around the catheter site. The patient may also have unexplained hyperglycemia, often an early warning sign of sepsis.

Metabolic complications

Metabolic complications include:
* hyperglycemia or hypoglycemia (high or low blood glucose level)
* hyperosmolar hyperglycemic nonketotic syndrome (HHNS)
* hyperkalemia or hypokalemia (high or low blood potassium level)
* hypomagnesemia (low blood magnesium level)
* hypophosphatemia (low blood phosphate level)
* hypocalcemia (low blood calcium level)
* metabolic acidosis
* liver dysfunction.

A glut of glucose

The patient may develop hyperglycemia if the formula's glucose concentration is excessive, the infusion rate is too rapid, or his glucose tolerance is compromised by diabetes, stress, or sepsis. Signs of hyperglycemia include fatigue, restlessness, and weakness. The patient may become anxious, confused and, in some cases, delirious or even comatose. He will be dehydrated and have polyuria and elevated blood and urine glucose levels.

A glimmer of glucose

Conversely, the patient may develop hypoglycemia if parenteral nutrition is interrupted suddenly or if he receives excessive insulin. Symptoms may include sweating, shaking, confusion, and irritability.

HHNS

An acute complication of hyperglycemic crisis, HHNS is caused by hyperosmolar diuresis resulting from untreated hyperglycemia. A patient with HHNS has a high serum osmolarity, is dehydrated, and has extremely high glucose levels — as high as 600 to 4,800 mg/dl. If untreated, he can develop glycosuria and electrolyte disturbances and even become comatose. Suspect HHNS if your patient becomes confused or lethargic or experiences seizures.

A plethora of potassium

Patients develop hyperkalemia because of too much potassium in the TPN formula, renal disease, or hyponatremia.

Look for skeletal muscle weakness, decreased heart rate, irregular pulse, and tall T waves.

A pittance of potassium

Patients develop hypokalemia because of too little potassium in the solution, excessive loss of potassium brought on by GI tract disturbances or diuretic use, or large doses of insulin. Look for muscle weakness, paralysis, paresthesia, and cardiac arrhythmias.

Magnesium mayhem

Hypomagnesemia results from insufficient magnesium in the solution. Suspect hypomagnesemia if your patient complains of tingling around the mouth or paresthesia in his fingers. He may also show signs of mental changes, hyperreflexia, tetany, and arrhythmias.

Phosphate funk

Hypophosphatemia results from insulin therapy, alcoholism, and the use of phosphate-binding antacids. Suspect hypophosphatemia if the patient shows irritability, weakness, and paresthesia. In extreme cases, coma and cardiac arrest can occur. Very rarely, a patient develops hyperphosphatemia. Patients with renal insufficiency are prone to hyperphosphatemia.

Calcium calamity

Hypocalcemia, a rare complication, results from too little calcium in the solution, vitamin D deficiency, or pancreatitis. The patient may develop numbing or tingling sensations, tetany, polyuria, dehydration, and arrhythmias.

Acid-base balance blues

Metabolic acidosis can occur if the patient develops an increased serum chloride level and a decreased serum bicarbonate level.

Last but not least, the liver

Increased serum alkaline phosphatase, lactate dehydrogenase, and bilirubin levels can indicate liver dysfunction.

Mechanical complications

Mechanical complications that can plague parenteral nutrition therapy include the following:
• air embolism

- venous thrombosis
- extravasation
- phlebitis.

Sounds like an air embolism

Suspect an air embolism if the patient develops apprehension, chest pain, tachycardia, hypotension, cyanosis, seizures, loss of consciousness, or cardiac arrest. Auscultation may also reveal the classic sign of an air embolism: a churning heart murmur.

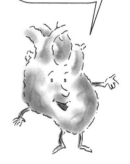

A churning heart murmur is a classic sign of air embolism.

Looks like thrombosis

Suspect thrombosis when you see redness or swelling at the catheter insertion site or swelling of the arm, neck, or face. Other signs and symptoms include pain at the insertion site and along the vein, malaise, fever, and tachycardia.

The risk of rushing

If TPN is infused too rapidly, the patient may feel nauseated, have a headache, and become lethargic. Heart failure is also a risk due to fluid overload.

An intimation of extravasation

If you observe swelling of the tissue around the insertion site, it may indicate extravasation. The patient may also complain of pain at the insertion site.

Feels like phlebitis

Pain, tenderness, redness, and warmth at the insertion site and along the vein path may indicate phlebitis.

Other complications

TPN and lipid emulsion administration pose distinct risks.

Particular PPN problems

Significant complications of PPN therapy include phlebitis, infiltration, and extravasation.

Lipid low points

Prolonged administration of lipid emulsions can produce delayed complications, including enlarged liver or spleen, blood dyscrasia (thrombocytopenia and leukopenia), and transient increases in results of liver function studies. A small number of patients receiving 20% I.V. lipid emulsion develop brown pigmentation due to fat pigmentation.

Discontinuing therapy

One major difference exists between the procedures for discontinuing TPN and PPN therapy. A patient receiving TPN should be weaned from therapy and receive some other form of nutritional therapy such as enteral feedings. When the patient is receiving PPN, therapy can be discontinued without weaning because the dextrose concentration is lower than in TPN. When discontinuing TPN therapy, you should wean the patient over 24 hours to prevent rebound hypoglycemia.

A patient receiving TPN should be weaned from therapy.

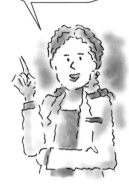

Quick quiz

1. The maximum amount of time that TPN solutions are permitted to infuse before the bag must be replaced is:
    A. 24 hours.
    B. 48 hours.
    C. 12 hours.
Answer: A. Don't allow TPN solutions to hang for more than 24 hours.

2. When administering TPN, one of the first signs of catheter-related sepsis is:
    A. hypothermia.
    B. pruritus.
    C. increased temperature.
Answer: C. When administering TPN, be alert for increased temperature, one of the earliest signs of catheter-related sepsis.

3. The first step in solving a clotted catheter is to:
    A. reposition the catheter.
    B. remove the catheter.
    C. stop I.V. infusion.
Answer: A. Reposition the catheter and attempt to aspirate the clot. If that doesn't work, instill urokinase to clear the catheter lumen.

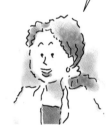

PPN therapy can be discontinued without weaning.

4. A commonly used anthropometric measurement that helps determine nutritional status is:

    A. biceps skinfold.

    B. lean body mass.

    C. midarm muscle circumference.

Answer: C. Weight, midarm muscle circumference, and triceps skinfold measurement are all anthropometric measurements that help to determine nutritional status.

5. Most of the calories in TPN are contributed by:

    A. fats.

    B. dextrose.

    C. amino acids.

Answer: B. Most calories in TPN solutions come from dextrose.

6. The type of solution usually used for TPN is:

    A. isotonic.

    B. hypotonic.

    C. hypertonic.

Answer: C. Solutions for TPN are hypertonic with an osmolarity of 1,800 to 2,400 mOsm/L.

Scoring

☆☆☆   If you answered six questions correctly, feel fulfilled. You've metabolized the chapter components and converted them to cerebral energy.

☆☆   If you answered four or five questions correctly, sit back and digest. Your mind has been well nourished.

☆   If you answered fewer than four questions correctly, have a snack and review this book. There's nothing wrong with enhancing your diet of knowledge with a fact-filled supplement.

All these puns are making me lose my appetite.

Appendices and index

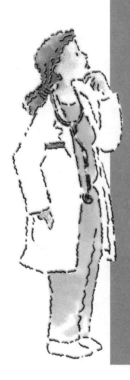

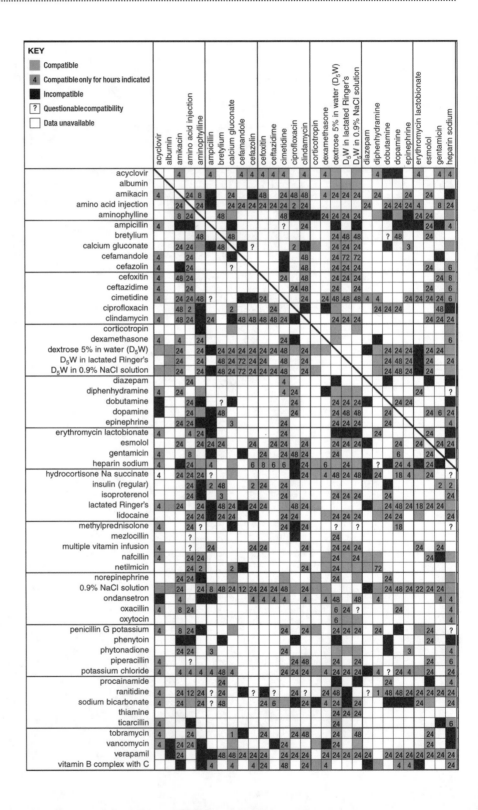

	hydrocortisone Na succinate	insulin (regular)	isoproterenol	lactated Ringer's	lidocaine	methylprednisolone	mezlocillin	multiple vitamin infusion	nafcillin	netilmicin	norepinephrine	0.9% NaCl solution	ondansetron	oxacillin	oxytocin	penicillin G potassium	phenytoin	phytonadione	piperacillin	potassium chloride	procainamide	ranitidine	sodium bicarbonate	thiamine	ticarcillin	tobramycin	vancomycin	verapamil	vitamin B complex with C
acyclovir	4			4		4		4	4	4		4		4		4			4	4		4	4		4		4	4	4
albumin																													
amikacin	24			24							24	24	4	8		8		24	24			24	24				24	24	
amino acid injection	24	24	24		24	24	?	?	24	24	24			24			24	24	?	4		12			24	24			
aminophylline	24			24	24	?			24	2		24									4		24	24				24	
ampicillin	?	2					24					8						3		4		?	?						4
bretylium		48	3	48	24							48							48	24	24	48					48		
calcium gluconate			24	24					2			24							4						1		48	4	
cefamandole												12															24		
cefazolin		2		24			24					24	4							?							24	4	
cefoxitin		24		24								24	4							24					24		24	24	
ceftazidime												24	4							?	6								
cimetidine		24	24		24	24						48	4		24		24		24								24	24	48
ciprofloxacin			48	24								24							24	24		24					24		24
clindamycin	24			24		24		24		24		24	4						48	24		?	24		48		24	24	
corticotropin																													
dexamethasone	4											4							4			24	4				24	4	
dextrose 5% in water (D5W)	48		24		24	?	24	24	24	24	24		48	6	6	24		24	24		48	24	24	24	24	24	24	24	24
D5W in lactated Ringer's	24		24		24			24				24		24		24			24			24			24			24	
D5W in 0.9% NaCl solution	48		24		24	?	24	24				48	?		24		24		24	24		24	24		48			24	
diazepam																						?						24	
diphenhydramine	24							72				4			24				4			4	1					24	
dobutamine			24	24	24							24							?	24	48						24		
dopamine	18			48	24	18						48		24						24		48					24	4	
epinephrine	4			24								24					3		4			24					24	4	
erythromycin lactobionate			18		24							22										24	24					24	
esmolol	24			24			24			24		24			24	24	24		24	24			24		24	24	24		
gentamicin		2		24			24					24	4							24							24		
heparin sodium	?	2	24		24	?						4	4	4		?	4	6	24	4	24	24		6			24	24	
hydrocortisone Na succinate		4	4	24		?						24	4	4		4	24		4	24		24						24	
insulin (regular)	4			24								2							4		24	3		2	2	2	48	4	
isoproterenol	4			24								24										24						24	
lactated Ringer's	24		24		24	?	72	24	24			24			24		24								24	24	24	24	
lidocaine		24		24					48			24					24		24	24								48	
methylprednisolone	?		?									?			24				?		48	2					24	?
mezlocillin			72									48																	
multiple vitamin infusion			24							24		24									24						24		
nafcillin			24	48								24					24			24		24					24		?
netilmicin									24			24																	
norepinephrine												24									?						24		
0.9% NaCl solution	24		24		24	?	48	24	24	24			48	24		24			24	24	24	48	24	24	24	48	24	24	
ondansetron	4											48							4		4				4		4		
oxacillin	4		24									24									4		24				24		4
oxytocin		2																	4				24				24	4	
penicillin G potassium			24		24							24										24					24		
phenytoin																						24					48		
phytonadione	4											24							4			24	4				24		4
piperacillin	24											24									24	4					24		
potassium chloride		4		24			24			24		24	4		4			4	24		4	48	24				24		
procainamide	4				24							24										24						48	24
ranitidine		24	24		24	48					?	48	4		24			4	48	24					24	24	24		
sodium bicarbonate	24	3		24	2		24	24				24				24	24		24										?
thiamine			24									24																24	
ticarcillin		2		24								24	4						24									24	
tobramycin		2		24								48										24						24	
vancomycin		2										24	4									24						24	
verapamil	24	48	24	24	48	24		24				24	24			24	24	48		24	24	48			24	24	24		24
vitamin B complex with C		4			?			?				4	4		4				4			24			?			24	

Glossary

active transport: movement of solutes from an area of lower concentration to one of higher concentration (The solutes are said to move against the concentration gradient.)

Add-a-line set: an I.V. administration set that can deliver intermittent secondary infusions through one or more additional Y-sites

aerosolization: dispersal of a solution into the air in an atomized form

agglutinization: clumping of red blood cells; part of the immune reaction that occurs with Rh incompatibility

air embolism: a systemic complication of I.V. therapy that occurs when air is introduced into the venous system and includes such signs and symptoms as respiratory distress, unequal breath sounds, weak pulse, increased central venous pressure, decreased blood pressure, and loss of consciousness

albumin: a protein that can't pass through capillary walls and that draws water into the capillaries by osmosis during reabsorption

aldosterone: a hormone secreted by the adrenal cortex that regulates sodium reabsorption by the kidneys (The renin-angiotensin system responds to decreased blood flow and decreased blood pressure to stimulate aldosterone secretion.)

alopecia: baldness that is partial or complete, local or general; in chemotherapy, caused by the destruction of rapidly dividing cells in the hair shaft or root

amino acids: in parenteral nutrition, nutrients that supply enough protein to replace essential amino acids, maintain protein stores, and prevent protein loss from muscle tissues

anaphylactic reaction (anaphylaxis): severe allergic reaction including flushing, chills, anxiety, agitation, generalized itching, palpitations, paresthesia, throbbing in the ears, wheezing, coughing, convulsions and cardiac arrest

anthropometry: an objective, noninvasive method of measuring overall body size, composition, and specific body parts that compares the patient's measurements with established standards (Commonly used anthropometric measurements include height, weight, ideal body weight, body frame size, skinfold thickness, midarm circumference, and midarm muscle circumference.)

antibody: an immunoglobulin molecule synthesized in response to a specific antigen

antidiuretic hormone (ADH): a hormone produced in the hypothalamus and stored in the posterior pituitary that responds to osmolarity and blood pressure changes, and promotes water reabsorption by the kidneys

anti-free-flow device: a device on an infusion pump that prevents inadvertent bolus infusions if the pump door is accidentally opened

antigen: a major component of blood that exists on the surface of blood cells and can initiate an immune response (A particular antigen can also induce the formation of a corresponding antibody when given to a person who doesn't normally have the antigen.)

arm board: a restraining device that helps prevent unnecessary motion that could cause infiltration or inflammation when an I.V. insertion site is near a joint or in the back of the hand

arrhythmia: heart rhythm irregularity that may occur during CV catheter insertion if the catheter enters the right ventricle and irritates the cardiac muscle (Arrhythmias usually abate when the catheter is withdrawn.)

autotransfusion: the collection and filtration of blood from a patient and the reinfusion of the blood to the same patient

backcheck valve: a device that prevents backflow of a secondary solution into a primary solution (In a primary line with a side Y port, a backcheck valve stops the flow from the primary line during drug infusion and returns to the primary flow after infusion.)

bacterial phlebitis: painful inflammation of a vein that can occur with peripherally inserted central catheters and usually occurs after a long period of I.V. therapy

biological response modifiers (BRMs): agents used in biological therapy that alter the body's response to cancer

biological safety cabinet (BSC): specialized work area for preparing chemotherapeutic drugs

blood products: the individual components that make up whole blood and are available for transfusion therapy to correct specific blood deficiencies; for example, red blood cells, plasma, platelets, granulocytes, immune globulin, albumin, and plasma protein

blood type: usually, one of the four blood types in the ABO system, including A, B, AB, and O, which is named for the antigens — A, B, both of these, or neither — that are carried on a person's red blood cells

body fluids: water and dissolved substances in the body (such as electrolytes) that help regulate body temperature, transport nutrients and gases throughout the body, carry wastes to excretion sites, and maintain cell shape

body surface area slide rule: a slide rule that's used to calculate a patient's body surface area when the patient's weight and height are known (Body surface area is expressed in square meters [m^2].)

butterfly needle: common name for a winged infusion set, which has flexible wings that lie flat after insertion and can be taped to the surrounding skin

capillary filtration: movement of fluid and solutes out through the capillary wall pores and into the interstitial fluid; caused by hydrostatic (or fluid) pressure and blood pressure against the walls of the capillaries

capillary reabsorption: the return of water and diffusible solutes to the capillaries that occurs when capillary blood pressure falls below colloid oncotic pressure

cell cycle: the reproductive and resting phases through which every cell, normal and malignant, passes

cellular elements: also called formed elements; make up about 45% of blood volume; include erythrocytes (red blood cells [RBCs]), leukocytes (white blood cells [WBCs]), and thrombocytes (platelets) (Commonly transfused cellular blood products include whole blood, packed RBCs, leukocyte-poor RBCs, WBCs, and platelets.)

central venous (CV) therapy: treatment in which drugs or fluids are infused directly into a major vein; used in emergencies, when a patient's peripheral veins are inaccessible, or when a patient needs infusion of a large volume of fluid, multiple infusion therapies, or long-term venous access (In CV therapy, a catheter is inserted with its tip in the superior vena cava, inferior vena cava, or right atrium of the heart.)

central venous pressure (CVP): an important indicator of circulatory function and the pumping ability of the right side of the heart; measured with a catheter placed in or near the right atrium of the heart

chemotherapeutic drugs: drugs used in chemotherapy that fall into categories, including alkylating agents, antimetabolites, hormones and hormone inhibitors, antibiotics, plant alkaloids, and enzymes, that are, in turn, grouped as cycle-specific (antimetabolites and plant alkaloids) and cycle-nonspecific (alkylating agents and most antibiotics); given alone or in various combinations, called protocols

chemotherapy: cancer treatment that requires effective delivery of a precise dosage of toxic drugs and typically employs more than one drug so that each drug can target a different site or take action during a different phase of the cell cycle (The challenge is to provide a drug dose large enough to kill the greatest number of cancer cells but small enough to avoid irreversibly damaging normal tissue or causing toxicity.)

chylothorax: puncture of a lymph node with leakage of lymph fluid

circulatory overload: an extremely large volume of fluid that the heart is incapable of pumping through the circulatory system (Symptoms include neck vein engorgement, respiratory distress, increased blood pressure, and crackles in the lungs.)

cold agglutinins: antibodies that could cause red blood cell clumping if cold blood is infused

colloid oncotic pressure (COP): the osmotic, or pulling, force of albumin in the intravascular space that draws water into the capillaries during reabsorption

colony-stimulating factors (CSFs): biological response modifiers that regulate hematopoietic growth and differentiation; for example, hematopoietic growth factors (erythropoietin), granulocyte colony stimulating factor, interleukin-3, macrophage colony stimulating factor, and thrombopoietin

compatibility: in transfusion therapy, typing and crossmatching the donor and recipient blood to minimize the risk of a hemolytic reaction (The most important compatibility tests include ABO blood typing, Rh typing, crossmatching, direct antiglobulin test, and antibody screening test.)

complement system: a group of enzymatic proteins (In a hemolytic transfusion reaction, an antibody-antigen reaction activates the body's complement system, causing red blood cell destruction [hemolysis], which releases hemoglobin [a red blood cell component] into the bloodstream and can damage renal tubules and lead to kidney failure.)

continuous delivery: in parenteral nutrition, delivery of an infusion over a 24-hour period

continuous I.V. therapy: administration of I.V. fluid over a prolonged period through a peripheral or central venous line, allowing careful regulation of drug delivery and enhancing the effectiveness of some drugs, such as lidocaine and heparin

controller: an electronic device that regulates the flow of I.V. solutions and drugs and is used when a precise flow rate is required

cooling cap: in chemotherapy, a device that is used to limit superficial blood flow to the scalp during drug administration, thus partially protecting the hair follicles and limiting alopecia

cross-sensitivity: hypersensitivity to similar I.V. drugs (If a patient is hypersensitive to a particular drug, he may be hypersensitive to other chemically similar drugs.)

cycle-nonspecific drugs: in chemotherapy, drugs that act independently of the cell cycle, allowing them to act on both reproducing and resting cells (During a single administration of a cycle-nonspecific chemotherapeutic drug, a fixed percentage of both normal and malignant cells die, while the others survive. Slower growing cancers, such as GI and pulmonary tumors, which have fewer cells undergoing division at any given moment, respond best to cycle-nonspecific drugs. Large tumors respond better to cycle-nonspecific drugs, but once the large tumor shrinks, the doctor may switch to a cycle-specific drug.)

cycle-specific drugs: in chemotherapy, drugs that are effective only during a specific phase of the cell cycle; designed to disrupt a specific biochemical process (When cycle-specific chemotherapy is administered, cells in the resting phase survive and eventually reproduce. Rapidly growing cancers, such as acute leukemias and lymphomas, respond best to cycle-specific chemotherapy. Generally, small tumors respond to drugs that affect DNA synthesis, especially cycle-specific drugs, because these tumors have a higher percentage of actively dividing cells than large tumors.)

cyclic delivery: in parenteral nutrition, delivery of the entire solution overnight; also used to wean a patient from total parenteral nutrition

cytokines: a type of biological response modifier — includes interferon, interleukins, tumor necrosis factor, and colony-stimulating factors

dextrose: a glucose solution that contributes most of the calories in parenteral nutrition solutions and can help maintain nitrogen balance

diffusion: movement of solutes from an area of higher concentration to one of lower concentration by passive transport (a fluid movement process that requires no energy)

diluent: a liquid used to reconstitute I.V. drugs that are supplied in powder form; for example, normal saline solution, sterile water for injection, dextrose 5% in water (Some drugs should be reconstituted with diluents that contain preservatives.)

direct injection: administration of a single dose (bolus) of a drug or other substance; sometimes called I.V. push

divalent cations: an electrolyte that carries two positively charged ions (such as Ca^{++}) (In I.V. medication therapy, a solution containing divalent cations has a higher incidence of incompatibility.)

double-chambered vial: container for some drugs in which the powder form of the drug is in a lower chamber and a diluent is in an upper one with a rubber stopper on top of the vial that is pressed to dislodge the rubber plug separating the compartments, thus mixing the diluent with the drug in the bottom chamber

drip controller: device used in CV therapy that permits infusion at low pressure; used most often with infants and children who could suffer serious complications from high-pressure infusion

electrolyte balance: the concentration levels of intracellular and extracellular electrolytes, which are about equal when balance is maintained

electrolytes: major components of body fluids — especially sodium, potassium, calcium, chloride, phosphate, and magnesium — that are involved in fluid balance and which dissociate into ions and conduct electric current that is necessary for normal cell functioning

emetogenic (vomit-inducing) potential: likelihood that a drug or drugs may cause nausea or vomiting (For example, cisplatin has a high emetogenic potential; more than 90% of patients receiving it will experience nausea and vomiting. Bleomycin has a low potential; only 10% to 30% of patients are affected. Other factors contributing to occurrence and severity include the combination of drugs, doses and routes of administration, rates of administration, treatment schedules, and patient characteristics.)

extension tubing: small-bore tubing that can be attached to any I.V. tubing to join it to the venipuncture device, allowing I.V. tubing to be changed away from the insertion site, thereby reducing the risk of contamination

extracellular fluid (ECF): any fluid in the body that isn't contained inside the cells, including interstitial fluid, plasma, and transcellular fluid

extravasation: infiltration of irritating fluids, resulting in damage to surrounding tissues; a medical emergency

fats: in parenteral nutrition, supplied as lipid emulsions; a concentrated source of energy that prevents or corrects fatty acid deficiencies; available in several concentrations to provide 30% to 50% of a patient's daily calories

febrile reaction: a possible complication of transfusion therapy; characterized by a temperature increase of 1.8° F with transfusion (for nonhemolytic febrile reactions), with no other known explanation and usually caused by antibodies directed against leukocytes or platelets; common in approximately 1% of transfusions within 2 hours after completion (Signs and symptoms of febrile reactions include fever, chills, headache, nausea and vomiting, hypotension, chest pain, dyspnea, nonproductive cough, and malaise.)

fistula: an abnormal passageway that may develop between the innominate vein and the subclavian artery due to perforation by a guide wire inserted into the vessel

flare reaction: an inflammatory response to infusion of an irritant; a local venous response with or without an accompanying skin reaction (The patient may complain of burning, pain, aching along the vein, or itching. You may observe redness surrounding the venipuncture site or along the vein path.)

flow regulator: a supplemental I.V. device that ensures accurate delivery of I.V. fluids by regulating the number of milliliters delivered per hour

fluid balance: constant and approximately equal distribution of fluids between the intracellular and extracellular fluid compartments

fluid movement: the process that helps regulate fluid and electrolyte balance between the major fluid compartments and transports nutrients, waste products, and other substances into and out of cells, organs, and systems

gamma globulin: the antibody-containing portion of plasma; obtained by chemical fractionation of pooled plasma; commonly used to prevent infectious hepatitis (type A), rubella, mumps, pertussis, and tetanus

gauge: diameter of a needle

gluconeogenesis: the conversion of protein to carbohydrates for energy (Essential visceral proteins [serum albumin and transferrin] and somatic body proteins [skeletal, smooth muscle, and tissue proteins] are converted to energy in starvation or severe nutrient deficiencies. When essential body proteins break down, a negative nitrogen balance results [more protein is used by the body than is taken in].)

glycogenolysis: in metabolism, the mobilization and conversion of glycogen to glucose in the body

granulocytopenia: a severely low granulocyte level

Groshong catheter: a common tunneled catheter, which has a pressure-sensitive valve in the catheter tip that keeps the lumen closed when not in use and opens inward during blood aspiration and outward during blood or fluid administration, eliminating the need to flush with heparin

guide wire: a device that stiffens a catheter to ease its advancement through a vein but can damage the vein if used incorrectly

hemapheresis: collecting and removing specific blood components from blood and then returning the remaining constituents to the patient

hematocrit: the percentage of red blood cells in whole blood

hematoma: bruising at venipuncture site as a result of bleeding in the area (Symptoms include a raised dark area around the site with accompanying tenderness and an inability to advance or flush the I.V. line.)

hemolytic reaction: a life-threatening reaction to transfusions that occurs as a result of incompatible ABO or Rh blood or improper blood storage

hemosiderosis: possible complication of transfusion therapy that typically results from multiple or massive transfusions; characterized by iron plasma level greater than 200 mg/dl (In hemosiderosis, an iron-containing pigment [hemosiderin] accumulates, causing red blood cell destruction.)

hemothorax: bleeding into the pleural cavity, a common complication of CV catheter placement; treated with the insertion of a chest tube for draining blood

heparin lock: an intermittent infusion device that is flushed with heparin

heparin: an anticoagulant

human leukocyte antigen (HLA): antigen that is essential to immunity; part of the histocompatibility system, which controls compatibility between transplant or transfusion recipients and donors (Generally, the closer the HLA match between donor and recipient, the less likely the tissue or organ will be rejected.)

hydrothorax: infusion of a solution into the chest

hyperglycemia: high blood glucose; a possible complication of parenteral nutrition; often an early warning sign of sepsis

hyperosmolar hyperglycemic nonketotic syndrome (HHNS): a possible complication of parenteral nutrition (The patient may develop confusion or lethargy, have seizures, or become comatose. Hyperglycemia, dehydration, or glycosuria can also occur.)

hypertonic solution: a solution with higher osmolarity (concentration) than the normal range of serum (275 to 295 mOsm/L), such as dextrose 5% in half-normal saline solution, dextrose 5% in normal saline solution, and dextrose 5% in lactated Ringer's injection

hypocalcemia: calcium deficiency (Signs and symptoms of calcium deficiency include tingling in the fingers, muscle cramps, nausea, vomiting, hypotension, cardiac arrhythmias, and seizures.)

hypodermoclysis: a method for accessing a peripheral vein, usually in infants and elderly patients, in which I.V. isotonic hydration fluids are delivered subcutaneously

hypoglycemia: low blood glucose; a possible complication of parenteral nutrition (Signs and symptoms may include sweating, shaking, and irritability.)

hypokalemia: low blood potassium; a possible complication of parenteral nutrition (Signs and symptoms include muscle weakness, paralysis, paresthesia, and cardiac arrhythmias.)

hypomagnesemia: low blood magnesium; a possible complication of parenteral nutrition. (Patient may complain of tingling around the mouth or paresthesia in the fingers and may show signs of mental changes, hyperreflexia, tetany, and cardiac arrhythmias.)

hypophosphatemia: low blood phosphates; a possible complication of parenteral nutrition (Patient may be irritable or weak and may have paresthesia. In extreme cases, coma and cardiac arrest can occur.)

hypotonic solution: a solution with lower osmolarity (concentration) than the normal range of serum (275 to 295 mOsm/L) — such as half-normal saline solution, 0.33% saline solution, or dextrose 2.5% in water — which hydrates cells while reducing fluid in the circulatory system

hypovolemic shock: shock due to loss of systemic volume; caused by internal bleeding, hemorrhage, or sepsis (Signs and symptoms include increased heart rate, decreased blood pressure, mental confusion, and cool, clammy skin.)

I.V. administration set: I.V. tubing set that may be vented or unvented and may come with various features such as ports for infusing secondary medications and filters

I.V. loop: a supplemental I.V. device made of small-bore tubing in a horseshoe shape that fits between the venipuncture device and I.V. tubing to enable the tubing to be changed away from the device and help stabilize the device

I.V. push: injection (usually of a drug) directly into a vein; also called direct injection

iatrogenic protein-energy malnutrition: a form of malnutrition, common during hospitalization, in which a patient's nutritional status deteriorates; most common in patients hospitalized longer than 2 weeks

idiosyncratic reaction: an inherent inability to tolerate certain therapeutic chemicals (For example, a tranquilizer may cause excitation rather than sedation in a particular patient.)

incompatibility: an adverse reaction to I.V. therapy that results when I.V. solutions, drugs, or blood products are mixed together (In I.V. medication therapy, the more complex the solution, the greater the risk of incompatibility. In transfusion therapy, incompatibility of donor and recipient blood can cause serious adverse effects.)

inferior vena cava: a central vein (Venous return from the legs enters the inferior vena cava and returns blood to the right atrium. Blood enters the inferior vena cava from the legs through the femoral venous system and accessory veins of the abdomen.)

infiltration: infusion of I.V. solution into surrounding tissues rather than the blood vessel (Symptoms include discomfort, decreased skin temperature around the site, blanching, absent backflow of blood, and slower flow rate.)

Infuse-A-Port: top-entry vascular access port, a surgically implanted venous access device

infusion control device: device used to maintain precise I.V. flow rates in drops per minute or milliliters per hour; for example, clamps, controllers, volumetric pumps, and rate minders

infusion pump: an electronic device that regulates the flow of I.V. solutions and drugs and is used when a precise flow rate is required; used in CV therapy when positive pressure is required; for example, when solutions are administered through a CV line at low flow rates or during intra-arterial infusion

in-line filter: a filter in the fluid pathway between the I.V. tubing and the venipuncture device that removes pathogens and particles and helps prevent air from entering the patient's vein

interferon: in chemotherapy, a type of biological response modifier subdivided into three major types: alpha, beta, and gamma, that inhibits viral replication and may also directly inhibit tumor proliferation (Hematologic cancers, including malignant lymphomas, cutaneous T-cell lymphoma, and chronic myelogenous leukemia as well as hairy-cell leukemia are responsive to interferon.)

intermittent I.V. therapy: administration of a solution at set intervals for a shorter period than continuous I.V. therapy; the most common and flexible method of administering I.V. drugs

intermittent infusion device: a device that maintains venous access in patients who must receive I.V. medications regularly or intermittently but don't require continuous infusion; commonly called a saline or heparin lock because a saline or heparin solution is flushed into it to keep the device patent

interstitial fluid (ISF): extracellular fluid that bathes all cells in the body; accounts for about 75% of extracellular fluid

intracellular fluid (ICF): fluid that's contained inside the cells of the body

intraosseous infusion: an emergency procedure for fluid resuscitation or for medication or blood infusion in children under age 6 in which an intraosseous needle is placed in the medullary cavity of a bone so that an I.V. solution can be infused directly into the cavity

intrathecal: within the spinal canal

intravenous (I.V.) therapy: treatment that involves introducing liquid solutions directly into the bloodstream

irritant: an agent that, when used locally, produces a local inflammatory reaction

isotonic solution: a solution with osmolarity that is within the range for serum (275 to 295 mOsm/L), such as lactated Ringer's injection and normal saline solution

kwashiorkor: a form of malnutrition that results from severe protein deficiencies without caloric deficit; occurs most often in children ages 1 to 3; usually secondary to malabsorption disorders, cancer and cancer therapies, kidney disease, hypermetabolic illness, and iatrogenic causes

lipid emulsions: in parenteral nutrition, used to prevent and treat essential fatty acid deficiency and provide a major source of energy

liposome: a vehicle for transmitting a chemotherapeutic drug directly to a cancerous tumor that consists of ring-shaped layers, usually phospholipids, with a space between the lipid rings that contains an aqueous solution (Drugs can be placed in the lipid layer or, if they're water-soluble, in the aqueous spaces and carried to specific tumor cells.)

loading dose: preliminary dose of a medication; usually given I.V. at the start of therapy

lock: see *intermittent infusion device*

lock-out interval: a time set on a patient controlled analgesia device during which the device can't be activated

luer-lock injection cap: a device, possibly attached to the end of an extension set, that contains a clamping mechanism to provide ready access for intermittent infusions, which reduces the discomfort of reaccessing the port and prolongs the life of the port septum by decreasing the number of needle punctures

lymphokines: in chemotherapy, a subset of cytokines that fight cancer by stimulating the production of T cells, activating the lytic (cell-destroying) mechanisms of macrophages, promoting the immigration of lymphoid cells from the bloodstream, and stimulating the release of other lymphokines, such as tumor necrosis factor and interferon gamma (Examples of lymphokines include interleukin-1 [IL-1] and interleukin-2 [IL-2].)

macrodrip delivery system: an I.V. administration set that delivers a solution in large quantities at rapid rates

maintenance dose: the amount of medication a patient requires to achieve an effective therapeutic effect

marasmus: a form of malnutrition involving prolonged and gradual wasting of muscle mass and subcutaneous fat that occurs most frequently in infants, ages 6 to 18 months, and in patients with postgastrectomy dumping syndrome, carcinomas of the mouth and esophagus, and chronic

malnutrition states; caused by inadequate intake of protein, calories, and other nutrients

mechanical phlebitis: painful inflammation of a vein; possibly the most common peripherally inserted central catheter complication, which may occur during the first 24 to 72 hours after insertion; more common in left-sided insertions and when a large-gauge catheter is used

Med-I-Port: a top-entry vascular access pump; surgically implanted venous device

metabolic acidosis: a possible complication of parenteral nutrition that can occur if the patient develops an increased serum chloride level and a decreased serum bicarbonate level

metacarpal veins: veins located on the back of the hand, formed by the union of digital veins between the knuckles

microaggregates: small particles formed from degenerating platelets, leukocytes, and fibrin strands after a few days of blood storage that may contribute to formation of microemboli (small clots that obstruct circulation) in the lungs (Microaggregates can pass through a 170-micron filter. A microaggregate filter removes smaller particles but costs more and may slow the infusion rate.)

microdrip delivery system: an I.V. administration set that delivers a small amount of solution with each drop and is used for pediatric patients and for adults who need small or closely regulated amounts of I.V. solution

micronutrients: also called trace elements; in parenteral nutrition solutions, used to promote normal metabolism; for example,

zinc, copper, chromium, iodide, selenium, and manganese

midline device: an extended peripheral catheter; often incorrectly called a peripherally inserted central catheter, but its tip rests in the axillary vein rather than in the central venous circulation

mucositis: inflammation of the mucous membranes

myelosuppression: the interference with and suppression of the blood-forming stem cells in the bone marrow; a possible complication of chemotherapy

nadir: the lowest point in some series of measurements, such as white blood cell, hemoglobin, or platelet levels

necrosis: tissue death

nomogram: a table for estimating body surface area when a patient's weight and height are known

noncoring needle: vascular access port needle with an angled or deflected point that slices the septum on entry, rather than coring it as a conventional needle does (When the noncoring needle is removed, the septum reseals itself.)

nontunneled catheter: type of central venous catheter usually designed for short-term use

nonvesicant: an agent that doesn't cause blisters

nutritional assessment: assessment of the relationship between nutrients consumed and energy expended, especially when illness or surgery compromises a patient's intake or alters his metabolic requirements;

includes a dietary history, physical assessment, anthropometric measurements, and diagnostic tests

occlusion: blockage that prevents ability to infuse fluids or flush a vein, due to the accumulation of blood materials, fibrin, platelets, or incompatible infusates that causes crystallization in the lumen of the infusion device or vein

osmolarity: the concentration of a solution expressed in milliosmols of solute per liter of solution

osmosis: the passive transport of fluid across a membrane from an area of lower concentration to one of higher concentration that stops when the solute concentrations are equal

over-the-needle catheter: the most commonly used device for peripheral I.V. therapy, which consists of a plastic outer tube and an inner needle (stylette) that is removed after insertion, leaving the catheter in place

oxygen-hemoglobin affinity: the tendency of hemoglobin to hold oxygen. (When oxygen's hemoglobin affinity increases, oxygen stays in the patient's bloodstream and isn't released into other tissues. Oxygen's hemoglobin affinity can increase during blood storage, causing oxygen to stay in a patient's bloodstream rather than being released into other tissues. Signs of this reaction include a depressed respiratory rate, especially in patients with chronic lung disease.)

parenteral: any route other than the GI tract by which drugs, nutrients, or other solutions may enter the body; for example I.V., I.M., or subcutaneously

parenteral nutrition: therapy that provides calories from dextrose and one or more nutrients that keep the body functioning; ordered when a nutritional assessment reveals a nonfunctional GI tract, increased metabolic need, or a combination of both; administered through either a peripheral or central venous infusion device (Solutions may contain one or more of the following: dextrose, proteins, lipids, electrolytes, vitamins, and trace elements.)

passive transport: fluid movement that requires no energy and in which solutes move from an area of higher concentration to one of lower concentration (This change is called moving down the concentration gradient and results in an equal distribution of solutes.)

patency: the state of being freely open (A patent vein is intact and without holes.)

patient-controlled analgesia (PCA): treatment that allows the patient to control I.V. delivery of an analgesic (usually morphine) and maintain therapeutic serum levels (The patient uses a specialized infusion device with a timing unit that delivers a dose of an analgesic at a controlled volume.)

peripheral central venous therapy: a variation of central venous therapy in which a catheter is inserted through a peripheral vein, with the catheter tip in the superior vena cava

peripheral parenteral nutrition (PPN): the delivery of nutrients through a short cannula inserted into a peripheral vein; generally provides fewer nonprotein calories than total parenteral nutrition because lower dextrose concentrations are used

peripherally inserted central catheter (PICC): a central venous access device that is inserted through a peripheral vein with the tip ending in the superior or inferior vena cava; generally used when patients need frequent blood transfusions or infusions of caustic drugs or solutions; especially useful if the patient doesn't have reliable routes for short-term I.V. therapy

phlebitis: painful inflammation along the venous path in which the cannula is placed; a common complication of I.V. therapy (Signs and symptoms of phlebitis include redness [erythema] at the site and along the vein, puffiness over the vein, firmness on palpation, and discomfort.)

physiologic pump: a mechanism that is involved in the active transport of solutes; for example, the sodium-potassium pump, which moves sodium ions out of cells to the extracellular fluid and potassium ions into cells from the extracellular fluid

piggyback infusion: use of an add-a-line administration set to add an I.V. drug into a primary line

piggyback line: an adjunct or secondary I.V. line attached to a primary line to deliver medications or solutions I.V.

plasma substitutes: may be used to maintain blood volume in an emergency, such as acute hemorrhage and shock (Plasma substitutes lack oxygen-carrying and coagulation properties. Examples include synthetic volume expanders, such as dextran in saline solution, and natural volume expanders, such as plasma protein fraction and albumin.)

plasma: the liquid component of blood that surrounds red blood cells, accounts for about 55% of blood volume, and consists of blood's noncellular components, including water (serum), protein (albumin, globulin, and fibrinogen), lipids, electrolytes, vitamins, carbohydrates, nonprotein nitrogen compounds, bilirubin, and gases (Commonly transfused plasma products include fresh frozen plasma, albumin, cryoprecipitate, and prothrombin complex. Plasma and plasma fractions are used in transfusion therapy to correct blood deficiencies, prevent disease, and control bleeding tendencies.)

platelets: cellular elements of blood that are infused to prevent or control bleeding (Platelet depletion may occur in patients with hematologic disease or those receiving antineoplastic therapy.)

pneumothorax: air in the thorax; the most common complication of central venous placement (Signs and symptoms may include chest pain, dyspnea, cyanosis, or decreased or absent breath sounds on the affected side. A thoracotomy should be performed and a chest tube inserted if the pneumothorax is large enough for intervention.)

Port-a-Cath: a top-entry vascular access port; a surgically implanted central venous access device

potassium intoxication: an increase in potassium levels after a transfusion that occurs because of blood cell maturation in stored blood components (Results of this transfusion reaction may include intestinal colic, diarrhea, muscle twitching, oliguria, renal failure, bradycardia that may proceed to cardiac arrest, and electrocardiogram changes with tall, peaked T waves.)

potentiate: to increase the potency of action (In chemotherapy, smaller doses of

different chemotherapeutic drugs are given in combination, the drugs potentiate each other, and the tumor responds as it would to a larger dose of a single drug.)

primary I.V. line: main I.V. line, usually used to deliver a continuous infusion of an I.V. solution

protein-energy malnutrition (PEM): a deficiency of protein and energy (calories); a spectrum of disorders that results from either prolonged, chronic, inadequate protein or caloric intake or high metabolic protein and energy requirements (Disorders that commonly lead to PEM include cancer, GI disorders, chronic heart failure, alcoholism, and conditions causing high metabolic needs, such as burns.)

protocol: a description of specific steps in patient care that may describe how to administer a medication

retrograde administration: administration method that allows a medication such as I.V. antibiotics to be given over a 30-minute period without increasing fluid volume

rhesus (Rh) system: in blood physiology, a major blood antigen system that consists of Rh-positive and Rh-negative groups (Rh-positive blood has a variant of the Rh antigen called a D antigen or D factor; Rh-negative blood doesn't have this antigen. A person with Rh-positive blood doesn't carry anti-Rh antibodies because they would destroy his red blood cells.)

S.E.A. Port: a side-entry vascular access port in which the needle is inserted almost parallel to the reservoir; a surgically implanted central venous access device

saline lock: an intermittent infusion device that is flushed with saline

scalp tourniquet: in chemotherapy, a device that is used to limit superficial blood flow to the scalp during drug administration, thus partially protecting the hair follicles from the circulating drug and reducing the risk of alopecia

scalp vein catheter: a small-diameter, winged over-the-needle catheter; the preferred venous access device for infants and young children

sclerosis: the hardening of a tissue or vessel

secondary set: I.V. tubing and infusion attached to the primary I.V. line; usually used for the administration of I.V. medication, also called piggyback infusion set

sepsis: infection of tissues with disease-causing microorganisms or their toxins (Signs and symptoms of sepsis include elevated temperature, glucose in the urine [glycosuria], chills, malaise, increased white blood cells [leukocytosis], and altered level of consciousness.)

sequential system: method used to document I.V. solutions throughout therapy in which each container is numbered sequentially

speed shock: shock caused by too-rapid direct injection of a drug (Most drugs must be given over a specific time period when using direct injection. To avoid speed shock, no drug should be injected in less than 1 minute, unless the order specifically requires it or the patient is in cardiac or respiratory arrest.)

stomatitis: inflammation of the mouth; in chemotherapy, painful mouth ulcers apparent 3 to 7 days after treatment begins, with symptoms ranging from mild to severe (Accompanying pain can lead to malnutrition and fluid and electrolyte imbalance if the patient is unable to chew and swallow adequate food and fluid. Treatment includes scrupulous oral hygiene and topical anesthetic mixtures.)

superior vena cava: a central vein (Venous return from the head, neck, and arms enters the superior vena cava before flowing into the right atrium. Blood enters the superior vena cava mainly through the subclavian, jugular, and innominate veins of the head, neck, and arms.)

syringe pump: a type of pump that is especially useful for giving intermittent I.V. medications to pediatric patients because it gives the greatest control over small-volume infusions; used with syringe sizes from 1 to 60 ml using low-volume tubing

T-connector: a supplemental I.V. device that is attached to I.V. tubing and into which another I.V. needle can be inserted, allowing simultaneous administration of fluids and drugs; also used as an intermittent infusion device

tension pneumothorax: type of pneumothorax in which air leaks into the lungs but can't escape, causing pressure in the lungs and eventually leading to lung collapse; a medical emergency in which the patient exhibits signs of acute respiratory distress, asymmetrical chest wall movement and, possibly, a tracheal shift away from the midline (A chest tube must be inserted immediately, before respiratory and cardiac decompensation occur.)

thrombocytopenia: blood platelet depletion

thrombogenic: a device or process that may cause or lead to thrombosis formation

thrombophlebitis: inflammation of the vein due to the formation of a blood clot

thrombosis: the development of a thrombus (blood clot)

through-the-needle catheter: a device for peripheral I.V. therapy with an introducer needle that must be guarded by an enclosed shield after insertion; generally used in long veins or when venous access is poor; kept in place for up to 4 weeks

time tape: a tape or preprinted strip marked in 1-hour increments; attached to an I.V. container and used to check the infusion rate

titration: gradual addition of a component to a solution that ends when no more of the component can be consumed by reaction in the solution (With I.V. therapy, you can accurately titrate medication doses by adjusting the concentration of the infusate and the administration rate.)

total nutrient admixture (TNA): also called 3:1 solution; daily allotments of total parenteral nutrition solution, including lipids and other parenteral solution components; commonly given in a single, 3-L bag

total parenteral nutrition (TPN): delivery of nutrients through a central line and usually through the subclavian vein with the tip of the catheter in the superior vena cava; usually indicated when parenteral nutrition is needed for more than 5 days

tourniquet: commonly, a soft rubber band 2″ (5 cm) wide that encircles a limb and traps blood in the veins by applying enough pressure to impede the venous flow

toxicity: the quality of being poisonous

transcellular fluids: a form of extracellular fluid that includes cerebrospinal fluid, lymph, and fluids in such spaces as the pleural and abdominal cavities

transfusion reaction: adverse reaction to transfusion therapy, the most severe of which is a hemolytic reaction, which destroys red blood cells and may become life-threatening (Signs of a transfusion reaction include fever, chills, rigors, headache, and nausea.)

transfusion therapy: the introduction of whole blood or blood components directly into the bloodstream; used mainly to restore and maintain blood volume, improve the oxygen-carrying capacity of blood, replace deficient blood components, or improve coagulation

treatment cycle: in chemotherapy, repeated drug doses, usually over several days, that is considered a single course of chemotherapy and is repeated on a cyclic basis, often every 3 to 4 weeks (Treatment cycles are carefully planned so normal cells can regenerate. Most patients require at least three treatment cycles before they show any beneficial response.)

Trendelenburg's position: position in which the head is low and the body and legs are on an inclined plane; used in central venous catheter insertion to distend neck and thoracic veins, thereby making them more visible and accessible

tumor resistance: the ability of a tumor to withstand the effects of chemotherapeutic drugs, either initially during treatment or developed after treatment

tunneled central venous catheter: central venous catheter with a cuff (usually made of Dacron) that encourages tissue growth at the exit site to anchor the catheter; designed for long-term use and usually made of silicone, which minimizes irritation or damage to the vein lining

universal donor: a person with group O blood, which lacks both A and B antigens and can be transfused in limited amounts in an emergency to any patient — regardless of the recipient's blood type — with little risk of adverse reaction

universal recipient: a person with AB blood type, which has neither anti-A nor anti-B antibodies (A person with AB blood may receive A, B, AB, or O blood.)

urokinase: a fibrinolytic agent used to dissolve clots

urticaria: a vascular reaction of the skin characterized by the eruption of hives and severe itching

Valsalva's maneuver: a maneuver, involving forced exhalation, that a patient can perform to help prevent air embolism whenever the catheter is open to the air; especially important when the patient is taking care of a catheter at home

vascular access port (VAP): a long-term central venous catheter that is implanted in a pocket under the skin with an attached indwelling catheter that is tunnelled through subcutaneous tissue so the catheter tip lies in a central vein; accessed with a specially designed, noncoring nee-

dle; typically used when an external catheter isn't suitable and also used for arterial access or implanted into the epidural space, peritoneum, or pericardial or pleural cavity; usually used to deliver intermittent infusions

vasoconstriction: narrowing of the lumen of a blood vessel

vasovagal reaction: sudden collapse of a vein during venipuncture, possibly caused by vasospasm due to anxiety or pain

vein dissection: a seldom-used way to access a peripheral vein in which a small incision is made in the vein to insert a plastic catheter that can remain in place for several days

venogram: radiographic examination of a vein filled with contrast medium; performed before catheter insertion to check the status of blood vessels, especially if the catheter is intended for long-term use

vesicant: an agent that causes or forms blisters

volume-control set: an I.V. administration set that is used to deliver small, precise amounts of fluids and medications and that may be attached directly to the venipuncture device or connected as a secondary infusion device at a Y-site

washed cells: blood from which 80% of the plasma is removed; rinsed with a special solution that removes white blood cells and platelets; for example, leukocyte-poor red blood cells

winged infusion set: an infusion set that has flexible wings that lie flat after insertion and can be taped to the surrounding skin; see also *butterfly needle*

Y-site: a secondary injection port on an I.V. administration set that allows separate or simultaneous infusion of two compatible solutions

Index

i refers to an illustration; t refers to a table.

i refers to an illustration; t refers to a table.

i refers to an illustration; t refers to a table.

i refers to an illustration; t refers to a table.

Lymphokines, cellular therapy and, 262
Lymphoma, chemotherapy protocols for, 261t

M

Macrodrip administration set, 24, 25i, 48
Magnesium, 9t
Maintenance dose, 328
Malignant lymphoma, chemotherapy protocol for, 261t
Marasmus, 290
Median antebrachial vein as venipuncture site, 58t
Medicaid policies, 35-36
Medicare policies, 35-36
Metabolic acidosis as TPN complication, 312t, 315
Metacarpal veins as venipuncture site, 58t
Metrisets (volume-control set), 47i, 49
Microaggregate filter, 229
Microaggregates, formation of, 229
Microdrip administration set, 24, 25i, 48
Micronutrients as parenteral solution component, 297t, 298
Midarm circumference, measuring, 292i
Midarm muscle circumference, measuring, 292i
Midline device, 109
Minerals as parenteral solution component, 296-297, 297t
Monoclonal antibodies, immunotherapy and, 259
Myelosuppression as chemotherapy complication, 280

N

Nadir, 328
Nausea and vomiting as chemotherapy complication, 279-280
Necrosis, 328
Needle and catheter gauges, 64t

Nerve damage as complication, 92t
Nomogram
    for adults, 176i
    for children, 175i
Noncoring needles, VAP and, 148, 148i
Nontunneled CV catheters, 99, 101
Nonvented bottle, attaching administration set to, 53
Nonvesicants, 268t
    administering, 271
    infiltration with, 273-274
    tissue damage potential for, 268t
Nurse practice acts, 34-35
Nutritional assessment, 290-291, 292-293i, 293, 294-295t, 295-296
Nutritional deficiencies, 288-290
    assessing for, 290-291, 292-293i
    diagnostic tests for, 294-295t
    signs of, 291

O

Occlusion as complication, 90t
Oncotic pressure, fluid movement and, 11-12
OneCath, 107i
Organ system dysfunction as chemotherapy complication, 282-283
Osmolarity, fluid balance and, 12
Osmosis, fluid movement and, 10-11
Over-the-needle catheter, 62i, 63
    positioning, for insertion, 70-71
Oxygen affinity for hemoglobin, increased, as transfusion complication, 246t, 249

PQ

Packed red blood cells, transfusion therapy and, 224, 226t
Pain
    at I.V. site as complication, 90t
    as PICC-specific complication, 143
Parenteral nutrition, 285-317
    additives to solutions for, 298

i refers to an illustration; t refers to a table.

i refers to an illustration; t refers to a table.

i refers to an illustration; t refers to a table.

i refers to an illustration; t refers to a table.

Notes...

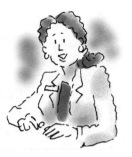

...notes...

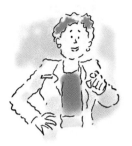

...notes...

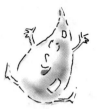

...more notes...

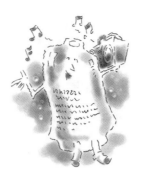

...and still more notes...

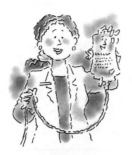